Social Indicators Research Series

Volume 90

This series provides a public forum for authored and edited volumes on social indicators research. It is a companion series to the journal Social Indicators Research. The book series deals with problems associated with the quality of life from a broad perspective. It welcomes research on a wide range of substantive areas, including health, crime, housing, education, family life, leisure activities, transportation, mobility, economics, work, religion and environmental issues. The topics represented in this series cover and involve a variety of segmentations, such as social groups, spatial and temporal coordinates, population composition, and life domains. The series presents empirical, philosophical and methodological studies that cover the entire spectrum of society and are devoted to giving evidence through indicators. It considers indicators in their different typologies, and gives special attention to indicators that are able to meet the need of understanding social realities and phenomena that are increasingly more complex, interrelated, interacted and dynamic. In addition, it presents studies aimed at defining new approaches in constructing indicators. An international review board for this series ensures the high quality of the series as a whole.

Available at 25% discount for International Society for Quality-of-Life Studies (ISQOLS).

Christian Suter • Jenny Chesters •
Sandra Fachelli
Editors

Well-being During the Pandemic

Comparative Perspectives from the Global North and South

Springer

Editors
Christian Suter
Institut de Sociologie
University of Neuchatel
Neuchâtel, Switzerland

Jenny Chesters
Youth Research Centre
University of Melbourne
Parkville, VIC, Australia

Sandra Fachelli
Department of Sociology
Pablo de Olavide University
Seville, Spain

ISSN 1387-6570 ISSN 2215-0099 (electronic)
Social Indicators Research Series
ISBN 978-3-031-63439-0 ISBN 978-3-031-63440-6 (eBook)
https://doi.org/10.1007/978-3-031-63440-6

Stiftung zur Förderung sozialwissenschaftlicher Forschung über die Weltgesellschaft

This Springer imprint is published by the registered company Springer Nature Switzerland AG
The registered company address is: Gewerbestrasse 11, 6330 Cham, Switzerland

Preface

In June 2023, the Research Committee 55 on Social Indicators (RC55) of the International Sociological Association (ISA) organized together with the Faculty of Education at the University of Melbourne an international pre-conference to the ISA World Congress in Melbourne on the topic of *The Impact of the 2020–2022 Pandemic on World Society*. The conference was supported by the *World Society Foundation (WSF)* based in Zurich, Switzerland, and took place at the University of Melbourne, hosted by the Faculty of Education.[1] This volume includes a selection of contributions focusing on the topic of the impact of the COVID-19 pandemic on well-being presented and discussed at the Melbourne conferences, both the RC55 pre-conference and the RC55 sessions of the ISA World Congress.

The pre-conference brought together 36 researchers from 22 different countries, including Australia, Bangladesh, Belgium, Estonia, France, Germany, Hong Kong, Indonesia, Israel, Italy, Japan, Lebanon, Mexico, Mongolia, Nigeria, the Philippines, Poland, Switzerland, Timor-Leste, the UK, and the USA. The presenters included highly regarded professors, scholars from outside the academy (international organizations, government institutions, private research institutions, foundations, and civil society institutions), postdoctoral researchers, and PhD students representing countries from both the Global North (58%) and the Global South (42%). With respect to academic rank, 47% of participants were faculty members, i.e., assistant, associate, or full professor; 31% were lecturers, research fellows, or postdocs; 8% were doctoral students; and 14% came from non-academic institutions. The gender distribution was quite balanced: 55% of participants were males and 45% were females.

[1] The *World Society Foundation* was established in 1982 by the Swiss sociologist Peter Heintz with the aim of encouraging and supporting scientific research on global structures and transformations. The pandemic with its profound economic, political, and social impacts all over the world has been one of the most important global events triggering new dynamics at all levels of global society. More details on the 2023 pre-conference in Melbourne, the World Society Foundation, and its sponsoring program are available on the WSF website at http://www.worldsociety.ch.

The conference was officially opened by Prof. Jim Watterston, Dean of the Faculty of Education. The conference program proceeded with the keynote lecture on "Managing Crisis After Financialization: Reflecting on 'novel' responses to COVID-19 and the 2008 Financial Crisis" (presented by Ben Spies-Butcher from Macquarie University Sydney) and eight sessions, each of which was dedicated to a particular theme: the pandemic, crisis management and policies, and their impact (2 parts); the pandemic and its impact on subjective well-being and life satisfaction; the pandemic, mental health, and social cohesion; the impact of the pandemic on children and youth; the impact of the pandemic on vulnerable and marginalized groups; the pandemic and social inequalities: class, race, ethnicity, and gender; and the pandemic, health, shift work, and addiction. Each of the researchers was selected to present at the conference after a rigorous selection process. The Organizing Committee, composed of the editors of this book, read more than 50 abstracts and invited the authors of 40 abstracts to submit their full paper, from which 25 were selected for presentation at the conference.

Many people have contributed to the realization of this volume and the 2023 Melbourne conference. First and foremost, the editors would like to thank the authors for their stimulating contributions and their patience during the reviewing and copyediting process. A large thank-you is due to Nadishka Weerasuriya, a PhD student in the Faculty of Education, for all of her work during the pre-conference, and to our colleagues from RC55 who contributed to the conference as session chairs and discussants. We would also like to thank the Faculty of Education and the University of Melbourne for their support of the conference and for providing the necessary infrastructure and conference facilities. Finally, we are very grateful to our main sponsor, the World Society Foundation, for providing generous financial support for the organization of the 2023 conference, for the travel grants provided to the invited speakers, and for the publication of this volume, particularly for making the book available in Open Access.

Neuchâtel, Switzerland	Christian Suter
Melbourne, Australia	Jenny Chesters
Seville, Spain	Sandra Fachelli
February 2024	

Acknowledgments

We are very grateful to the World Society Foundation, Zurich, Switzerland (www.worldsociety.ch), for providing generous financial support for the Open Access version of this publication.

Contents

About the Editors and Contributors

About the Editors

Christian Suter is Professor Emeritus of Sociology at the University of Neuchâtel (Switzerland). After receiving his PhD in sociology from the University of Zurich, he was Visiting Scholar at the Colegio de México, Visiting Professor at the Friedrich-Schiller University Jena, Assistant Professor of Sociology at the Swiss Federal Institute of Technology, Zurich, and Full Professor of Sociology at the University of Neuchâtel. He is currently doing research on social indicators and quality of life and on globalization and world society. Earlier research has focused on social and economic inequalities and poverty, sovereign debt and global debt crises, social and political transformations in Latin America, and social support and health. He has published and edited more than 40 books and special issues, as well as many articles in international social sciences journals, encyclopedias, and volumes. His most recent publications include *The Global Politics of Census Taking* (Routledge 2024), *Measuring Gender Equality* (Springer 2023), *African-Asian Relations* (LIT 2022), *Measuring and Understanding Complex Phenomena* (Springer 2021), *The Middle Class in World Society* (Routledge 2020), and *Wealth(s) and Subjective Well-Being* (Springer 2019). He is the winner of the *Book Award of the American Sociological Association, Political Economy of the World-System Section* (1993; for *Debt Cycles in the World-Economy*, Westview 1992), and he has been awarded the *Fritz Thyssen Prize* for articles in social sciences journals (1998) and the Research Fellow Award 2020 from the *International Society for Quality-of-Life Studies* for substantial contribution to quality-of-life research (2020).

Personal website: http://www2.unine.ch/socio/page-42993.html

Jenny Chesters is Associate Professor in the Faculty of Education at the University of Melbourne. Her PhD was awarded by the University of Queensland in 2009. She is currently coordinating the Capstone subject for the Master of Education and is Chief Investigator of the Australian Research Council-funded Life Patterns project. She is a board member of RC55 "Social Indicators" of the

International Sociological Association. Her recent publications include "School-to-work transition and subjective well-being in Australia" (2021, *British Journal of Sociology*) and "Cross-national comparison of age and period effects on levels of subjective well-being in Australia and Switzerland during volatile economic times (2001–2016)" (2020, *Social Indicators Research*). She is also the editor of the *Research Handbook on Transitions into Adulthood* published in 2024 (Edward Elgar) and a sub-section editor for the *Child and Youth Studies Handbook* (Second Edition) (2023, Springer). Her research interests include comparative perspectives on subjective well-being, social stratification, and transitions between education and employment throughout the life course.

Sandra Fachelli is Associate Professor of the Department of Sociology of Pablo de Olavide University. She has Postdoctorate in Social Science from the University of Buenos Aires (UBA), PhD in Sociology from the Autonomous University of Barcelona (UAB), Diploma of Advanced Studies in Sociology, Master's in Introduction to Research in Sociology (UAB), and Master's in Design and Management of Policies and Social Programs (FLACSO Argentina). She is teaching coordinator and professor of the Master's program in Applied Social Research Techniques (TISA) that is co-coordinated by UAB and Barcelona University. She is currently President of the Research Committee 06 "Inequality and Social Stratification" of the Spanish Federation of Sociology (FES) and Vice-president of RC55 "Social Indicators" of the International Sociological Association. Her most recent books are *Measuring Gender Equality* (Springer 2023), *Towards a Comparative Analysis of Social Inequalities Between Europe and Latin America* (2021), and *Perspectivas y fronteras en el estudio de la desigualdad social: movilidad social y clases sociales en tiempos de cambio* (2020). Her main lines of research include inequality, stratification and social mobility, higher education, and work.

Personal web: https://investiga.upo.es/investigadores/158663/detalle

Contributors

Md Fakhrul Alam Shahjalal University of Science and Technology, Sylhet, Bangladesh

Shireen AlAzzawi Santa Clara University, Santa Clara, CA, USA

Bijoy Krishna Banik University of Rajshahi, Rajshahi, Bangladesh

Catherine White Berheide Skidmore College, Saratoga Springs, NY, USA

Marc Callens Ghent University, Ghent, Belgium

Megan A. Carpenter St. Lawrence University, Canton, NY, USA

Jenny Chesters University of Melbourne, Melbourne, Australia

David A. Cotter Union College, Schenectady, NY, USA

Sandra Fachelli Pablo de Olavide University, Seville, Spain

Gour Gobinda Goswami North South University, Dhaka, Bangladesh

Haridhan Goswami Manchester Metropolitan University, Manchester, UK

Anja Gvozdanović Institute for Social Research, Zagreb, Croatia

Vladimir Hlasny Ewha Womans University, Seoul, Korea

United Nations Economic and Social Commission for Western Asia (UN ESCWA), Beirut, Lebanon

M. Ibrahim Khalil Government Brojomohun College, Barishal, Bangladesh

Eileen McNeely Harvard University, Cambridge, MA, USA

Oliver Nahkur University of Tartu, Tartu, Estonia

Indera Ratna Irawati Pattinasarany Universitas Indonesia, Depok, Indonesia

Gonzalo A. Saraví Center for Research and Graduate Studies in Social Anthropology (Ciesas), Mexico, Mexico

Regina Skiba Jagiellonian University, Cracow, Poland

Joonmo Son National University of Singapore, Singapore, Singapore

Dragan Stanojević University of Belgrade, Belgrade, Serbia

Pildoo Sung Hong Kong Baptist University, Kowloon Tong, Hong Kong

Christian Suter University of Neuchâtel, Neuchâtel, Switzerland

Benjamin Tay National Volunteer & Philanthropy Centre, Singapore, Singapore

Bojan Todosijević Institute of Social Sciences, Belgrade, Serbia

Dries Verlet Ghent University, Ghent, Belgium

Dorota Weziak-Bialowolska Kozminski University, Warsaw, Poland

Karoliine Zarina Tallinn University, Tallinn, Estonia

Chapter 1
Introduction: Threats to Well-Being During the COVID-19 Pandemic

Christian Suter, Jenny Chesters, and Sandra Fachelli

1.1 Comparative Perspectives on the Pandemic Experiences in the Global North and South

In the beginning of 2020 a novel coronavirus, COVID-19, spread from China to firstly Europe and then the rest of the world provoking a global health and economic crisis threatening well-being and quality of life in all countries across the globe. Governments introduced restrictions, in some cases, quite severe ones, to try to curb the spread of the virus. Researchers scrambled to identify the genetic makeup of the virus so that vaccines could be developed. Pharmaceutical companies reallocated their research resources to develop and test new classes of vaccines. Meanwhile, fear among the general population increased as daily death counts mounted.

According to the World Health Organization (WHO), by the end of December 2020, the official death toll from COVID-19 was 1.8 million. However, based on estimates of excess mortality, the WHO has concluded that there were 3.4 million deaths associated with the virus (WHO 2023). Excess mortality, the difference between the number of deaths during the pandemic and the deaths expected under normal (non-pandemic) conditions, resulted in a general reduction of life expectancy, reversing or interrupting the previous secular trends towards higher life expectancy in most countries of the world. Worldwide, on average, in 2019 life expectancy at birth was 72.8 years and in 2021, it had declined to 71.4 years (UNDP 2020, 2022).

C. Suter (✉)
University of Neuchâtel, Neuchâtel, Switzerland
e-mail: christian.suter@unine.ch

J. Chesters
University of Melbourne, Melbourne, VIC, Australia

S. Fachelli
Pablo de Olavide University, Seville, Spain

C. Suter et al. (eds.), *Well-being During the Pandemic*, Social Indicators Research Series 90, https://doi.org/10.1007/978-3-031-63440-6_1

Restrictions on contact and movement varied from country to country, and in some cases between regions within countries. For example, in Australia, state governments determined which restrictions to implement as well as when and where to implement them. Furthermore, the national border was closed for 2 years. In contrast, Mexico did not restrict travel or close its borders, however, educational institutions across the country were closed for around 18 months.

Despite its global reach, how the pandemic impacted on people was heavily reliant on the economic, political, social and cultural context in place before and during the pandemic. High-income countries in the Global North were, in general, better placed to control the spread through the implementation of travel restrictions between and within their borders. They were also able to quickly respond by adopting and adapting supplementary welfare programs and payments to support people (and companies) who were adversely impacted by the restrictions to work, travel and trade (for instance by short-term compensation or unemployment benefits). In contrast, low-income countries in the Global South often depended on export income derived from labor intensive industries and the wages earned by migrant workers based in higher income countries and repatriated home. Without fully established welfare schemes, it was hardly possible for low-income countries in the Global South to provide financial support for their citizens and/or companies. Furthermore, within countries, high-income households were better placed to isolate at home and order in essentials such as food and medicines and working remotely whereas low-income households and individuals had to keep working (on site) despite the threat of contracting the virus.

This considerable variety of COVID-19 experiences across and within countries is confirmed by a comparative analysis of the experiences during the first year of the pandemic, including several indicators measuring the COVID-19 related health situation (notably COVID-19 deaths, number of new COVID-19 cases, change of mortality rate between 2019 and 2021), the health measures and restrictions implemented by governments (stringency of COVID-19 measures), and the general socio-economic conditions (e.g. GDP per capita, poverty, health expenditures). Preliminary analysis suggests two main factors explaining 67% of the variance in these societal conditions across countries: firstly, and most important, the socio-economic conditions (poverty), and secondly, the incidence of COVID-19 (Fachelli et al. 2024). A cluster analysis including 214 countries finds three different groups of country experiences: a first group of highly affected countries of both the Global North (notably UK, and Southern and Eastern European countries like Italy, Spain, Portugal, Poland, the Baltic, Croatia, Romania) and the Global South (notably Latin American and Maghrebian countries), a second group of moderately affected countries mostly of the Global North (like the U.S., Western and Northern European countries, Australia, New Zealand, and Singapore) and a large third group of less affected countries of the Global South (notably African and Asian countries). This evidence shows the importance of delving deeper into the relationship between countries' socio-economic conditions and COVID-19 status, as it does not seem that there is a unidirectional relationship. Adopting a comparative perspective is particularly useful to explore both this relationship and to go beyond a view limited to considerations based on simple COVID-19 incidence and the related health situation. This volume, therefore, includes a considerable variety of countries, in particular countries of both the Global North and the Global South representing different structural contexts and COVID-19 experiences, but also various population groups within countries including those suffering particularly from adverse socio-economic conditions, like refugees, adolescents in poor neighborhoods, or informal workers.

1.2 Well-Being: Concepts and Measures

The concept of well-being has become increasingly popular over the past decades, both in research, policy and official statistics. Although there are different understandings of well-being, most researchers conceptualize well-being as multidimensional phenomenon that may refer both to the individual and societal level, and includes the "objective" living conditions covering various life domains (like education, employment, income and wealth, housing situation, health, social contacts, work and leisure time, environmental conditions, political participation) and different aspects of "subjective" well-being (Ehrler et al. 2016; Maggino 2023; Noll 2002). Three components of subjective well-being are often distinguished: cognitive well-being referring to general and domain-specific life satisfaction; hedonic well-being referring to the emotional dimension like positive feelings (happiness, pleasure) and negative feelings (fear, sadness); and eudemonic well-being covering the psychosocial dimension of well-being including interpersonal relatedness and positive social relationships, personal growth and "flourishing" (Seligman 2011).

A wide range of instruments have been suggested over the past decades for measuring well-being and certain standards have been developed. The most widely used measures are summarized in the OECD (2013) handbook, including the measures of general (and domain-specific) life satisfaction (cognitive subjective well-being), happiness (hedonic subjective well-being), and flourishing (eudemonic well-being)—measures which will be also used in the chapters of this volume (see also Maggino 2023). According to Veenhoven (1996, 6), measures of life satisfaction provide an indication of how much an individual "positively evaluates the overall quality of his/her life" whereas Headey et al. (2013) posit that levels of life satisfaction are the result of an individual's ability to achieve their life goals. Diener et al. (2013) posit that levels of subject well-being vary according to personal factors such as marital status and health as well as by the societal context such as labor market conditions and the distribution of income and wealth.

More recently, researchers have begun to examine whether the efficacy of measures of subjective well-being vary according to cultural context (Headey et al. 2022; Krys et al. 2023). For example, Krys et al. (2023) argue that traditional measures of subjective well-being are based on an assumption that definitions of life satisfaction and/or happiness are stable across cultures. They developed a new culturally sensitive measure and tested it on a sample recruited from 49 countries, including participants from both the Global North and the Global South. Krys et al. (2023) concluded that conceptualisations of life satisfaction and happiness do, in fact, vary according to culture. Headey et al. (2022) also found that cultural differences, such as variations in family, prosocial, political, religious and materialistic values, influence conceptualisations of life satisfaction. Consequently, researchers conducting international comparisons of levels of subjective well-being may need to factor in the effect of cultural differences.

1.3 Well-Being in Times of Crisis

The COVID-19 pandemic provoked, in addition to the health crisis, considerable economic and financial turmoils. Some economic sectors (like transportation, tourism, hospitality and personal services, commerce) were severely affected by the travel and contact restrictions. Global GDP collapsed in 2020 by about –8%—significantly more than during previous economic crises, like the Global Financial Crisis of 2008 or the dot-com crisis of 2002. International trade and investment slowed down as result of the disruption of global production and supply chains in the wake of the COVID-19 pandemic and Russia's invasion of the Ukraine. These combined and overlapping health, economic, financial, and political crises negatively impacted on quality of life and well-being.

The relationships between economic crisis (and/or economic growth) and well-being have been widely studied, both within and across countries. Empirical evidence based on earlier economic crises demonstrates that quality of life (i.e. "objective" indicators of well-being like income, poverty, material deprivation) often declined significantly during recessions. Thus, empirical research investigating the impact of the 2008 Global Financial Crisis and the subsequent Great Recession reports recession-induced increases in poverty and deprivation rates (e.g. Addabbo et al. 2012; Gábos et al. 2015; Guardiola and Guillen-Royo 2015; Keeley and Love 2010), in particular, for vulnerable and disadvantaged groups (e.g. Simona-Moussa and Ravazzini 2019; Smeeding et al. 2011).

The impact of economic crises on *subjective* well-being, however, is less clear and empirical evidence shows mixed results. Thus, Parker et al. (2016) found that the Global Financial Crisis negatively impacted on the levels of subjective well-being of young people in Australia aged 19–22 years and Deaton (2011) shows that mean happiness considerably decreased in the United States during the Global Financial Crisis and the subsequent Great Recession. Similar results are reported for transition countries (Russia, Baltic states) and, regarding financial satisfaction, for Latin American countries (see Easterlin et al. 2010). A recent study conducted by Burger et al. (2023) shows that levels of subjective well-being declined during periods of economic crises in Brazil. They linked this decline to changes in economic circumstances (including greater risk of unemployment, falling incomes, increasing debt) at the individual level. Conversely, Chesters et al. (2021) found that the Global Financial Crisis and the Great Recession did not depress levels of subjective well-being in Australia. This aligns with the results of Callens (2017) showing that the Great Recession in 2008 did not impact on levels of life satisfaction in Flanders (Belgium). Clark and Heath (2014) found that subjective well-being declined during the Global Financial Crisis in both the UK and the United States.

Differences in the effects of economic crises may be due to differences between short- and long-term impacts (see Easterlin 2015) and are likely to be related to cultural contexts and institutional arrangements. For example, although Morgan and Connor's (2022) examination of levels of subjective well-being in 23 European countries during the Great Recession showed that levels of subjective well-being declined between 2007 and 2009, population characteristics and labor market policies mediated the impact of the economic crisis. Their results indicate that increased support for the unemployed reduced the negative impact of the Great Recession. With regards to age, young people aged less than 25 years experienced the largest decline in subjective well-being. Compared to their counterparts with university level education, people with lower levels of education experienced larger declines in subjective well-being during the Great Recession.

1.4 Predictors and Correlates of Well-Being

Research conducted in societies of the Global North indicates that levels of well-being vary according to several demographic characteristics such as gender, age and level of education, however Gerling and Diener (2020) argue that demographic characteristics have a relatively small influence with effect sizes being marginal. Although there is a general agreement that the association between age and subjective well-being forms a U-shaped curve (Ambrey and Fleming 2014; Fritjers and Beatton 2012; Iglesias et al. 2017), Toshkov (2022) found that the relationship between age and subjective well-being varies according to income. He found that the U-shaped curve according to age was clearly visible for those on low incomes but flattened out completely for those on high incomes. Other factors, such as family type, employment status, income, socio-economic status and health status have been found to be strong predictors (Ambrey and Fleming 2014; Blanchflower and Oswald 2005; Chesters et al. 2021; Fleche et al. 2021; Gerling and Diener 2020; Headey and Muffels 2018; Kuhn and Brulé 2018; Layard et al. 2014; Manning et al. 2016; Oesch and Lipps 2013; Suter et al. 2015; Toshkov 2022). For example, in their analysis of data collected by the Gallup World Poll across 166 countries, Gerling and Diener (2020) found that income was positively associated with subjective well-being. Handa et al.'s (2023) analysis of data from young people aged 15–24 years across 150 countries confirmed this finding. Furthermore, they found that levels of life satisfaction were higher in the highest income quintiles regardless of regional location.

The association between education and subjective well-being is less clear with some researchers finding that levels of subjective well-being increase as levels of education increase (Blanchflower and Oswald 2005; Callens 2017; Fukuda 2013;

Gerling and Diener 2020; Yang 2008) but other researchers find a negative association (Ambrey and Fleming 2014; Clark and Oswald 1996; Manning et al. 2016; Veenhoven 1996). These contradictions appear to be related to differences in datasets and countries. For example, analysis of Household Income and Labour Dynamics in Australia (HILDA) data show that higher levels of education are strongly associated with lower levels of subjective well-being (Manning et al. 2016), whereas analysis of Swiss data indicates that the highly educated report higher levels of subjective well-being (Oesch and Lipps 2013; Suter et al. 2015).

Negative life events, such as divorce or unemployment, experiences of poverty and material deprivation have consistently been found to be associated with lower levels of subjective well-being (Brulé and Suter 2019; Callens 2017; Connelly and Garling 2022; Fleche et al. 2021; Gerling and Diener 2020; Headey and Muffels 2018; Iglesias et al. 2017; Kuhn and Brulé 2018; Layard et al. 2014; Suter and Iglesias 2005). For example, Gerling and Diener (2020) found that married people reported higher levels of subjective well-being than those who were divorced and that the effect size for life satisfaction was medium-to-large. In their examination of the impact of unemployment on levels of life satisfaction in Australia, Denmark, the UK, the US and Sweden, Connelly and Garling (2022) found that the unemployed reported lower levels of life satisfaction and emotional well-being than their employed counterparts. Several researchers have concluded that divorce and unemployment continue to depress levels of subjective well-being over the life course (Bell and Blanchflower 2011; Chesters et al. 2021; Kuhn and Brulé 2018). There is also evidence of an intergenerational transfer of levels of well-being with Headey et al. (2014) finding a strong correlation between parental well-being and an individual's well-being even after controlling for the factors known to impact on well-being in adulthood.

Examinations of the correlates and predictors of subjective well-being in the Global South are a relatively recent phenomenon. Given the disparate contexts it is not surprising that researchers based in the Global South have also argued that the measurement of well-being and life satisfaction requires a more nuanced approach (Katumba et al. 2022). Cultural differences between countries and between regions within countries, make the measurement of well-being far more complicated than in the Global North. Katumba et al. (2022) developed a Reflective Quality of Life Index for the South African context. Their analysis indicates that race and to a lesser extent, gender are predictors of life satisfaction. In their qualitative study based in the Eastern Cape Province in South Africa, Moller et al. (2015) found that levels of life satisfaction were associated with material well-being, with a focus on access to money and living conditions.

Burger et al.'s (2022) examination of levels of subjective well-being in Colombia also showed that location was an important factor with people living outside of major cities reporting lower levels of happiness. Furthermore, their findings show that marital status, migrant status, religion and civic engagement were either not associated with subjective well-being or were only marginally associated.

The association between employment status and levels of subjective well-being is clearly illustrated in the research conducted by Rodrıguez-Puello et al. (2022) in

Chile. They found that there was a strong negative association between being underemployed and levels of subjective well-being. Other predictors of lower subjective well-being include having young children at home, living in an urban area and being employed in manual work. On the other hand, being in a long-term relationship, having a relatively high income, having higher levels of education and working in a highly skilled occupation were positively correlated with well-being (Rodrıguez-Puello et al. 2022). Another study in Chile conducted by Ditzel et al. (2022) examined levels of life satisfaction and happiness of children aged 9–14 years. Their results indicate that boys reported higher levels of subjective well-being than girls. These results differ from those of Savahl et al. (2023) who examined levels of subjective well-being of children aged 10–12 years in South Africa. Their results show that gender and location were not associated with levels of well-being.

1.5 Overview of Parts and Chapters

This edited collection includes 13 chapters examining the impact of COVID-19 on various aspects of well-being during the pandemic. Although the novel coronavirus, COVID-19, continues to mutate and waves of the pandemic continue to wash across the globe, we focus on the 2020–2022 period when it had its greatest impact. Adopting a global, comparative perspective, including both the experiences of countries from the Global North and the Global South, the volume brings together insights from different angles and diverse cultural, social, political and economic backgrounds. Societies from all regions of the world are included in the analyses of the 13 chapters: Europe, North America, Australia/Oceania, Asia, Africa, and Latin America.

The COVID-19 pandemic generated an abundance of research regarding the health, medical and epidemiological impacts of the virus and the measures taken to curtail its spread. However, there has been less attention paid to its impact on (subjective) well-being and happiness, including the various sub-domains of well-being and the pandemic experiences of specific population groups. Therefore, the chapters of this volume are clustered around four themes: Firstly, the impact of COVID-19 on subjective well-being (life satisfaction and happiness), based on comparative and/or longitudinal studies; secondly, the impact of COVID-19 on employment, workers' well-being, and work-life balance; thirdly, sociability, civic participation and solidarity during the COVID-19 pandemic; and fourthly, the well-being impact of COVID-19 on children, a population group that has been most severely affected by the pandemic.

The three chapters included in the first part conduct analysis of population data to examine the evolution of subjective well-being (life satisfaction/happiness) during the pandemic adopting a comparative cross-national perspective. Research examining the impact of economic crises on levels of subjective well-being indicate that personal circumstances have the potential to limit the impact of economic shocks on subjective well-being. As demonstrated above in Sect. 1.3, research on earlier crises shows mixed results concerning the crisis impact on subjective well-being. A comparison of the COVID-19 pandemic with earlier crises, is, therefore, of particular interest.

The chapter contributed by Marc Callens and Dries Verlet tracks trends over time in subjective well-being in eight European countries (Denmark, France, former West-Germany, Great-Britain, Ireland, Italy, the Netherlands, and Belgium) using cross sectional data from the Eurobarometer survey collected between 1973 and 2022. Distinguishing between age, period and cohort effects, the study finds that period effects dominate cohort effects, except in France. The chapter demonstrates that past severe economic recessions have had a significant and lasting (negative) impact on life satisfaction and concludes that the COVID-19 crisis and the early 1980s economic crisis have comparable short-term effects on life satisfaction, but that the latter crisis has a deeper and longer-lasting effect.

Using data from two cross-sectional surveys conducted in Indonesia, Indera Pattinasarany examines the impact of the pandemic on levels of happiness. Her results indicate that COVID-19 infection rates were associated with levels of happiness in that people living in areas with higher levels of infection reported having lower levels of happiness. Giving regular and occasional donations is associated with increased self-reported happiness. Conversely, a negative moderation effect indicates that making regular and occasional donations diminishes the link between COVID-19 severity and self-reported happiness. Ultimately, the pandemic's severity diminishes the positive influence of donations on happiness.

Based on data from the European Social Survey, the final chapter of this first part, co-authored by Dragan Stanojević, Bojan Todosijević, and Anja Gvozdanović, investigates the relationship between social ties, labour market integration, and levels of subjective well-being of 15–35 year olds during the COVID-19 pandemic in 31 European countries. The chapter demonstrates the positive impact of employment and informal networks on subjective well-being. Interestingly, young people who worked in offices reported lower levels of satisfaction compared to those who predominantly worked from home. The chapter also shows that income inequality exhibits negative associations with levels of subjective well-being of young people. As income inequality increases between countries, the significance of informal social contacts becomes greater for subjective well-being. This finding suggests that personal informal networks compensate for structural inequalities.

In the second part, three chapters examine the impact of COVID-19 on the well-being of workers (including depression, health) and their work-life balance. During the early phase of the pandemic, large proportions of workplaces were either shut down or subject to density restrictions. Consequently, unemployment dramatically increased and large proportions of the workforce were forced to work from home. Becoming unemployed during the pandemic was particularly devastating as businesses were either shutdown or struggling to survive. Even the businesses which were able to continue to operate engaged in a hiring freeze. For those working remotely, balancing work and home and/or separating work *from* home became increasingly difficult.

The chapter co-authored by Shireen AlAzzawi and Vladimir Hlasny draws on data from the Economic Research Forum (ERF) COVID-19 MENA Monitor to examine the impact of COVID-19 on employment outcomes in four of the five countries in the Middle East and North Africa (MENA): Egypt, Jordan, Morocco, and Tunisia. Young workers and women were more disadvantaged than older workers and men. Informal workers were seen to exit the labor market in greater numbers than formal workers. Among economically inactive workers, women faced an extreme risk (95%) of remaining inactive or unemployed, while the risk was somewhat lower (around 80%) among men. Meanwhile, formal private-sector workers—particularly from older cohorts, faced a distinctly lower risk of becoming inactive or unemployed. In general, the results indicate that the pandemic exacerbated inequality by increasing already high levels of informal employment.

The chapter co-authored by Catherine White Berheide, Megan Carpenter, and David Cotter examines levels of well-being reported by academic staff from three colleges in New York State. Their results show that the pandemic exacerbated existing gender inequalities and worsened what little work-life alignment parents had achieved prior to the pandemic. While all three colleges gave untenured faculty the option to delay going up for tenure, that policy may not be enough to address the way differences in demands and resources affected faculty productivity. Among the group of workers studied, women and parents experienced a greater decline in levels of life satisfaction; and assistant and associate professors reported lower levels of satisfaction with their work-life balance than full professors.

In the final chapter in this part, Regina Skiba, Eileen McNeely, and Dorota Weziak-Białowolska conduct analysis of data from the Longitudinal Worker Well-being Survey to compare levels of life satisfaction between shift workers and regular workers in Poland. Shift work, as a job performed in unfavorable conditions due to disruption of day and night rhythms, could be associated with negative consequences. Their results indicate that shift workers, mainly manual workers, reported lower levels of general health, mental health and satisfaction with their relationships.

The three chapters included in the third part of this collection focus on sociability, civic participation and solidarity during the COVID-19 pandemic. Levels of sociability refer to the quality of social relations, most of which were severely impacted during the pandemic. When restrictions to movement were implemented, families were confined to their homes and interactions with extended family and friends switched from face-to-face to virtual. Public spaces were emptied and public activities, like traditional volunteering were restricted. Even people who had a legitimate reason to be outside their homes were reluctant to engage in incidental social interaction. In other words, the restrictions implemented during the pandemic affected sociability through its impact on social relationships with friends, colleagues and peers, family relationships, and the use of public space.

The first chapter in this part, contributed by Gonzalo Saraví examines the relationship between sociability and well-being of young people during the pandemic lockdown in Mexico where schools were closed for almost 2 years. His findings highlight how young people living in poorer neighborhoods in Mexico City had to endure their confinement in contexts of social precariousness and economic limitations, which negatively impacted on their socio-emotional well-being. Many of the socio-emotional discomforts experienced by these adolescents during the pandemic, such as anxiety, depression, or sadness, may be associated with an inconsistency between a stopped biographical time and a chronological time that kept moving forward.

The chapter of Joonmo Son, Pildoo Sung, and Benjamin Tay deals with volunteering during the pandemic by investigating how satisfaction in organized volunteering impacted on donative behavior. Using data from the Individual Giving Study in Singapore including detailed information on various aspects of volunteer satisfaction the chapter identifies five groups of volunteers showing different levels and patterns of volunteer satisfaction. The results of the analysis demonstrate that volunteer satisfaction is positively related to donative behavior. Interestingly, not all aspects of volunteer satisfaction similarly impact on donation. Satisfaction with the organization's efficacy and satisfaction with the social relationships and the mutual bonding among volunteers, in particular, turn volunteers into donors.

In his chapter, Fakhrul Alam presents his findings from semi-structured interviews conducted with 49 Rohingya refugees and 42 front-line service providers in Bangladesh. His findings show that movement restrictions in the refugee camps severely impacted Rohingya's income, food consumption, education, and opportunities to access health services. The action of volunteers in disseminating information about COVID-19 symptoms, testing, treatment, isolation, and quarantine, made people aware of rumors and misconceptions, and counseled refugees with symptoms to attend the available health services. The study concludes that volunteers made a significant contribution to developing civic responsibilities among the refugees, which encouraged them to participate in COVID-19 related health programs.

The three chapters in the final part of this volume, Part IV, focus on the impact of COVID-19 on levels of well-being of children and young people. Although people of all ages experienced dramatic changes in their social, cultural and physical environments, children and young people were more severely impacted because they have little control over their living arrangements and conditions. Furthermore, children and young people were isolated from their friends due to being confined to their homes and being unable to go to school or engage in extracurricular activities.

In the first chapter of this part, Haridhan Goswami, Bijoy Banik, Gour Goswami, and M. Ibrahim Khalil focus on school children aged 10–12 years in Bangladesh. Their analysis of data from the Children's Worlds COVID-19 Special Survey, using 12 indicators that reflect different aspects of life, shows that rural children were significantly less satisfied with several aspects of their lives during the pandemic including their home, area of living, safety, learning at school, and future. A gendered aspect was observed where boys reported significantly lower satisfaction with their material possessions and how adults listened to them. Girls reported experiencing lower levels of satisfaction with time use and learning at home during the pandemic than boys.

The chapter of Oliver Nahkur and Karoline Zarina provides an analysis of data collected by the International Children's Worlds COVID-19 Supplement Survey from children aged 9–13 years from 16 countries in 2021. Although experiences of social distancing was not an important correlate of children's subjective well-being decline in most of the countries, it influenced children's subjective well-being indirectly through other factors. Across countries, pandemic-related school anxiety consistently negatively impacted on children's subjective well-being decline, and in many countries the lack of psychological need(s) fulfilment also helped to explain the decline. Negative outcomes of school closures and the social distancing of the whole population outweigh its positive aspects.

In the final chapter of the collection, Jenny Chesters draws on data from the Household, Income and Labour Dynamics in Australia panel study to compare levels of subjective well-being between 2001 and 2020 of young people aged 15–17 years. Adolescence is the period when young people develop their own social networks, thus, peer relationships become increasingly more important. During the pandemic, young people were isolated from their friends at school, extra-curricular activities were disrupted and life became increasingly uncertain. Thus, the COVID-19 pandemic further complicated an already complex process. Her analysis reveals that young people reported similar levels of subjective well-being in 2001, 2005, 2010, 2015 and 2020 suggesting that age effects trumped period effects. However, within the 2020 cohort, levels of subjective well-being were negatively associated with concerns of catching COVID-19.

Table 1.1 presents the main features of each chapter mapping the scope of the volume and highlighting the sources of data and methods of analysis employed by the authors.

Table 1.1 Well-being and quality of life during the pandemic in the Global North and Global South: Main features of the chapters

Author/s	Title	Topic	Analysis unit	Spatial delimitation	Temporal delimitation	Data source	Methodology/ Main techniques
Part I: The impact of COVID-19 on life satisfaction and happiness: comparative and longitudinal perspectives							
Marc Callens & Dries Verlet	The impact of COVID-19 on life satisfaction: A cross-national, long term perspective	Impact of COVID-19 on life satisfaction	Adult population	Denmark, France, West-Germany, Great Britain, Ireland, Italy, the Netherlands, and Flanders (Belgium)	1973–2022	Eurobarometer (EU) $n = 585{,}154$	Quantitative: Regressions
Indera Ratna Irawati Pattinasarany	Happiness trends before and during the COVID-19 pandemic in Indonesia	Impact of COVID-19 on happiness	Adult population	Indonesia	2017 & 2021	Surveys on Happiness $n = 137{,}958$	Quantitative: Multilevel mixed-effects ordered logistic model
Dragan Stanojević, Bojan Todosijević, & Anja Gvozdanović	The well-being of young people in Europe during the pandemic	Well-being of young people	Young people (15–35 years old)	Europe: 31 countries	2020–2022	European Social Survey $n = 14{,}435$	Quantitative: Multi-level random intercept linear models
Part II: The impact of COVID-19 on employment and workers' well-being							
Shireen AlAzzawi & Vladimir Hlasny	Employment vulnerabilities of female and young adults in Arab countries	Youths' employment	Young people (17–29 years old) and other adults (30–59 years)	Egypt, Jordan, Morocco & Tunisia	February 2020 to September 2021	Economic Research Forum (ERF) COVID-19 Survey (MENA Monitor)	Quantitative: Transition matrices and multinomial logit models
Catherine White Berheide, Megan A. Carpenter, & David A. Cotter	The effect of the COVID-19 pandemic on faculty well-being: A study of academic staff at three colleges in New York	Well-being of academic staff	3 private colleges	New York	2020	Survey of tenured academics $n= 204$	Quantitative: OLS regressions

Regina Skiba, Eileen McNeely, & Dorota Weziak-Bialowolska	Limited social contact at work during the COVID-19 pandemic and shift worker's health and well-being	Worker's health and well-being	Garment factories workers	Poland	2019, 2020 & 2021	Longitudinal Worker Well-being Survey $n = 631$	Quantitative: OLS regressions
Part III: Sociability, civic participation and solidarity during the pandemic							
Gonzalo A. Saraví	The pandemic effects on sociability and well-being of low-income adolescents in Mexico	Sociability and well-being	Children and young people (low-income sectors)	Mexico	2020–2021	61 adolescents	Qualitative: participatory-research
Joonmo Son Pildoo Sung, & Benjamin Tay	The latent classes of the volunteer satisfaction index and donation during the pandemic in Singapore	Volunteerism, altruistic values, donation behaviors	Adult volunteers	Singapore	2021	Individual Giving Survey	Quantitative: Latent Class Analysis
Md. Fakhrul Alam	COVID-19 and community-based volunteerism	Volunteerism	Rohingya refugees	Bangladesh	Oct-2020 to Jan 2021	49 refugees, 42 organizations	Qualitative: in depth face-to-face interviews
Part IV: The impact of COVID-19 on children's well-being							
Haridhan Goswami, Bijoy Krishna Banik, Gour Gobinda Goswami & M. Ibrahim Khalil	Children's well-being during the COVID-19 pandemic	Well-being in childhood	Children aged 10–12 years	Bangladesh	2020	Children's Worlds COVID-19 Special Survey $n = 1370$	Quantitative: Univariate and bivariate statistical techniques

(continued)

Table 1.1 (continued)

Author/s	Title	Topic	Analysis unit	Spatial delimitation	Temporal delimitation	Data source	Methodology/ Main techniques
Oliver Nahkur & Karoline Zarina	Children's profiles of subjective well-being change during the COVID-19 pandemic and its correlates: A multi-national study	Subjective well-being in childhood	Children aged 9–13 years	Germany, Turkey, Bangladesh, Italy, Albania, Romania, Chile, Wales, Colombia, Taiwan, Belgium, Algeria, Israel, South Korea, Indonesia, and Estonia.	2021	International Child Well-being. COVID supplement Survey	Quantitative: Non parametric test and logistic regression analysis
Jenny Chesters	The impact of COVID-19 on young people's levels of subjective well-being: Evidence from HILDA 2001–2020	Subjective well-being in youth	Young people aged 15–17 years	Australia	2001, 2005, 2010, 2015 & 2020	Household Income and Labour Dynamics in Australia	Quantitative: Multiple regression models

References

Addabbo, T., R. García-Fernández, C. Llorca-Rodríguez, and A. Maccagnan. 2012. Poverty and unemployment: The cases of Italy and Spain. In *Social exclusions*, ed. G. Parodi and D. Sciulli, 199–219. Berlin: Springer.

Ambrey, C.L., and C.M. Fleming. 2014. Life satisfaction in Australia: Evidence from ten years of the HILDA survey. *Social Indicators Research* 115: 691–714.

Bell, D.N., and D.G. Blanchflower. 2011. Young people and the Great Recession. *Oxford Review of Economic Policy* 27 (2): 241–267.

Blanchflower, D.G., and A.J. Oswald. 2005. Happiness and the human development index: The paradox of Australia. *Australian Economic Review* 38 (3): 307–318.

Brulé, G., and C. Suter, eds. 2019. *Wealth(s) and subjective well-being*. Cham: Springer Nature.

Burger, M.J., M. Hendriks, and E.I. Ianchovichina. 2022. Happy but unequal: Differences in subjective well-being across individuals and space in Colombia. *Applied Research in Quality of Life* 17: 1343–1387.

———. 2023. Economic crises. Subjective well-being, and vote switching: The case of Brazil's 2018 presidential election. *Journal of Happiness Studies* 24: 2831–2583.

Callens, M. 2017. Long term trends in life satisfaction, 1973-2012: Flanders in Europe. *Social Indicators Research* 130: 107–127.

Chesters, J., J. Simona, and C. Suter. 2021. Cross-national comparison of age and period effects on levels of subjective well-being in Australia and Switzerland during volatile economic times (2001–2016). *Social Indicators Research* 154 (1): 361–391.

Clark, T., and A. Heath. 2014. *Hard times: The divisive tool of the economic slump*. New Haven, CT: Yale University Press.

Clark, A.E., and A.J. Oswald. 1996. Satisfaction and comparison income. *Journal of Public Economics* 61: 359–381.

Connelly, F.F., and T. Garling. 2022. Mediators of differences between employed and unemployed in life satisfaction and emotional well-being. *Journal of Happiness Studies* 23: 1637–1651.

Deaton, A.S. 2011. *The financial crisis and well-being of Americans. NBER Working Paper Series 17128*. Cambridge, MA: National Bureau of Economic Research. http://www.nber.org/papers/w17128.

Diener, E., R. Inglehart, and L. Tay. 2013. Theory and validity of life satisfaction scales. *Social Indicators Research* 112 (3): 497–527.

Ditzel, L., F. Casas, J. Torres-Vallejos, and A. Villarroel. 2022. The subjective well-being of Chilean children living in conditions of high social vulnerability. *Applied Research in Quality of Life* 17: 1639–1660.

Easterlin, R.A. 2015. Happiness and economic growth—The evidence. In *Global handbook of quality of life: Exploration of well-being of nations and continents*, ed. W. Glatzer, L. Camfield, V. Moller, and M. Rojas, 283–299. Dordrecht: Springer.

Easterlin, R.A., L.A. McVey, M. Switek, O. Sawangfa, and J.S. Zweig. 2010. The happiness-income paradox revisited. *Proceedings of the National Academy of Sciences* 107: 22463–22468.

Ehrler, F., F. Bühlmann, P. Farago, F. Höpflinger, D. Joye, P. Perrig-Chiello, and C. Suter, eds. 2016. *Swiss social report 2016: Wellbeing*. Zürich: Seismo.

Fachelli, S., C. Suter, and J. Chesters. 2024 (forthcoming). *An empirical exploration of COVID in the world*. Unpublished manuscript. Sevilla: Pablo de Olavide University.

Fleche, S., W.N. Lekfuangfu, and A.E. Clark. 2021. The long-lasting effects of family and childhood on adult wellbeing: Evidence from British cohort data. *Journal of Economic Behaviour and Organization* 181: 290–311.

Fritjers, P., and T. Beatton. 2012. The mystery of the U-shaped relationship between happiness and age. *Journal of Economic Behaviour & Organization* 82: 525–542.

Fukuda, K. 2013. A happiness study using age-period-cohort framework. *Journal of Happiness Studies* 14: 135–153.

Gábos, A., R. Branyiczki, B. Lange, and I. György Tóth. 2015. *Employment and poverty dynamics in the EU countries before, during and after crisis.* ImPRovE working papers, 15(06). Antwerp: Herman Deleeck Centre for Social Policy.

Gerling, D.M., and E. Diener. 2020. Effect size strengths in subjective well-being research. *Applied Research in Quality of Life* 15: 167–185.

Guardiola, J., and M. Guillen-Royo. 2015. Income, unemployment, higher education and wellbeing in times of economic crisis: Evidence from Granada (Spain). *Social Indicators Research* 120: 395–409.

Handa, S., A. Pereira, and G. Holmqvist. 2023. The rapid decline of happiness: Exploring life satisfaction among young people across the world. *Applied Research in Quality of Life* 18: 1549–1579.

Headey, B., and R. Muffels. 2018. A theory of life satisfaction dynamics: Stability, change and volatility in 25-year life trajectories in Germany. *Social Indicators Research* 140: 837–866.

Headey, B., R. Muffels, and G.G. Wagner. 2013. Choices which change life satisfaction: Similar results for Australia, Britain and Germany. *Social Indicators Research* 112: 725–748.

———. 2014. Parents transmit happiness along with associated values and behaviors to their children: A lifelong happiness dividend? *Social Indicators Research* 116: 909–933.

Headey, B., G. Trommsdorff, and G.G. Wagner. 2022. Alternative recipes for life satisfaction: Evidence from five world regions. *Applied Research in Quality of Life* 17: 763–794.

Iglesias, K., P. Gazareth, and C. Suter. 2017. Explaining the decline in subjective well-being over time in panel data. In *Metrics of subjective well-being: Limits and improvements*, ed. G. Brulé and F. Maggino, 85–105. Dordrecht: Springer.

Katumba, S., J. de Kadt, M. Orkin, and P. Fatti. 2022. Construction of a reflective quality of life index for Gauteng province in South Africa. *Social Indicators Research* 164 (1): 373–408.

Keeley, B., and P. Love. 2010. *From crisis to recession: The causes, course and consequences of the Great Recession*. Paris: OECD.

Krys, K., B.W. Haas, E.R. Igou, A. Kosiarczyk, A. Kocimska-Bortnowska, A. Kwiatkowska, et al. 2023. Introduction to a culturally sensitive measure of well-being: Combining life satisfaction and interdependent happiness across 49 different cultures. *Journal of Happiness Studies* 24: 607–627.

Kuhn, U., and G. Brulé. 2018. Buffering effects for negative life events: The role of material, social, religious and personal resources. *Journal of Happiness Studies* 20: 1397–1417. https://doi.org/10.1007/s10902-018-9995-x.

Layard, R., A. Clark, F. Cornaglia, N. Powdthavee, and J. Vernoit. 2014. What predicts a successful life? A life-course model of wellbeing. *The Economic Journal* 124: 720–738.

Maggino, F., ed. 2023. *Encyclopedia of quality of life and well-being research.* Cham: Springer. https://doi.org/10.1007/978-3-031-17299-1.

Manning, M., C.L. Ambrey, and C.M. Fleming. 2016. A longitudinal study of indigenous wellbeing in Australia. *Journal of Happiness Studies* 17: 2503–2525.

Moller, V., B. Roberts, and D. Zani. 2015. The personal wellbeing index in the South African IsiXhosa translation: A Qualitative focus group study. *Social Indicators Research* 124: 835–852.

Morgan, R., and K.J. O'Connor. 2022. Labor market policy and subjective well-being during the Great Recession. *Journal of Happiness Studies* 23: 391–422.

Noll, H.H. 2002. Towards a European system of social indicators: Theoretical framework and system architecture. *Social Indicators Research* 58: 47–87. https://doi.org/10.1023/A:1015775631413.

OECD (Organization for Economic Co-operation and Development). 2013. *OECD guidelines on measuring subjective well-being*. Paris: OECD.

Oesch, D., and O. Lipps. 2013. Does unemployment hurt less if there is more of it around? A panel analysis of life satisfaction in Germany and Switzerland. *European Sociological Review* 29 (5): 955–967.

Parker, P.D., J. Jerrim, and J. Andres. 2016. What effect did the global financial crisis have upon youth wellbeing? Evidence from four Australian cohorts. *Developmental Psychology* 42 (4): 640–651.

Rodrıguez-Puello, G., A. Arcos, and B. Jara. 2022. Would you value a few more hours of work? Underemployment and subjective well-being across Chilean workers. *Applied Research in Quality of Life* 17: 885–912.

Savahl, S., S. Adams, and P. Hoosen. 2023. The subjective and psychological well-being of children in South Africa: A population-based study. *Applied Research in Quality of Life* 18: 2315–2347.

Seligman, M. 2011. *Flourishing: A visionary new understanding of happiness and well-being*. New York: Free Press.

Simona-Moussa, J., and L. Ravazzini. 2019. From one recession to another: Longitudinal impacts on the quality of life of vulnerable groups. *Social Indicators Research* 142 (3): 1129–1152.

Smeeding, T.M., J.P. Thompson, A. Levanon, and E. Burak. 2011. Poverty and income inequality in the early stages of the Great Recession. In *The great recession*, ed. D.B. Grusky, B. Western, and C. Wimer, 82–126. New York: Russell Sage Foundation.

Suter, C., and K. Iglesias. 2005. Relative deprivation and well-being: Switzerland in a comparative perspective. In *Contemporary Switzerland: Revisiting the special case*, ed. H. Kriesi, P. Farago, M. Kohli, and M. Zarin-Nejadan, 9–37. Houndmills: Palgrave Macmillan.

Suter, C., K. Iglesias, and J. Moussa. 2015. From dissonance to well-being and adaptation? Quality of life in Switzerland over the past decades. In *Global handbook of quality of life: Exploration of well-being of nations and continents*, ed. W. Glatzer, L. Camfield, V. Moller, and M. Rojas, 685–714. Dordrecht: Springer.

Toshkov, D. 2022. The relationship between age and happiness varies by income. *Journal of Happiness Studies* 23: 1169–1188.

UNDP (United Nations Development Programme). 2020. *Human Development Report 2020. The next frontier Human development and the anthropocene*. New York: UNDP. https://www.undp.org/belarus/publications/next-frontier-human-development-and-anthropocene. Accessed 17 Feb 2024.

———. 2022. *Human Development Report 2020/2021. Uncertain times, unsettled lives: Shaping our future in a transforming world*. New York: UNDP. https://hdr.undp.org/system/files/documents/global-report-document/hdr2021-22pdf_1.pdf. Accessed 17 Feb 2024.

Veenhoven, R. 1996. Developments in satisfaction-research. *Social Indicators Research* 37 (1): 1–46.

WHO (World Health Organization). 2023. *The true toll of COVID-19: Estimating global excess mortality*. https://www.who.int/data/stories/the-true-death-toll-of-covid-19-estimating-global-excess-mortality. Accessed 21 Jan 2024.

Yang, Y. 2008. Social inequalities in happiness in the United States, 1972 to 2004: An age-period-cohort analysis. *American Sociological Review* 73 (2): 204–226.

Christian Suter is Professor Emeritus of Sociology at the University of Neuchâtel (Switzerland). He is currently doing research on social indicators, quality of life, globalization and world society. His most recent publications include *The Global Politics of Census Taking* (Routledge 2024), *Measuring Gender Equality* (Springer 2023), and *The Middle Class in World Society* (Routledge 2020). He is currently a Board member and has been a former President of RC55 "Social Indicators" of the International Sociological Association. He is a winner of a *Book Award of the American Sociological Association* (1993) and of the Research Fellow Award from the *International Society for Quality-of-Life Studies* (2020).

Jenny Chesters is Associate Professor in the Faculty of Education, at the University of Melbourne, Australia. She is a CI on the Life Patterns Research Project—a longitudinal mixed methods study tracking 3 cohorts of school leavers over time. Her research interests focus on transitions between education and employment throughout the life course and inequality in educational attainment. She is a Board member of RC55 "Social Indicators" of the International Sociological Association. Her recent publications include the *Research Handbook on Transitions into Adulthood* (Edward Elgar 2024).

Sandra Fachelli is Associate Professor at the Department of Sociology of Pablo de Olavide University, Sevilla, Spain. She is subcoordinator of the INCASI2 International Network for Comparative Analysis of Social Inequalities, an European project (GA 101130456). She is currently President of the Research Committee 06 "Inequality and Social Stratification" of the Spanish Federation of Sociology (FES) and Vice-president of RC55 "Social Indicators" of the International Sociological Association. Her most recent books are *Measuring Gender Equality* (Springer 2023), *Towards a Comparative Analysis of Social Inequalities between Europe and Latin America* (2021), and *Perspectivas y fronteras en el estudio de la desigualdad social: movilidad social y clases sociales en tiempos de cambio* (2020).

Part I
The Impact of COVID-19 on Life Satisfaction and Happiness: Comparative and Longitudinal Perspectives

Chapter 2
The Impact of COVID-19 on Life Satisfaction: A Cross-National, Long Term Perspective

Marc Callens and Dries Verlet

2.1 Introduction

Early 2020 a novel coronavirus, COVID-19, took the world in surprise. It disrupted the daily lives of billions of people, and confronted societies with an unprecedented health crisis that provoked economic turmoil worldwide.

Several studies, based on survey or social media data, have extensively documented on the immediate negative impact of the COVID crisis on several domains, including individual well-being. However, being pressed to deliver insights in a timely manner, most research designs used tend to bypass somehow sound methodological rigor. Some studies use non-probability samples and hence findings might be impacted by selectivity issues; other studies lack a sound comparative and/or longitudinal perspective: they are confined to a single country, or they are cross-sectional in nature.

The central theme in this chapter is the impact of the COVID-19 crisis on subjective well-being, more specifically *happiness* in the form of *general life satisfaction*. To assess the impact of the COVID-19 crisis on life satisfaction adequately, it is important to take both a long-term and a comparative perspective into account. By doing so, we can put the effects of the COVID-19 crisis into perspective by comparing with previous (economic) crises, such as the unemployment/inflation crisis (early eighties) or the Great Recession (2007–2008).

However, in human societies, time is a complex phenomenon as three subdimensions are simultaneously at work: next to historical time (period, trend) also birth cohort (generation) and age (life cycle) play a role. With each of these three time dimensions, different theoretical explanations can be associated. Age effects represent age-related developmental changes through the life cycle. In principle, life

M. Callens (✉) · D. Verlet
Department of Public Governance & Management, Ghent University, Campus Rommelaere, Ghent, Belgium
e-mail: marc.callens@ugent.be; dries.verlet@ugent.be

C. Suter et al. (eds.), *Well-being During the Pandemic*, Social Indicators Research Series 90, https://doi.org/10.1007/978-3-031-63440-6_2

cycle effects are more general in nature and apply regardless of time and birth cohort. Period and birth cohort effects refer to exogenous contextual changes in broader social conditions. Period effects occur as a result of cultural and economic societal changes that are unique to specific time periods (e.g., a severe economic recession, a health crisis like the COVID-19 crisis) and thus apply to everyone regardless of age. Cohort effects are the essence of social change, not just determined by the time of birth as such, but also by cumulatively going through the same historical and social factors.

The main research questions in this chapter are: (1) what is the relative impact of age, period, birth cohort, GDP and unemployment rate on general life satisfaction in the long-term (1973–2022) and across eight West-European countries; (2) compared with previous large economic crises after 1972, how important is the impact of the COVID-19 crisis (2000–2022) on general life satisfaction across eight West-European countries (1973–2022).

To answer these questions, most earlier (cross-sectional) study designs are inadequate because they focus on only one temporal dimension and thereby thus assume that the other two temporal dimensions have no effects. A solution to this problem, proposed by Yang and Land (2013) is to apply Hierarchical Age-Period-Cohort Regression (HAPC-regression), to a set of pooled repeated cross-sectional surveys thereby making it possible to estimate the net trend, life cycle and generation effects. We apply this technique to a combined set of Eurobarometer survey data (n = 585,154) covering half a century (1973–2022) for eight countries that were already part of the European Union in 1973: Denmark, France, former West Germany, Great Britain (i.e., excluding Northern Ireland), Ireland, Italy, the Netherlands and Belgium (Flanders only).

The study indicates that period effects dominate cohort effects. Moreover, severe economic recessions and the COVID-19 crisis have both a significant but different impact on life satisfaction levels. The remainder of the chapter is as follows: Sect. 2.2 provides an overview of the literature and gives the context. Section 2.3 presents the data and our empirical strategy. In Sect. 2.4, we describe the results of the analysis, and we conclude in Sect. 2.5.

2.2 Literature Review

Subjective well-being refers to an individual's own assessment of their life and encompasses both cognitive (perceptive) and affective (emotional) aspects. (Sirgy 2021; Verlet and Callens 2010). The extent to which someone feels good is referred to as the "hedonic feeling level" or "happiness" (Veenhoven 2002). General Life Satisfaction is a conscious cognitive judgement with life as a whole (Huebner and Dew 1996), while happiness is the affective component that measures how a person feels about their life (Veenhoven 2002). According to Diener et al. (1985, 71), life satisfaction is described as a mental evaluation process that relies on comparing one's circumstances with a perceived standard of what is considered appropriate.

The closer the perception of life achievements aligns with the standard, the higher the individual's life satisfaction will be. People can evaluate their life intellectually by comparing wishes and reality, and by estimating the likelihood of their wishes being fulfilled (Veenhoven 2002).

In recent years, the use of happiness (life satisfaction) as an alternative measure of social progress in contrast to the traditional measure of Gross Domestic Product (GDP) has been debated in various circles (Commission of the European Communities 2009; Stiglitz et al. 2009). The criticism of GDP includes that it does not accurately reflect social and ecological dimensions. On the other hand, while GDP can detect economic fluctuations quite well, change of happiness seems to vary substantially in the long run in only some developed countries (Easterlin and O'Connor 2023). Moreover, general life satisfaction research seems to reveal only limited variation along socio-economic strata (Verlet and Callens 2010). International comparisons, on the other hand, show that developed countries do indeed seem to differ from each other (Pittau et al. 2010), even though it cannot be excluded that these differences are partly due to measurement issues.

The main focus of this chapter is to examine the effect of the COVID-19 pandemic on subjective well-being, measured as general life satisfaction. To get a complete understanding of how the crisis has affected life satisfaction, it is crucial to consider both a long-term and a cross-national perspective. This will enable us to compare the impact of the COVID crisis with that of previous economic downturns, such as the unemployment/inflation crisis of the early 1980s and the Great Recession (2007–2008) and to consider possible explanations for heterogeneity among countries.

To determine the impact of such crises, it is important to distinguish three time dimensions: age (life cycle), historical time (period, trend), and birth cohort. Age effects represent age-related developmental changes over the life cycle (e.g., health: Gove et al. 1989). Period and cohort effects refer to exogenous contextual changes in broader social conditions. According to Ryder (1965), cohort effects form the essence of social change. Thus, a birth cohort is not only determined by the time of birth as such, but also by cumulatively experiencing the same kind of social experiences: the social conditions in early life, formal education, the same historical and social factors. Period effects arise as a result of cultural and economic changes that are unique to specific time periods (e.g., the COVID-19 crisis, the Great Recession, …) and thus apply to everyone regardless of age.

We found that in Flanders trend fluctuations are stronger than life-cycle effects with little to no generation effects, while some other countries exhibit signs of a generational change with few trend fluctuations (Callens 2017). It was also found that the international differences in life satisfaction are stronger than the temporal differences. As Callens (2017) mainly focused on the effect of social stratification variables (including across time and cohort) only, it remained unclear as to what macro-level factors can explain the long-term trends in the data.

The present chapter complements an earlier analysis in Callens (2017), which was focused on social stratification differentials, by adding macro-economic context variables (GDP, unemployment rate) and by extending the reference period to also include the effects of the COVID-19 pandemic (1973–2022). During this era, Western Europe faced several major economic crises (Eichengreen 2008) including the 1973 oil crisis, the 1981–1982 recession, the 1989–1991 recession, the 2007–2008 financial recession and more recently the 2009–2012 Eurozone Debt Crisis (Collignon 2012) and the COVID-19/Ukraine crisis. In addition, there were also other smaller recessions and economic difficulties during this period.

The 1973 oil crisis was a period of high inflation and economic recession caused by the sudden increase in oil prices by the Organization of the Petroleum Exporting Countries (OPEC). In 1981–1982, a global recession was caused by a combination of oil price increases, inflation and high unemployment. The late 1980s and early 1990s recession was a period of economic slowdown in Europe caused by declining competitiveness, high government debt and slow growth. The 2007–2008 global financial crisis started with the collapse of the US housing market and spread to Europe; this crisis led to widespread bank failures and a global recession. The Eurozone Debt Crisis began in 2009 and was a result of the high sovereign debt levels of several European countries, which led to a crisis in the eurozone.

More recently, the COVID-19 health crisis (2020–2022) has had far-reaching and profound consequences, both globally and at the individual level. The direct impact on health and mortality was high as the virus infected a large number of people who then became very sick, leading to increased healthcare costs and a significant strain on healthcare systems globally. But the COVID-19 isolation measures (social distancing, travel restrictions, …) imposed to prevent illness in the absence of an effective vaccine, had also very negative consequences on the economy and the (mental) well-being of people.

Economically, the pandemic resulted in widespread job losses, business closures, supply chain disruptions and decreased mobility, … resulting in a significant decline in the global economy. Many individuals and businesses have faced financial difficulties as a result. However, the economy recovered strongly from 2021 into early 2022 following the introduction of effective COVID-19 vaccines. By the end of 2022, raising inflation (partly due to the energy crisis caused by the Ukraine-Russia war), led central banks to raise interest rates, thereby increasing recession risks.

Levels of life satisfaction first dropped considerably during the early stages of the pandemic and then showed high volatility along the different waves (Brülhart and Lalive 2020; Recchi et al. 2020). The major question from a long term perspective is then whether life satisfaction levels will fully recover from pre-pandemic levels; however this is not an easy question to answer as the ending phase of the COVID-crisis meanwhile overlaps with a new crisis (Ukraine-Russia war, energy crisis, high levels of inflation).

How has overall subjective well-being evolved in recent decades: has it increased or decreased? Veenhoven and Kregel (2022) report average happiness in more than 50 nations worldwide for periods ranging from 1997–2018 (Peru) up to 1946–2017 (USA). For change of average happiness expressed in a ten points scale, they report an average rise of 0.652 (50 studies) and an average decline of –.582 (30 studies) in life satisfaction over the various study periods considered. Over the period 1973–2019 Eurobarometer data show a rise for Denmark (+0.70), Italy (+0.20), the

Netherlands (+0.60) and France (+0.30), United Kingdom (+0.46) and West Germany (+0.46; 1990–2019) but declines in Belgium (–0.59) and Ireland (–0.40). However, trend studies based on average life satisfaction levels, do not control for age or other relevant individual covariates. So, it is very much in question whether such trends are robust enough against statistical control at the individual level.

The research literature, using panel data or time series also shows mixed findings, that often contradict findings in reported average happiness or that are based on cross-sectional data (e.g., Easterlin and O'Connor (2023). Easterlin (1995) finds little or no empirical support for an increase in subjective well-being. In the US, there has even been a slight decrease (Blanchflower and Oswald 2004). On the other hand, Easterlin and O'Connor (2023) found between 1981–1982 and 2017–2018 considerable variation for the change in happiness among nine European countries. Spain, Italy and France increased up to 10% of the scale used, but Denmark and Sweden decreased 3%. Easterlin and O'Connor (2023) concluded in their analyses that generous welfare programs are the main driver for changes in happiness. Based on panel data for Australia and Switzerland between 2001 and 2016, Chesters et al. (2021) found no evidence for negative period effects due to the Great Recession.

Does increased prosperity over the past decades have a positive effect on general life satisfaction. The relative utility theorists (e.g., Davis 1984) predict that, despite increased prosperity, there will not be an increase in overall subjective well-being: not the absolute standard of living of an individual is important, but rather their relative position, either compared to others (reference thesis) or to their own past (adaptation thesis). According to the proponents of the absolute utility theory (e.g., Hagerty and Veenhoven 2003), increased prosperity leads to the fulfillment of more needs and therefore subjective well-being increases.

What is the relationship between unemployment and general life satisfaction? It is a well stated finding that unemployment reduces well-being considerably. For the UK, Clark and Oswald (1994) found that joblessness depressed well-being more than other negative experiences such as a divorce. Unemployment has a negative effect on people that are unemployed themselves, but also on people who are not personally affected by unemployment (Di Tella et al. 2003). However, sensitivity of subjective well-being to fluctuations in unemployment rates is much lower in the public than in the private sector. Civil servants, who are protected the most against economic shocks do not worry about job security, the opposite is the case for workers in the private sector who worry about losing their job, especially in high unemployment rate conditions (Luechinger et al. 2010).

In summary, we can say that there are frequent indications of social, temporal, and international gradients in the field of subjective well-being. Since both theory and empirics are partly characterized by contradictory elements, it is not possible to formulate precise research hypotheses in the current state of affairs. The research questions are therefore necessarily of a more general, exploratory nature: (1) over the long haul (1973–2022) and across eight West-European countries, what is the relative effect of age, period, birth cohort, GDP, and unemployment rate on overall life satisfaction; (2) in comparison to previous significant economic crises after

1972, what is the impact of the COVID-19 crisis (2000–2022) on general life satisfaction across the same eight West-European countries (1973–2022).

2.3 Data and Method

2.3.1 Variables

In this chapter we use individual level data from a series of Standard Eurobarometer surveys going back to 1973. The Standard Eurobarometer survey, conducted by the European Commission's Directorate-General for Communication, is a periodic, standardized survey that covers a range of topics including citizens' attitudes towards the EU, their political and social values, and their beliefs and perceptions on issues such as immigration, the economy, and the environment.

Only part of these surveys is available in a harmonized form as the so-called Mannheim Eurobarometer Trend File (doi: 10.4232/1.0074) including data from the European Communities Studies 1970 up to Eurobarometer 57.2 in 2002. This trend file contains information of 1,134,384 respondents from, in total 82 waves and 145 variables (Schmitt et al. 2008, 2009). To cover the 2003–2022 period, we standardize Eurobarometer Survey data as available by the end of January 2023 up to Eurobarometer 98.1 (European Commission 2022). The data for Eurobarometer 98.1 were collected in June/July 2022.

The early Eurobarometer surveys were held in only six countries (the then Member States of the EU). As the EU gradually grew, so did the number of participating countries in the Eurobarometer surveys. At present, in addition to the twenty-seven member states, also candidate countries, the United Kingdom, Norway, Switzerland and other territories are also included, in total more than forty territorial units. In this chapter, the focus is on the long term and for this reason the analysis includes only seven countries (Denmark, France, West Germany, Great Britain, Ireland, Italy, the Netherlands), and the region of Flanders (Belgium). The total sample size for the pooled dataset (1973–2022) is 585,154 persons of 15 years and older (no age limit) and residing in the EU. Country total sample size ranges from 75,551 for Ireland to 79,038 for the United Kingdom; for the Flemish Region the sample size is significantly lower: 42,851. Typically, the sample size per country per individual survey is thousand units.

The collection of Standard Eurobarometer data, currently spanning half a century, can be regarded as a set of repeated cross-sectional surveys,[1] a type of research design where a population is repeatedly sample surveyed at different points in time (typically once a year). Ideally, each Standard Eurobarometer survey uses the same survey design (questionnaire, sample design, survey mode, …) so that the data

[1] Note however that in such a design, as opposed to in a panel design, it is not possible to follow individuals over time.

obtained from a cross-section of the population are comparable. Such a design allows us to track changes in the population over time and make comparisons between different time points.

Although the majority of trend questions concern people's knowledge of and opinion about the EU, several other social, economic, and political topics (e.g. overall life satisfaction) are also included. In addition, various background variables such as: age, gender, education, marital status, region, income, subjective social class, occupation … are available.

The key variable of interest in this study is overall life satisfaction. This variable measures how people evaluate their life as a whole rather than their current feelings: the focus of overall life satisfaction is the life one leads in general, whereby the time frame is undefined. The question used in the Eurobarometer is: "On the whole, are you very satisfied, fairly satisfied or not at all satisfied with the life you lead? Would you say you are …?". The respondents report this themselves by means of a verbal four-point scale: "Very satisfied (1), satisfied (2), not satisfied (3), not very satisfied (4)." We reverse this scale in the analysis so that the "not very satisfied"-category corresponds to the lowest score (1), and the "very satisfied"-category to the highest score (4). In this way, achieving a high score corresponds to a high degree of life satisfaction.

We explicitly include the three different dimensions of time: Age, Period and Cohort (APC). Age is operationalized by age of the respondent (in years); Period by historical time (calendar year) and Cohort by birth cohort of the respondent (grouped in 5 year birth cohorts). Age of the respondent (in years, 15–98 years) is centered around the average age in the pooled dataset (45.02 years). In the multivariate analysis, age is specified in quadratic form (age + age squared; see below). Historical time includes each calendar year between 1973 and 2022, but not *1974* and *1996* as in both these years the question about overall life satisfaction was not included in the Standard Eurobarometer surveys. To avoid identification issues with age, birth cohort of the respondent is operationalized as 23 5-year birth cohorts: *until 1899*, *1900–1904*, ..., *2000–2004*, and *from 2005*. Note that the pooled dataset includes respondents that were born in three different centuries.

As stratification variables we include: gender, country (or region), educational level and marital status. Unfortunately, because of their fairly to extremely high item-nonresponse, other relevant variables such as income, occupation, (subjective) social class, the number of members in the household, … could not be included in the analysis. The inclusion of these variables in our dataset, especially in combination, would lead to a high dropout and an unwanted selectivity.

In more recent years, gender in the Eurobarometer surveys also includes the non-binary category. However for reasons of comparability with older Eurobarometer surveys, we dropped the non-binary cases and assigned *female* as the reference category. Educational level, defined as the age when finishing education has four levels: *still studying*, *15 years and less*, *16–19 years* (reference category), and *more than 20 years*. Marital status consists of four categories: *single*, *divorced*, *widowed* and *married* (reference category).

We also include in the analysis a number of variables at the country/region level: *change in gdp per capita* and *unemployment rate*. *Change in gdp per capita* is measured in chained dollars in 2015 prices and derived from the National Accounts Main Aggregates Database (United Nations 2023). Measurement in chained dollars adjusts real dollar amounts for inflation. To measure *unemployment rate* we use the Annual Macro-economic Database (AMECO) of the European Commission's Directorate General for Economic and Financial Affairs (ECFIN 2023). ECFINs version of unemployment rate is survey-based and agrees with the definition by the International Labor Organization. When the Region of Flanders is analyzed on its own, alternative data are used based on administrative data. These data, which are more robust than data based on surveys, are produced by the Federal Planning Bureau of Belgium (Federaal Planbureau 2022).

2.3.2 Method

The combined Eurobarometer data provide a unique opportunity to disentangle trend, age and cohort effects using Age-Period-Cohort (APC) analysis. APC analysis distinguishes three types of variations related to time: variations associated with age group (life cycle), historical period (trend), and birth cohort (generation). It is a valuable tool to understand the underlying causes of these variations, which can be internal (due to age) or external (due to historical events or birth cohort experiences) (Ryder 1965). If life cycle effects dominate the other two time dimensions, then the explanatory basis is often to be found internally (for example, diseases increase with age and it can be expected that overall life satisfaction decreases accordingly). Trends and birth cohort differences are based on external causes (e.g., the COVID-19 crisis) or thalidomide used by pregnant women to cure morning sickness (cohort). The COVID-19 crisis affected all individuals regardless of their age, while thalidomide only affected the children of a generation of pregnant women (until the drug was taken out of circulation).

However, the three time processes involved are linearly related to each other (cohort = period – age) which poses a challenging problem that is difficult to solve. The classic APC analysis method is controversial and suffers from the identification problem (Mason et al. 1973) where the estimated regression coefficients are not unique, leading to difficulties in estimation (Mason et al. 1973). Efforts have been made to solve this problem but with limited success (Glenn 1976, 2005).

A different situation arises when the researcher (as in the case of the Eurobarometer data) has access to microdata in the form of (a sufficient number of) repeated cross-sectional surveys. In a series of articles, Yang (2008) and Yang and Land (2006, 2013) propose a number of innovations in the analysis of repeated cross-sectional data, offering a solution to the identification problem using different temporal groups for period and cohort and a non-linear transformation of age. In this chapter we use single year for age (thereby applying a quadratic transformation), year of survey for period, and 5-year intervals for birth cohort.

Conceptually, the data structure of the Eurobarometer data is a cross-classified hierarchy: respondents (level 1) are hierarchically clustered in a cross-classified classification of two social contexts (level 2) defined by birth cohort and time period. In other words, all respondents are simultaneously members of exactly one birth cohort and one time period. The core idea is then to consider birth cohort and time period as social contexts (Yang and Land 2006).

To model the impact of period and birth cohort, two alternative strategies can be used: a fixed effects or a random effects model. The fixed effects approach is achieved through an Analysis of Covariance repeated cross-sectional regression model, where the effect of birth cohort and time period is controlled by the inclusion of dummy variables. However, this approach has limitations such as underestimating the significance level of covariate regression coefficients and the inability to introduce intercepts and covariates at the birth cohort and time period level.

In a random effects model the variability in general life satisfaction associated with individuals, birth cohorts, and time periods can be specified as random intercepts with variance parameters (Goldstein 2003; Raudenbush and Bryk 2002; Snijders and Bosker 2012). The interpretation of the β-parameters is that of a regression coefficient in a classic multiple regression model. According to Ferrer-i-Carbonell and Frijters (2004), it should make little or no difference whether scores for life satisfaction are ordinal or cardinal. Therefore, we prefer to work with a linear specification for general life satisfaction instead of ordered logits; the latter still posing many estimation problems, including non-convergence (Callens 2004).

How to model the impact of country/region? Besides the two previously mentioned social contexts birth cohort and time period, we also consider country/region as a social context. As outlined in Callens (2010), there are three modeling strategies for specifying country/region as a social context: separate regressions, ANCOVA regression, and multilevel regression. The use of multilevel models is elegant but cannot be applied here because the number of available countries/regions is too small. For this reason, we use separate regressions per country/region. The disadvantage of separate regressions is that time-constant explanatory variables at the country level cannot be included in the analysis.

2.4 Results

2.4.1 Flanders

In Table 2.1 the results for four cross-classified random effects age-period-cohort regression models for general life satisfaction in Flanders (1973–2022) are presented. For the fixed effects, unstandardized regression coefficients and for the random effects, variances are used. Interpreting the fixed effects is straightforward: life satisfaction is rated on a scale of 1–4, therefore a fixed effect of 0.1 for a particular independent variable indicates a 3.33% increase in life satisfaction per 1 unit

Table 2.1 General life satisfaction, results for four sub-models of cross-classified random-effect age-period-cohort regressions, Flanders, 1973–2022

Fixed effects	**Model 1**	**Model 2**	**Model 3**	**Model 4**
	Beta	Beta	Beta	Beta
Intercept	3.2382***	3.2043***	3.1879***	3.5317***
Age		–.0022***	–.0013***	–.0011**
Age²		0.0001***	0.0001***	0.0001***
Male			–.0034	–.0046
Education (ref = 16–19 yr.)				
Education (14–15 yr.)			–.0462***	–.0464***
Education (20–22 yr.)			0.0881***	0.0877***
Still studying			0.0760***	0.0764***
GDP-Cap-Ch				–.0000
Unemployment rate				–.0242***
Random effects	**Model 1**	**Model 2**	**Model 3**	**Model 4**
	Variance	Variance	Variance	Variance
Period effect	0.0101***	0.0097***	0.0098***	0.0067***
Cohort effect	0.0026*	0.0021**	0.0022*	0.0020*
Individual variance	0.4098***	0.4089***	0.4069***	0.4080***
Goodness of fit	79,708	79,642	79,463	77,768

* $p < 0.05$, ** $p < 0.01$, *** $p < 0.001$

Source: Standard Eurobarometer Survey Data (1973–2022), GESIS

increase on that variable's scale. For categorical independent variables, the fixed effect represents the difference in life satisfaction between the selected subgroup and a reference group.

Model 1, a so-called empty model, shows three variance estimates (period, cohort and individual variance) but no fixed estimates. Both time-level variances are small but significant. We therefore prefer a multilevel approach over a fixed effect (ANCOVA) one. The share of the period variance in the total variance is 2.5%, that of the cohort variance barely 0.5%; the individual variance (97%) clearly dominates the two other (time-related) variance components. In Model 2, the net overall effects for respectively age, cohort and period are given. Age is represented as a fixed estimate (Beta) and cohort and period as variances of random effects. We present the results of Model 2 in more detail in Figs. 2.1, 2.2, and 2.3 (see below).

In Model 3, the results for independent variables at the individual level (i.e., gender and educational level[2]) are presented. While the effect for gender is not statistically significant, the effect for educational level is: the higher the educational level, the higher the life satisfaction. Finally, in Model 4, we present the results for independent variables at the country level. The negative effect for unemployment, in

[2] We omitted in Table 2.1 the results for the interaction effects between social stratification variables and across cohort/period. The results are similar to these found in Callens (2017).

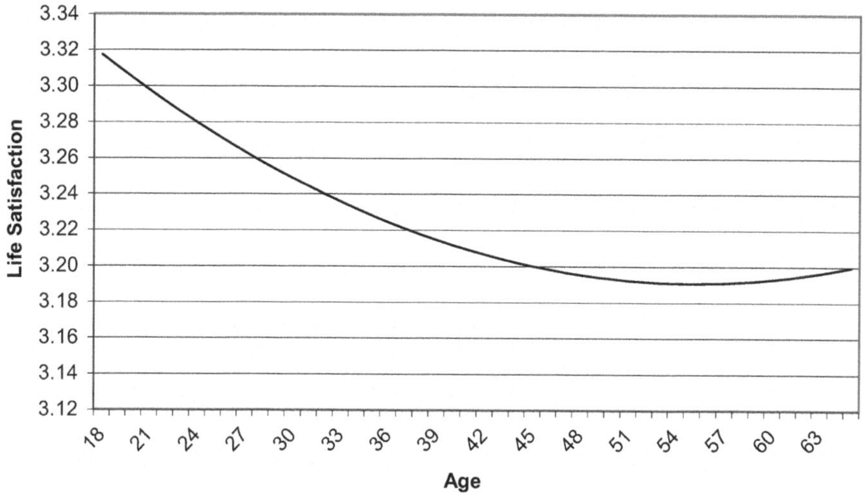

Fig. 2.1 Overall effect of age on general life satisfaction, Flanders, 1973–2022. *Source*: Standard Eurobarometer Survey Data (1973–2022), GESIS

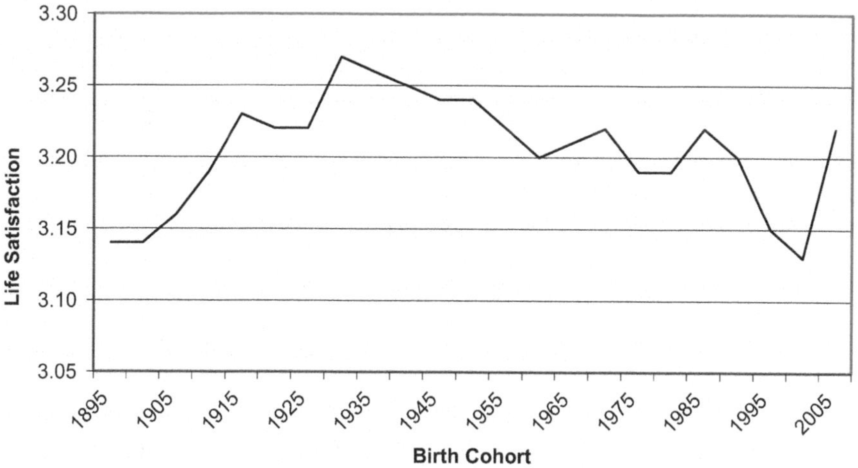

Fig. 2.2 Overall effect of (5 year) birth cohort on general life satisfaction, Flanders, 1973–2012. *Source*: Standard Eurobarometer Survey Data (1973–2022), GESIS

line with theoretical expectations, is clearly significant. The effect for Change in GDP per capita, on the other hand is not significant.

According to the findings of Model 2 shown in Fig. 2.1, there is a significant impact of age on life satisfaction after accounting for random period and cohort

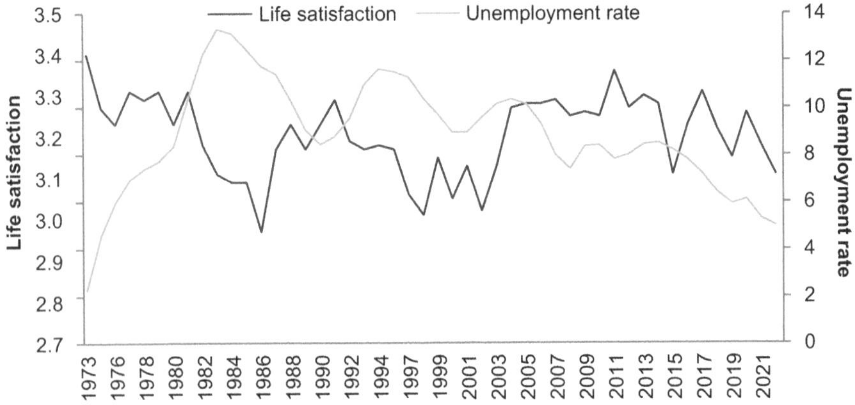

Fig. 2.3 Overall effect of period on general life satisfaction (series 1) and observed unemployment rates (series 2), Flanders, 1973–2022. *Source*: Standard Eurobarometer Survey Data (1973–2022), GESIS and HERMREG, Federal Planning Bureau

effects. The decrease in life satisfaction is modest, with an average of 0.0022 units per year. This decline is not constant, but rather gradually slows down as one ages until the age of 56, and then begins to reverse. Over a full professional working life span (18–65 years), the difference adds up to a reduction of 0.12 units or 4%.

These results do not support the maturity hypothesis (Gove et al. 1989), which predicts that life satisfaction increases with age due to positive psychological adaptation processes such as increased self-confidence. In Flanders, after the happy years as a teenager/young adult, life satisfaction gradually decreases in middle age and then slowly reverses at the age of 56. The dynamics behind this pattern are possibly due to the demands of combining family and work during (early) middle age.

Figure 2.2 displays the estimated random effects (controlled for age and period) for 23 different 5-year birth cohorts (born before 1995 up to born after 2005). In comparison with age (see Fig. 2.1) and period, (see Fig. 2.3), only relatively weak predicted cohort effects are found (maximum deviation from the average cohort is 0.08, only 2.7% in terms of the life satisfaction scale): one peak at around (1930–1934 cohort: +0.07) and two troughs (1900–1904 cohort: –0.07 and 2000–2004 cohort: –0.07). The four 5-year cohorts after the 1930–1934 cohort also show significantly positive deviations from the average (ranging from 0.03 to 0.05). A possible explanation here is that despite facing hardships during their childhood and adolescence, these generations were able to benefit from the economic growth following World War II in the 1950s and 1960s, leading to—against their own initial expectations—ultimately a positive evaluation of their lives.

The three eldest cohorts deviate on average –0.06 from the average cohort. This negative impact might be due to the experience of cumulative hardships during the World War I, the depression in the 1930s and World War II. Finally, the 2000–2004 cohort experienced a –0.08 deviation from the average cohort. A possible explanation might be that the COVID-19 crisis—taking place during the formative years of this generation—had a much larger impact on the 2000–2004 cohort than the older generations.

In Fig. 2.3 we show the predicted period effects (in deviations from the average trend)[3] in Flanders in the last 50 years. The peak level is situated at the start of the observations in 1973 (+0.20 above the average trend). Then follows a period with significantly positive effects until 1981 (on average +0.075 above the average trend). A second positive period is found between 2004 and 2014 (on average +0.078). In between these two periods, there is a deep trough in 1986 (–0.23), the lowest life satisfaction of a negative period that started in 1983 (average of –0.125). A second longer trough is situated between 1997 and 2003 (–0.20 in 1998; on average –0.135). In between the two troughs, the life satisfaction trend predictions hover around the average trend, except in 1991 (+0.09). Recently there are two negative trend years, in 2015 (–0.09) and 2022 (–0.10). Surprisingly, 2021 is the only negatively impacted trend year in the recent 3-year COVID-period (2020–2022). However, compared with the three previous years (2017–2019), the 3 years impacted by the COVID-19 crisis (2020–2022), on average saw a decline in predicted life satisfaction levels by –0.08. Compared with other crisis periods in the last 50 years, the impact of the COVID-crisis on life satisfaction in Flanders seems to be rather limited based on this analysis.

The net predicted trends for life satisfaction over the 1973–2022 period roughly correlate with the unemployment rate in the same period (see Fig. 2.3): a peak in life satisfaction seems to coincide with a trough in unemployment rate (e.g., 1973, 1991) and vice versa (mid-eighties, mid-nineties). However, from 2008 onwards, this negative link between unemployment rate (reaching again low levels) and life satisfaction seems to gradually have weakened.

2.4.2 Europe

This section compares the general life satisfaction in Flanders to seven other European countries, Denmark, the Netherlands, Ireland, Great Britain, West Germany, France, and Italy. Based on eight separate random intercept models average life satisfaction for each country, roughly shows a north-south gradient with Denmark (3.57) and the Netherlands (3.37) on the top and France (2.89) and Italy (2.74) on the bottom. In between we have Flanders (3.21), Ireland (3.19), Great Britain (3.15) and West Germany (3.06). The difference between the lowest and highest life satisfaction level, about a quarter of the scale range, is fairly large.

[3] The predicted period effects for life satisfaction are net period effects, controlled for the average age (45 years) and the average birth cohort.

Table 2.2 General life satisfaction, variance components and ranking, results for eight separate cross-classified random effects age-period-cohort regressions, Flanders, and seven European countries, 1973–2022

	Period		Cohort		Individual		Total
Country/region	Variance	Rank	Variance	Rank	Variance	Rank	Variance
Denmark	0.006***	6	0.000	7	0.335***	8	0.342***
The Netherlands	0.004***	8	0.001*	3	0.391***	7	0.395***
Flanders	0.010***	4	0.002*	2	0.409***	5	0.421***
Ireland	0.011***	3	0.000*	7	0.525***	2	0.536***
Great Britain	0.005***	7	0.001*	3	0.506***	4	0.511***
West Germany	0.012***	2	0.001**	3	0.406***	6	0.419***
France	0.005***	5	0.016*	1	0.517***	3	0.539***
Italy	0.014***	1	0.001*	3	0.528***	1	0.542***

* $p < 0.05$, ** $p < 0.01$, *** $p < 0.001$
Source: Standard Eurobarometer Survey Data (1973–2022), GESIS

Table 2.2 gives the variance components (period, cohort and individual variance) and the total variance. In all countries, the individual (residual) variance is significantly larger than the other two variance components. In most countries the trend fluctuations clearly dominate the cohort variance; except in France, where cohort fluctuations are stronger than the period variance. In general, cohort variance is (very) low (0.001–0.002) to non-existing (Denmark and Ireland), except in France (0.016). For period variances there are two groups, one with low variances: the Netherlands, France, Great Britain and Denmark (0.004–0.006) and one with high variances: Flanders, Ireland, West Germany and Italy (0.010–0.014).

The age effect takes different functional forms. The dominant functional form is negative quadratic (Denmark, Flanders, and Italy); in the Netherlands, the age effect is also negative, but linear. In Ireland and Great Britain, we see a positive quadratic relationship. Finally, in France and in West Germany there seems to be no effect of age. Why the overall life satisfaction increases through the life cycle in one country and decreases in another, is an open question.

Not surprisingly, as already could be inferred from the mostly (very) low levels of the country-specific cohort variances presented in Table 2.2, the predicted yearly cohort effects in Table 2.3, are also quite low, not exceeding absolute values of 0.08 (in Flanders) and 0.06 (in Italy). One exception however is France, where negative deviations up to –0.11 (cohorts 1915–1960) and positive deviations up to +0.27 (cohorts 1980–2005) are found. The contrast between these older and younger generations is very clear in France. One possible explanation is that, due to external immigration in recent decades, the composition of younger cohorts has changed such that the typical negative cultural attitude towards happiness of the French (Senik 2014), is now mixed with a more positive cultural attitude of the younger (and larger) immigrant cohorts. In the other countries we do not find any such clear patterns. The finding for Flanders that the 2000–2004 5-year cohort deviates negatively from the average cohort, is not confirmed in other countries. More generally, country patterns across cohorts seem to be mostly country specific.

Table 2.3 General life satisfaction and estimated cohort effects, results for eight separate cross-classified random effects age-period-cohort regressions, Flanders, and seven European countries, 1973–2022

	Denmark	The Netherlands	Flanders	Ireland	Great Britain	West Germany	France	Italy
Cohort	Beta	Beta	Beta	Beta	Beta	Beta	Beta	Beta
1895								
1900			–.07*					
1905								
1910								0.05**
1915					–.03*		–.07*	
1920		–.03**					–.07*	
1925		–.03*					–.09**	
1930		–.03*	0.07***				–.11***	–.03*
1935			0.05**			0.02*	–.11***	
1940	0.02*		0.04**			0.04***	–.11***	
1945	0.02**		0.03*			0.03**	–.11***	
1950	0.02*		0.04**	–.02*			–.11***	–.04***
1955				–.02*		–.03**	–.11***	–.06***
1960				–.02*		–.03**	–.08**	–.04***
1965					–.03**	–.03**		
1970								
1975		0.04**						
1980		0.03*					0.09**	
1985					0.03*		0.12**	
1990					0.04*		0.23***	
1995							0.20***	0.05*
2000		–.01	–.08*		–.03	–.01	0.27***	0.01
2005		0.00	0.01		–.01	0.00	0.22**	0.03

* $p < 0.05$, ** $p < 0.01$, *** $p < 0.001$
Source: Standard Eurobarometer Survey Data (1973–2022), GESIS

In Table 2.4, we show the results for the predicted period effects of eight countries. In the context of this chapter, it is not possible to analyse the eight country-specific profiles in detail. Therefore, we restrict the analysis to two periods: the 1983–1986 economic crisis and the 2020–2022 COVID-crisis, comparing them also with their pre-crisis periods (respectively 1979–1982 and 2017–2018).

During the 1983–1986 economic crisis, the trend effect, is consistently and clearly present in all eight countries/regions. Averaged over the eight countries and for the 4-year period, the estimated deviation from average life satisfaction amounts to –0.08. When applying the same calculus to the COVID-19 era, the estimated deviation is +0.045; a remarkable difference (0.125). However, from a short term perspective, compared with the 3 years preceding the COVID-19 era, we see on average a 0.05 drop during the COVID-19 crisis. This is comparable with the 1983–1986 shock, which showed on average a 0.04 drop from the previous period (of 4 years).

Table 2.4 General life satisfaction and estimated period effects, results for eight separate cross-classified random effects age-period-cohort regressions, Flanders, and seven European countries, 1973–2022

	Denmark	The Netherlands	Flanders	Ireland	Great Britain	West Germany	France	Italy
Year	Beta	Beta	Beta	Beta	Beta	Beta	Beta	Beta
1979	–.13***	0.03	0.10***	–.06*	–.08**	0.03	–.12***	–.18***
1980	–.08***	0.05*	0.03	–.03	0.01	–.06*	–.11***	–.10***
1981	–.05	–.02	0.10**	–.07*	–.05*	–.13***	–.08**	–.03
1982	–.06**	0.00	–.02	0.00	0.01	–.07**	0.01	–.05*
1983	–.08***	–.09***	–.09***	–.15***	–.06**	–.12***	–.05**	–.08**
1984	–.06***	–.02	–.11***	–.09***	–.02	–.06**	–.07***	–.06*
1985	–.04**	–.11***	–.11***	–.16***	–.05**	–.11***	–.07***	–.06*
1986	–.05**	–.08***	–.23***	–.17***	–.06**	–.04	–.05*	0.00
2017	0.11***	0.08***	0.10***	0.18***	0.12***	0.21***	0.07**	–.07*
2018	0.10***	0.10***	0.02	0.13***	0.11***	0.16***	0.07**	–.06*
2019	0.12***	0.10***	–.05	0.12***	0.12***	0.18***	0.04	0.06
2020	0.12***	0.12***	0.05	0.07*	0.03	0.23***	0.04	0.00
2021	–.07***	0.03*	–.03	–.05*	–.05*	0.20***	0.01	–.05*
2022	0.02	0.05**	–.10***	0.20***	0.00	0.17***	–.02	0.05*
A	0.02	0.07	–.03	0.07	–.01	0.20	0.01	0.00
B	0.11	0.09	0.02	0.15	0.12	0.18	0.06	–.02
C	–.09	–.02	–.05	–.07	–.13	0.02	–.05	0.02
D	–.19	–.08	–.08	–.12	–.08	–.02	–.03	–.05

* $p < 0.05$, ** $p < 0.01$, *** $p < 0.001$
Note: A: Covid average (2020, 2021 and 2022); B: pre-Covid average (2017, 2018, 2019); C: difference between A and B; D: difference between 2021 and 2020
Source: Standard Eurobarometer Survey Data (1973–2022), GESIS

It is remarkable that, on average, 2020 (the first pandemic year) compared with 2019, does not show any decline in life satisfaction levels. However, in the second year of the pandemic (2021), average life satisfaction levels clearly decline (–0.08) to rebound again (+0.05) in 2022, compensating more than half the drop in the previous year (2021), but clearly not yet at pre-pandemic levels. But recovery is not yet on its way in all countries: in Flanders, West Germany and Italy, life satisfaction is still declining (slightly) in 2022. Finally, the change of life satisfaction in the COVID-19 era, compared with the previous 3-year period varies considerably across countries, from a decline of –0.13 in Great Britain, to a small rise of 0.02 in West Germany and Italy.

To conclude, the short term-effect of the economic crisis of the early eighties and the COVID-crisis on life satisfaction is comparable in size, but seen on the long-term, the life satisfaction trough in the eighties was much deeper and (probably) longer, than the trough caused by the COVID-crisis.

Finally, in Table 2.5, we present the effect of two macro-variables on life satisfaction, change in GDP per capita and unemployment rate. For the GDP-variable used

Table 2.5 General life satisfaction, GDP change per capita and unemployment rate, results for eight separate cross-classified random effects age-period-cohort regressions, Flanders, and seven European countries, 1973–2022

	Denmark	The Netherlands	Flanders	Ireland	Great Britain	West Germany	France	Italy
Variable	Beta	Beta	Beta	Beta	Beta	Beta	Beta	Beta
Change in GDP/capita	0.000	0.000	0.000	0.000	0.000	0.000	0.000	0.000
Unemployment rate	0.008	–.003	–.017*	–.012***	0.000	–.023***	0.009	0.008

* $p < 0.05$, ** $p < 0.01$, *** $p < 0.001$
Source: Standard Eurobarometer Survey Data (1973–2022), GESIS

in the analysis, no (statistical) significant effect has been found.[4] These findings are in line with the relative utility thesis (Davis 1984). For unemployment, no (statistical) significant effect has been found for the group of low trend variance countries (Denmark, the Netherlands, Great Britain and France) and Italy. In three out of four high trend variance counties, the effect is—in line with theoretical expectations—negative: West Germany (–0.023), Flanders (–0.017) and Ireland (–0.012). This means that a 1% rise in unemployment rate on average induces a decrease of the life satisfaction level of –0.76% in West Germany, –0.56% in Flanders and –0.4% in Italy.

2.5 Discussion and Conclusion

In this chapter, we apply several Hierarchical Age-Period-Cohort regressions on Eurobarometer survey data combined with economic time series, to assess the relative impact of age, period, cohort and economic variables (GDP and unemployment) on general life satisfaction. We thereby use a long-term (1973–2022) and cross-national perspective: Denmark, the Netherlands, Ireland, Great Britain, West Germany, France, Italy, and Belgium (Flanders only). A second analytic goal is to compare the impact of the COVID-19 crisis on general life satisfaction levels with the impact of previous severe economic crisis (since 1973), across the same eight West-European countries.

Based on the empirical results (see Sect. 2.4), some general conclusions can be made. Although countries show considerable heterogeneity in the results: different functional forms of the age effects, variation in the size of the cohort and trend variances, partly country-specific predicted period effect trends, …; we also see some regularities both from a long-term and a cross-national perspective.

When time variance levels (period or cohort) for a country are relatively large, subsequent analysis of the predicted trend, respectively cohort variances can reveal important insights. In general, period effects dominate cohort effects. However,

[4] Neither did GDP nor GPD per capita.

France is an exception here. In France, a negative cultural attitude towards happiness is responsible for comparatively low life satisfaction levels. In recent French generations we clearly see systematically growing life satisfaction levels, probably due to a growing influx of immigrants that have a more positive cultural attitude towards life satisfaction.

In high period variance countries such as West Germany, Ireland, and the region of Flanders, the effect of the unemployment rate on life satisfaction is clearly negative, as predicted on theoretical grounds. Not a single statistically significant period effect is found for various included GDP-based variables. Therefore, we conclude that the relative utility theorist position (e.g., Davis 1984) is confirmed once more and no evidence is found for the absolute theorist position (e.g., Hagerty and Veenhoven 2003).

Another systematic finding is that the impact of severe economic recessions is systematically and clearly visible in the predicted period effects for general life satisfaction for all eight countries. The take-away message is clear here: at least when the economic conditions are highly fluctuating, life satisfaction measures can pick up such changes in society; but for minor external changes, this seems far less the case, comparable with the limited sensitivity of life satisfaction towards socio-demographic variables.

The chapter also compares the predicted period effects of the 2020–2022 COVID-19 crisis with these of the severe 1983–1986 economic crisis. The results indicate that the economic crisis and the COVID-crisis have comparable short-term effects on life satisfaction, but the life satisfaction trough in the eighties economic crisis was much deeper and longer-lasting. The predicted period results of the eighties economic crisis are consistently present in all eight countries; this is not always the case for COVID-19, where the results vary to some extent across countries, probably reflecting different cultural attitudes (e.g., towards fear) and country-specific coping mechanisms in society at large.

This brings us to an important take-away message for further long-term cross-national research in this field: next to economic factors, other societal and cultural factors must also be included in the empirical analysis.

References

Blanchflower, D., and A. Oswald. 2004. Well-being over time in Britain and the USA. *Journal of Public Economics* 88: 1359–1386.

Brülhart, M., and R. Lalive. 2020. Daily suffering: helpline calls during the COVID-19 crisis. *Covid Economics CEPR Press* 19: 143–158.

Callens, M. 2004. *Essays on multilevel logistic regression*. PhD dissertation. Leuven: Faculteit Economische en Toegepaste Economische Wetenschappen, Katholieke Universiteit Leuven.

———. 2010. *Contextuele regressiemethoden voor internationaal vergelijkend onderzoek*. Brussel: Studiedienst Vlaamse Regering.

———. 2017. Long term trends in life satisfaction, 1973–2012: Flanders in Europe. *Social Indicators Research* 130: 107–127.

Chesters, J., J. Simona, and C. Suter. 2021. Cross-national comparison of age and period effects on levels of subjective well-being in Australia and Switzerland during volatile economic times (2001–2016). *Social Indicators Research* 154: 361–391. https://doi.org/10.1007/s11205-020-02567-6.

Clark, A.E., and A.J. Oswald. 1994. Unhappiness and unemployment. *Economic Journal* 104 (424): 648–659.

Collignon, S. 2012. Europe's debt crisis, coordination failure, and international effects (July 12, 2012). *ADBI working paper no. 370*. https://doi.org/10.2139/ssrn.2103987.

Commission of the European Communities. 2009. *GDP and beyond. Measuring progress in a changing world*. https://eur-lex.europa.eu/LexUriServ/LexUriServ.do?uri=COM:2009:0433:FIN:en:PDF. Accessed 20 Jan 2023.

Davis, J.A. 1984. New money, an old man/lady and 'two's company': Subjective welfare in the NORC general social surveys, 1972–1982. *Social Indicators Research* 15: 319–350.

Diener, E., R.A. Emmons, R.J. Larsen, and S. Griffin. 1985. The satisfaction with life scale. *Journal of Personality Assessment* 49 (1): 71–75. https://doi.org/10.1207/s15327752jpa4901_13.

Di Tella, R., R.J. MacCulloch, and A.J. Oswald. 2003. The macroeconomics of happiness. *The Review of Economics and Statistics* 85 (4): 809–827.

Easterlin, R. 1995. Will raising the income of all increase the happiness of all? *Journal of Economic Behaviour and Organisation* 27: 35–48.

Easterlin, R., and K.J. O'Connor. 2023. Explaining happiness trends in Europe. *Discussion paper series no 15904*. IZA Institute of Labor Economics.

ECFIN. 2023. Ameco online (Version 2022-11-11 11:00). https://dashboard.tech.ec.europa.eu/qs_digit_dashboard_mt/public/sense/app/667e9fba-eea7-4d17-abf0-ef20f6994336/sheet/2f9f3ab7-09e9-4665-92d1-de9ead91fac7/state/analysis, https://economy-finance.ec.europa.eu/economic-research-and-databases/economic-databases/ameco-database_en.

Eichengreen, B. 2008. *The European economy since 1945*. Princeton, NJ: Princeton University Press.

European Commission. 2022. Brussels: *Eurobarometer 97.5, June-July 2022*. Kantar Public, Brussels [Producer]; GESIS, Cologne [Publisher]: ZA7902, dataset version 1.0.0. https://doi.org/10.4232/1.14010. Accessed 25 Jan 2023.

Federaal Planbureau. 2022. *Regionale economische vooruitzichten 2022–2027*. https://www.plan.be/uploaded/documents/202207180948360.FOR_HermReg_2022_12671_N.pdf. Accessed 27 Jan 2023.

Ferrer-i-Carbonell, A., and P. Frijters. 2004. How important is methodology for the estimates of the determinants of happiness? *Economic Journal* 114: 641–659.

Glenn, N.D. 1976. Cohort analysts' futile quest: statistical attempts to separate age, period, and cohort effects. *American Sociological Review* 41: 900–905.

———. 2005. *Cohort analysis*. 2nd ed. Thousand Oaks, CA: Sage.

Goldstein, H. 2003. *Multilevel statistical models*, Kendall's library of statistics. 3rd ed. London: Arnold.

Gove, W.R., S.T. Ortega, and C. Brigss Style. 1989. The maturational and role perspectives on aging and self through the adult years: an empirical evaluation. *American Journal of Sociology* 94: 1117–1145.

Hagerty, M.R., and R. Veenhoven. 2003. Wealth and happiness revisited—growing national income does go with greater happiness. *Social Indicators Research* 64: 1–27.

Huebner, E.S., and T. Dew. 1996. The interrelationships of positive affect, negative affect and life satisfaction in an adolescent sample. *Social Indicators Research* 38 (2): 129–137.

Luechinger, S., S. Meier, and A. Stutzer. 2010. Why does unemployment hurt the employed? Evidence from the life satisfaction gap between the public and the private sector. *Journal of Human Resources* 45: 998–1045.

Mason, K.O., W.M. Mason, H.H. Winsborough, and K.W. Poole. 1973. Some methodological issues in cohort analysis of archival data. *American Sociological Review* 38: 242–258.

Pittau, M.G., R. Zelli, and A. Gelman. 2010. Economic disparities and life satisfaction in European regions. *Social Indicators Research* 96 (2): 339–361.

Raudenbush, S.W., and A.S. Bryk. 2002. *Hierarchical linear models: Applications and data analysis methods*. 2nd ed. Thousand Oaks, CA: Sage.

Recchi, E., E. Ferragina, E. Helmeid, S. Pauly, M. Safi, N. Sauger, and J. Schradie. 2020. The "Eye of the hurricane" paradox: An unexpected and unequal rise of well-being during the COVID-19 lockdown in France. *Research in Social Stratification and Mobility* 68: 100508. https://doi.org/10.1016/j.rssm.2020.100508. Accessed 29 Jan 2023.

Ryder, N.B. 1965. The cohort as a concept in the study of social change. *American Sociological Review* 30: 843–861.

Schmitt, H., E. Scholz, I. Leim, and M. Moschner. 2008. *The Mannheim eurobarometer trend file 1970–2002 (ed. 2.00)*. European Commission [Principal investigator]. Cologne: GESIS Data Archive. ZA3521 Data file Version 2.0.1.

———. 2009. *The Mannheim eurobarometer trend file 1970–2002. Data set edition 2.01. Codebook and unweighted frequency distributions. Updated version*. Cologne: GESIS Data Archive.

Senik, C. 2014. The French unhappiness puzzle: The cultural dimension of happiness. *Journal of Economic Behavior & Organization* 106: 379–401.

Sirgy, M.J. 2021. *The psychology of quality of life: Wellbeing and positive mental health*, Social indicators research series. Vol. 89. Berlin: Springer.

Snijders, T.A.B., and R.J. Bosker. 2012. *Multilevel analysis: An introduction to basic and advanced multilevel modeling*. London: Sage.

Stiglitz, J. E., A. Sen, and J.-P. Fitoussi. 2009. *Report by the Commission on the measurement of economic performance and social progress*. https://ec.europa.eu/eurostat/documents/8131721/8131772/Stiglitz-Sen-Fitoussi-Commission-report.pdf. Accessed 26 Jan 2023.

United Nations. 2023. *National accounts main aggregates database*. https://unstats.un.org/unsd/snaama/Basic. Accessed 25 Jan 2023.

Veenhoven, R. 2002. Het grootste geluk voor het grootste aantal. *Sociale Wetenschappen* 4: 1–43.

Veenhoven, R., and S. Kregel. 2022. *Trend report average happiness in nations 1946–2021, World database of happiness*. Erasmus Happiness Economics Research Organization EHERO, Erasmus University Rotterdam, The Netherlands. https://worlddatabaseofhappiness.eur.nl/wp-content/uploads/TrendReport-AverageHappinessInNations1946-2021-4.pdf.

Verlet, D., and M. Callens. 2010. De contente vlaming. Algemene levenstevredenheid bij de doorsneebevolking in Vlaanderen. In *De kwaliteit van het leven: een mozaïek van het dagelijks leven*, ed. D. Verlet and M. Callens, 36–66. Brussel: Studiedienst van de Vlaamse Regering.

Yang, Y. 2008. Social inequalities in happiness in the United States, 1972 to 2004: An age-period-cohort analysis. *American Sociological Review* 73: 204–226.

Yang, Y., and K.C. Land. 2006. A mixed models approach to the age-period-cohort analysis of repeated cross-section surveys, with an application to data on trends in verbal test scores. *Sociological Methodology* 36: 75–97.

———. 2013. *Age-period-cohort analysis: New models, methods, and empirical applications*. New York: Chapman & Hall/CRC Press.

Marc Callens holds a PhD on multilevel logistic regression (KULeuven, 2004). He also obtained a Master of Statistics (KULeuven, 2000) and a Master Degree in Sociology (VUB, 1989). Since 2022, he is visiting Professor of Statistics and Methodology at the department of Public Governance and Management at Ghent University. Marc Callens held various positions in public administration (1990–2023): he started his career as a Researcher at the Population and Family Study Centre, was Director of Research at the Research Centre of the Flemish Government and Head of Data and Methods at Statistics Flanders.

Dries Verlet holds a PhD on measurement of subjective well-being and political attitudes (2003). Since 2006 he is visiting professor at the Department of Public Governance and Management, Faculty of Economics and Business Administration, Ghent University (Belgium). Besides, Dries Verlet is active in public administration. In the period 2007–2016 he was advisor policy evaluation for the Research Centre of the Flemish Government. Since 2016 he is advisor on methodology for Statistics Flanders as regional statistical authority.

Chapter 3
Happiness Trends Before and During the COVID-19 Pandemic in Indonesia: Assessing the Influence of Charitable Donations and Pandemic Severity

Indera Ratna Irawati Pattinasarany

3.1 Introduction

The global COVID-19 pandemic has spurred extensive research efforts to comprehend its multifaceted effects on individuals and societies worldwide (see, for example, Brodeur et al. 2021; Faghih and Forouharfar 2022; Hai-Anh and Toan 2022; Indrawati et al. 2022; Kuah et al. 2023; Morgan 2021). Against this setting, Indonesia, the fourth most populous country in the world, known for its generosity (Charities Aid Foundation 2022) and profoundly impacted by the pandemic,[1] stands out as a compelling focal point for in-depth investigations. In this context, a distinctive opportunity exists to explore several crucial facets, encompassing the dynamics of happiness, the prevalence of charitable endeavors, and the nationwide impact of the pandemic's severity. A study of these dimensions within the Indonesian context has the potential to furnish valuable insights into how a populous and compassionate nation addresses the complexities arising from a global health crisis.

The World Happiness Report (WHR), an annual report on happiness across countries, relies on three well-being indicators: life evaluation, positive affect, and negative affect. Countries are ranked based on life evaluation because this indicator is stable in measuring people's quality of life. The ranking of the life evaluation among World Happiness Report countries serves as a benchmark for a country's social and economic progress. Furthermore, the report outlines the factors that determine these three well-being indicators, utilizing six key variables: income,

[1] Like many other nations, Indonesia has faced significant challenges during the pandemic. According to Worldometer (2023), as of February 23, 2023, Indonesia stood as the 20th country in the world with the highest number of reported COVID-19 cases and the 11th country with the highest number of COVID-19-related deaths.

I. R. I. Pattinasarany (✉)
Universitas Indonesia, Depok, Indonesia
e-mail: indera.pattinasarany@ui.ac.id

C. Suter et al. (eds.), *Well-being During the Pandemic*, Social Indicators Research Series 90, https://doi.org/10.1007/978-3-031-63440-6_3

health, a reliable social support network, the perception of freedom to make important life choices, generosity, and the absence of corruption.[2] Concerning the generosity covariate, the World Happiness Report analysis suggests that the impact of generosity on life evaluations is predominantly mediated by its influence on the positive affect of individuals.[3] In other words, when people engage in acts of generosity or encounter generosity in their social interactions, it tends to elevate their positive affect. Such heightened positive affect, in turn, plays a pivotal role in shaping an individual's overall life evaluation. The greater the positive affect experienced by individuals, the more likely they are to report heightened life satisfaction and an enhanced sense of well-being (Helliwell et al. 2020, 2022, 2023).

Generosity is of particular interest and very relevant to Indonesia's achievements in giving. The World Giving Index (WGI) named Indonesia as the most generous country in the world for 2018–2022 (Charities Aid Foundation 2022). World Giving Index comprises three indicators: helping strangers in need, donating money to charity, and volunteering time for organizations. In Indonesian society, generosity is closely related to ingrained social actions: *sedekah* and *gotong royong*. *Sedekah* refers to voluntary religious donations focusing on aiding the less fortunate.[4] *Gotong royong* is a fundamental social ethos viewed as complementary to generosity.[5] Given Indonesia's global recognition as the most generous nation, it is essential to understand the relationship between giving donations and happiness.

The objective of this study is to examine the dynamics of generosity and its influence on individual well-being during the COVID-19 pandemic in Indonesia. Specifically, the study aims to investigate how the act of making regular (at least once a month) and occasional *sedekah* moderates the associations between COVID-19 severity and self-reported happiness. This study addresses a critical gap in the existing literature by examining the interplay between charitable behavior, pandemic conditions, and individual well-being. While there is a growing body of research on the impacts of COVID-19, there needs to be more research that explores the role of donations as moderators in this context. By investigating potential

---

[2] The generosity indicator in WHR is generated from the question, "Have you donated money to a charity in the past month?"

[3] Positive affect is measured as the mean of individual responses to three questions about whether specific emotions were experienced on the previous day: laughter, enjoyment, and engagement in learning or something interesting.

[4] The term *sedekah* initially described voluntary donations made within the Muslim community. However, over time, its usage has broadened to the extent that it now encompasses not only followers of Islam but a wider range of people.

[5] *Gotong royong* is a core social principle in Indonesia, directly interpreted as "jointly bearing burdens" (Geertz 1985). This term embodies the idea of people coming together to work collaboratively, extending assistance to one another, or engaging in mutual support. In numerous Indonesian villages, crucial public amenities like irrigation systems, roads, and places of worship (such as mosques or churches) are customarily constructed through *gotong royong*, where funds and construction materials are gathered collectively.

moderation effects, the study seeks to shed light on whether engagement in donations enhances or buffers self-reported happiness in the face of pandemic-related challenges. This insight can have implications for both public health and philanthropic efforts aimed at promoting well-being during crises.

The study objective will be further elaborated through the following four research questions:

- Research question 1: In what ways has the severity of COVID-19 impacted self-reported happiness? Assessing the connection between COVID-19 severity at the provincial level and self-reported happiness is essential in providing insights into the broader impact of the pandemic on individual well-being. By exploring this relationship, the study directly addresses its objective to examine how sociological factors, such as regional disparities in COVID-19 severity, shape the well-being of people in Indonesia during the pandemic.
- Research question 2: How does engaging in acts of charity (*sedekah*) affect self-reported happiness? Investigating the impact of regular and occasional *sedekah* on self-reported happiness addresses how different forms of giving contribute to well-being during a global crisis. This research question helps elucidate the multifaceted nature of generosity and its role in individual welfare, which is integral to understanding the study's sociological dynamics.
- Research question 3: To what extent does engaging in acts of generosity, such as making *sedekah*, moderate the relationship between COVID-19 severity and self-reported happiness? This inquiry investigates the moderating influence of donations, exploring how both regular and occasional acts of *sedekah* shape the connection between the severity of COVID-19 and individuals' reported happiness. Understanding whether *sedekah* amplifies or diminishes the impact of the pandemic on happiness reveals the vital role of generosity during a crisis, aligning directly with the study's objective to examine the sociological dynamics of generosity in the context of the pandemic.
- Research question 4: Do the contextual factors surrounding individuals impact how individuals assess their happiness levels? This question broadens the scope to consider economic conditions and inequality at the provincial level and their association with self-reported happiness.

These research questions are vital instruments of inquiry, tightly woven into the study's objective. They offer a comprehensive perspective on how generosity, regional disparities, and contextual factors jointly shape the well-being of individuals during the COVID-19 pandemic in Indonesia.

This chapter comprises six sections. Section 3.2 provides an overview of previous research pertinent to the central themes of this study. Section 3.3 outlines the methodology and models applied in the analysis, and Sect. 3.4 provides insights into the data used. The analysis and discussion of the estimation results are presented in Sect. 3.5. Subsequently, Sect. 3.6 summarizes the findings and presents policy recommendations.

3.2 Literature Review

3.2.1 Warm Glow Theory of Giving

In this research, we apply the warm glow theory of giving to shed light on the practice of giving *sedekah* and its impact on individuals' reported happiness. The theory posits that when people contribute to a public good, such as charitable causes, they are primarily driven by two key motivations, as initially proposed by Andreoni (1989, 1990). The first motivation is altruism, driven by a genuine desire to improve the availability of the public good, often called "pure altruism." The second motivation involves individuals deriving personal satisfaction and private benefits from giving, akin to experiencing a heartwarming or "warm glow" sense of fulfillment. This duality of motivation is termed "impure altruism" and provides a simple yet robust framework for understanding charitable behavior, closely aligning with real-world observations.

In a study encompassing over 200,000 survey participants from 136 countries, Aknin et al. (2013) revealed a global correlation between prosocial spending and an enhanced sense of subjective happiness. This effect was evident in economically disadvantaged and affluent nations, although the strength and significance of this relationship displayed variations across individual countries. Nonetheless, the detectability of this association across diverse global regions bolsters the idea that the warm glow of giving can be considered a functional universal. Ugur's (2018) study aims to quantify the extent of the warm-glow phenomenon by employing subjective well-being indicators within the longitudinal datasets from the Netherlands. After accounting for major happiness-influencing events, including changes in marital status, income, and employment, the research reveals that individuals engaged in charitable giving tend to experience higher happiness levels, thereby suggesting a warm glow effect.

3.2.2 Studies on Giving Donations and Happiness

Aknin et al. (2019) reviewed research on the motivations behind donating time and money to assist others. They found a positive association between donating funds and increased well-being. Nevertheless, causality remains uncertain due to potential reverse causality and confounding factors such as wealth. Researchers are using experimental evidence to tackle this issue, with evidence suggesting that using money to benefit others enhances happiness.

This study employs national longitudinal data from face-to-face interviews to examine how giving donations moderates the relationship between COVID-19 severity and self-reported happiness. Therefore, the studies reviewed in this section primarily concentrate on non-experimental empirical research that relies on longitudinal survey data.

The collective findings from the reviewed studies consistently affirm a positive connection between donating money and self-reported happiness. Furthermore, in addition to the research mentioned earlier (Aknin et al. 2013; Helliwell et al. 2020, 2022, 2023; Ugur 2018), global studies have echoed similar conclusions. For instance, a study conducted in Indonesia by Utama et al. (2021), revealed that individuals who directed more resources toward prosocial activities were more likely to feel financially secure, experience happiness, and express satisfaction with their lives.

In Thailand, individuals who followed the five precepts of Buddhism reported elevated levels of happiness (Winzer et al. 2018). Within these precepts, one emphasizes making donations. In connection with charitable giving, the study observed that individuals who actively made donations were more inclined to perceive themselves as happy than those who infrequently or never participated in such acts of generosity.

A study conducted in China established that individual donation behavior directly impacts happiness levels (Wu et al. 2021). In light of the potential variations in individual autonomy concerning donation choices, this study deploys an autonomy questionnaire to classify individual donation behaviors into three categories: "fully voluntary," "semi-voluntary," and "mandatory." The results reveal that, although fully voluntary donation behaviors might not exhibit the same degree of autonomy as non-voluntary ones, they are associated with a significantly more pronounced enhancement in happiness levels when compared to the other two categories. Similar studies, such as those by Ren and Ye (2017) and Zheng et al. (2021) in China; Pholphirul (2015) in Thailand; Jun et al. (2022) and Song et al. (2019) in Korea, also found a positive connection between donating money and self-reported happiness.

In contrast, a study conducted in Japan by Tiefenbach and Kohlbacher (2014) did not confirm the link between happiness and donations. This result can be ascribed to the connection between donations and involvement in volunteer activities. Those who contribute donations are more likely to engage in volunteer work and vice versa. The coefficients achieve statistical significance when solely employing a binary variable accounting for donation behavior. Nevertheless, when both variables are considered, it becomes apparent that the primary correlation is between participation in volunteering activities and happiness.

Finally, with regard to causality, a research study carried out in Germany by Boenigk and Mayr (2016) explored the connections between charitable giving and happiness and offered a different viewpoint. Their investigation scrutinized the causal relationship between charitable giving and happiness to identify the predominant causal direction: whether giving leads to happiness or happiness motivates giving. The outcomes of their study confirm two fundamental findings: first, a positive correlation exists between happiness and giving, and second, they support the idea that the primary causal flow originates from happiness, propelling individuals toward charitable acts.

3.3 Methodology

3.3.1 *Addressing the Limitations of Prior Studies by Employing Enhanced Data Sources*

Despite the numerous studies that have investigated the impact of the pandemic on subjective well-being in Indonesia (Borualogo and Casas 2022; Dwidienawati et al. 2021; Halimatussadiah et al. 2021; Iskandarsyah et al. 2022; Rahmanita et al. 2021; Tjahjana et al. 2021), none of these studies have explicitly delved into the effect of donations on happiness. Furthermore, these studies are afflicted by one or more of the following limitations: a focus on specific population segments (e.g., healthcare workers, students), reliance on single-point data collection, participants selected through convenience sampling, online survey administration, restricted data observations, dependence on respondents' retrospective reports of pre-pandemic conditions.

We overcome these limitations because we use data from national-level cross-sectional surveys from two different samples collected at two different points in time. First, our survey data covers the period before and during the pandemic, thus providing an opportunity to study changes in self-reported happiness levels associated with the pandemic. To our benefit, using survey data with a total observation of 137,958 respondents gives this study sufficient statistical power to examine changes in happiness levels across time with better precision.

Second, our survey data was collected via face-to-face interviews, whereby the respondents were selected using a rigorous sampling method. Online surveys cannot adequately describe the selected sample's distribution and respondents with biases selecting themselves into the sample (Andrade 2020). Therefore, conclusions drawn from studies based on online surveys should be tentative.

Third, in this study, the self-reported happiness levels are made at two different points in time to represent the happiness level with more accuracy. Our study avoids using self-reported happiness levels collected retrospectively, thus eliminating or minimizing recall bias (Hyman 2013; Tadic et al. 2014).

3.3.2 *Multilevel Mixed-Effects Ordered Logistic Model*

In this chapter, we utilize a multilevel mixed-effects ordered logistic model that addresses nesting while considering the categorical nature of the dependent variables. This approach also provides adjusted standard errors, enhancing the precision of the coefficients (Mehmetoglu and Jakobsen 2017; Snijders and Bosker 2012). Our study involves observations of individuals (level 1) nested within provinces (level 2). We employ multilevel regressions with random intercepts for each province to account for varying pandemic impacts across provinces and to acknowledge potential similarities among respondents within the same province. An ordered logistic model's choice is based on the dependent variable's ordered nature (Rabe-Hesketh and Skrondal 2022).

We postulate a latent variable (y^*) to represent an individual's underlying happiness. This study estimates two models: the "main" model (the Main Model) and the "with interaction terms" model (the Interaction Model). In the Main Model, the latent variable is associated with individual characteristics such as gender, age, marital status, education, and making donations. It also includes household characteristics like residence type and household income, as well as provincial contextual variables such as the Gini coefficient of per capita expenditures, Gross Regional Domestic Product (GRDP) per capita, and the total COVID-19 cases per 100,000 population. The latter serves as a measure of the severity of the COVID-19 pandemic. The Interaction Model encompasses the Main Model and further introduces interaction variables between donations and the severity of the COVID-19 pandemic.

The Main Model is specified as follows:

$$y_{ij}^{*} = x1_{ij}\beta 1 + x2_{j}\beta 2 + COVID_{j}\beta 4 + z_{ij}u_{j} + \epsilon_{ij}$$

while the Interaction Model is specified as follows:

$$y_{ij}^{*} = x1_{ij}\beta 1 + x2_{j}\beta 2 + Donations_{ij} \times COVID_{j}\beta 3 + COVID_{j}\beta 4 + z_{ij}u_{j} + \epsilon_{ij}$$

$$y_{ij} = \begin{cases} 0 if\ y_{ij}^{*} \le \kappa_1 \\ 1 if\ \kappa_1 < y_{ij}^{*} \le \kappa_2 \\ 2 if\ \kappa_2 < y_{ij}^{*} \le \kappa_3 \\ 3 if\ \kappa_3 < y_{ij}^{*} \le \kappa_4 \\ 4 if\ \kappa_4 < y_{ij}^{*} \le \kappa_5 \\ 5 if\ \kappa_5 < y_{ij}^{*} \end{cases}$$

where:

y_{ij}^{*}	is the unobserved happiness for individual i who resides in province j (latent variable)
$x1_{ij}$	is thc individual (including making donations) and household characteristics for individual i living in province j
$x2_{j}$	is the provincial contextual variables for province j
$COVID_{j}$	is the COVID-19 pandemic severity measure for province j
$Donations_{ij} \times COVID_{j}$	is the interaction terms of gender and type of residence covariates with COVID-19 severity measure
z_{ij}	is the covariates corresponding to the random effects; as this model follows a random-intercept model, z_{ij} is simply the scalar 1
u_{j}	is the random effects and
ϵ_{ij}	is the errors, distributed as logistic with mean 0 and variance $\pi^2/3$ and are independent of u_j

This model, $x1_{ij}$ and $x2_{j}$ do not contain a constant term because its effect is absorbed into the cutpoints (κ).

We conduct model estimation with Stata 17.0 using the meologit procedure (StataCorp. 2021). This procedure is employed to estimate an ordered logistic regression model that includes fixed effects (specifically $x1_{ij}$ and $x2_j$ along with their interaction terms) as well as random effects (denoted as u_j).

3.4 Data

The primary data source for this study is the Happiness Level Measurement Survey (SPTK) 2017 and 2021 (Badan Pusat Statistik 2017, 2021).[6] SPTK was administered by the Badan Pusat Statistik (BPS), which is the Central Statistics Agency of Indonesia, and was simultaneously carried out in all *kabupaten* (regencies) and *kota* (municipalities) across all 34 provinces. The 2021 wave of SPTK fieldwork took place from July 1 to August 27, 2021, during Indonesia's peak of the COVID-19 pandemic.

The unit of analysis comprises randomly selected households, chosen using a two-stage, one-phase sampling approach (Badan Pusat Statistik 2021). Within each selected household, either the head of the household or the spouse (wife or husband) of the head is designated as the respondent, representing the entire household. This study is centered on 137,958 respondents aged between 25 and 80 years who are actively employed or primarily engaged in household responsibilities. In addition to assessing happiness levels, the SPTK provided data at both individual and household levels.

In this study, the provincial-level data is sourced from various channels. Specifically, the information regarding COVID-19 exposure, i.e., the total number of positive COVID-19 cases, was obtained from KawalCOVID19. The macroeconomic data on the Gini coefficient of expenditures per capita and Gross Regional Domestic Product (GRDP) per capita measuring income inequality per capita is collected from BPS.

3.4.1 Self-Reported Level of Happiness

Happiness levels are assessed through the Cantril ladder, a visualization where respondents envision themselves on a scale with steps numbered from zero at the bottom to ten at the top. They are then prompted to gauge their overall life satisfaction by responding to the question, "How happy are you with life as a whole?" The

[6] The SPTK is a repeated cross-sectional survey administered in 2012, 2013, 2014, 2017, and 2021. The survey has seen notable enhancements in its conceptual and methodological framework over the years. To ensure comparability, we will focus on the most recent two waves of data. We must emphasize that the 2021 SPTK does not aim to investigate the impact of the pandemic on happiness levels.

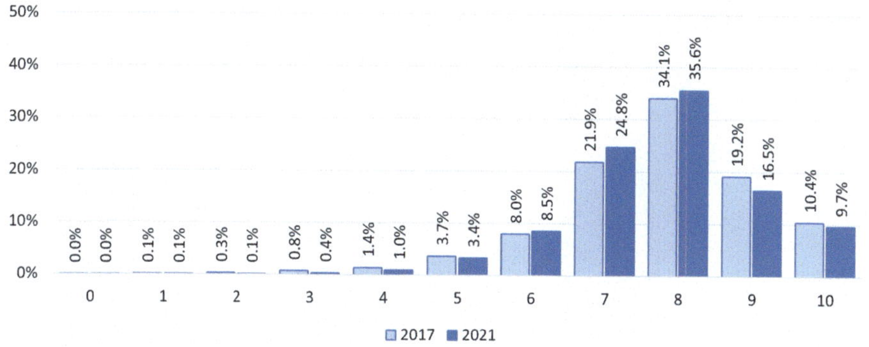

Fig. 3.1 Distribution of self-reported happiness, 2017 and 2021. Notes: Calculated from SPTK

possible answers span from 0 (indicating very unhappiness) to 10 (very happy). As illustrated in Fig. 3.1, the distributions of happiness display a leftward skew. Most respondents place themselves on the eighth rung (accounting for 34.1% in 2017 and 35.6% in 2022). In 2017, the national average was calculated at 7.78; in 2021, it slightly decreased to 7.76.

As a comparison, the Social Well-Being Survey in Asia 2018 covers seven provinces in Indonesia and solicits respondents' happiness evaluation using a 0–10 Cantril ladder evaluation. The survey results also show that happiness is skewed to the left, with an average of 7.67 (Pattinasarany 2018).

We recoded the happiness levels to facilitate the estimation of multilevel mixed-effects ordered logistic models. Given the limited number of respondents rating their happiness between zero and five, we combined these five responses to create a more balanced distribution. Additionally, the recoding process aligns with the requirements of the ordered logistic method, ensuring that each category contains at least three percent of the observations.

3.4.2 *The Act of Giving Donations*

The SPTK asks, "Have you/your spouse made a *sedekah* from some of your assets, in terms of money/goods, in the past year?". The question has three answer choices: "Yes, at least once a month," "Yes, not every month," and "Did not donate."[7] Figure 3.2 shows that from 2017 to 2021, the percentage of individuals offering charitable contributions experienced a slight decline, dropping from 91.0

[7] In the 2017 SPTK, following this question, respondents were asked, "What is the main reason for you or your spouse to make *sedekah*?" The question offered four answer options that were not read aloud: "Grateful for God's sustenance/blessing" (chosen by 45.4% of respondents), "Because of religious guidance, particularly to receive rewards from God" (selected by 32.0%), "To help or share with others" (endorsed by 21.4%), and "Other (open answer)" (picked by 1.2%). Overall,

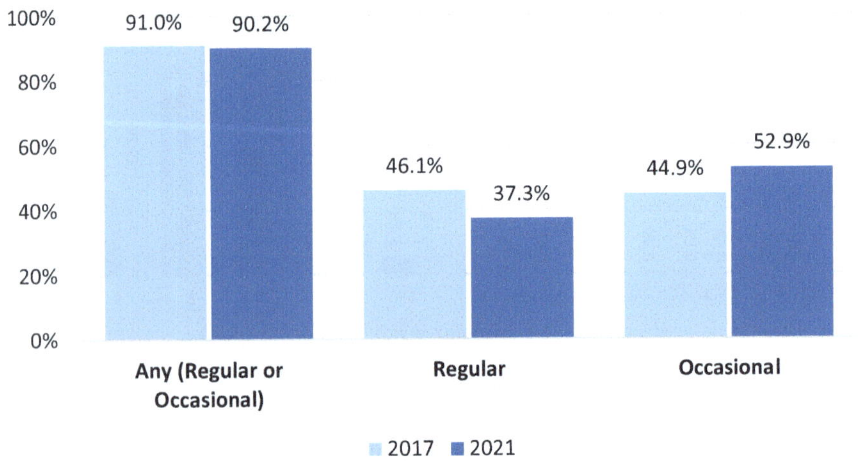

Fig. 3.2 *Sedekah* giving by type, 2017 and 2021. Notes: Calculated from SPTK

to 90.2%. Concurrently, the frequency of regular *sedekah* (defined as giving *sedekah* at least once a month) decreased notably, from 46.1 to 37.3%. Conversely, the proportion of occasional *sedekah* exhibited a significant increase, rising from 44.9 to 52.9%.

The pandemic may have caused disruptions in daily routines, financial challenges, and heightened uncertainty, all of which can impact altruistic behavior, thereby attributing the decline in the percentage of individuals making regular *sedekah* and the rise in those opting for occasional *sedekah*. When faced with economic hardships, individuals often feel compelled to reassess their spending priorities, potentially reducing regular donation commitments. On the contrary, a combination of immediate crisis response, heightened empathy, spontaneous acts of kindness, community and social influence, and flexible financial situations can be attributed to the increase in occasional donations during the COVID-19 pandemic. These factors collectively contributed to a surge in occasional acts of generosity as individuals responded to the unique challenges and needs presented by the crisis. Moreover, philanthropic actors in Indonesia have adeptly shifted from traditional to digital fundraising platforms (Filantropi Indonesia 2021). They have successfully overcome pandemic-related challenges such as social distancing and restrictions, thereby minimizing their impact on philanthropic activities.

Table 3.1 presents the mean and standard deviation of all the variables used in this study, categorized by year.

---

these insights highlight the intrinsic role of religious beliefs in shaping the charitable actions of the surveyed individuals.

Table 3.1 Mean and standard deviation of data

	2017		2021	
Variable	Mean	Std dev	Mean	Std dev
Individual and household characteristics	***N* = 67,450**		***N* = 70,508**	
Self-reported Happiness (0–10)	7.78	(1.43)	7.76	(1.33)
Self-reported Happiness (0–5)	2.83	(1.30)	2.79	(1.24)
Male [reference]	0.486	(0.500)	0.487	(0.500)
Female	0.514	(0.500)	0.513	(0.500)
Age (in years)	46.4	(12.25)	47.5	(12.46)
Not Married [reference]	0.166	(0.372)	0.180	(0.384)
Married	0.834	(0.372)	0.820	(0.384)
Education:				
– Up to Primary [reference]	0.219	(0.414)	0.183	(0.387)
– Completed Primary	0.276	(0.447)	0.301	(0.459)
– Completed Junior Secondary	0.159	(0.366)	0.172	(0.377)
– Completed Senior Secondary	0.234	(0.423)	0.242	(0.428)
– Tertiary	0.111	(0.315)	0.102	(0.303)
Household Work [reference]	0.226	(0.418)	0.258	(0.437)
Currently Working	0.774	(0.418)	0.742	(0.437)
Rural [reference]	0.581	(0.493)	0.571	(0.495)
Urban	0.419	(0.493)	0.429	(0.495)
Household income				
– Low: up to IDR 1.8 million/month [reference]	0.314	(0.464)	0.277	(0.447)
– Lower-middle: IDR >1.8-3.0 million/month	0.292	(0.455)	0.315	(0.465)
– Upper-middle: IDR >3.0-4.8 million/month	0.190	(0.393)	0.206	(0.404)
– High: IDR >4.2 million/month	0.204	(0.403)	0.203	(0.402)
Giving donations (*Sedekah*)				
– Did not Donate [reference]	0.090	(0.286)	0.098	(0.298)
– Regular Donations	0.461	(0.498)	0.373	(0.484)
– Occasional Donations	0.449	(0.497)	0.529	(0.499)
Province contextual characteristics	***N* = 34**		***N* = 34**	
Gini of Expenditures per capita (0–1)	0.364	(0.034)	0.355	(0.036)
log (GRDP per capita)	17.28	(0.44)	17.35	(0.44)
log (total COVID-19 cases per 100,000 population)	0.00	–	6.34	(0.58)

Source: SPTK, KawalCOVID19, and BPS
Notes: The number of COVID-19 cases in 2017 was zero, but the logarithmic values are assigned as zeros

3.5 Estimation Results and Discussions

Table 3.2 displays the estimated happiness levels obtained from a multilevel mixed-effects ordered logistic analysis, encompassing the Main Model (Models [1]–[2]) and the Interaction Model (Models [3]–[4]). The Null Model, a model that does not include any predictors, estimates reveal an Intraclass Correlation Coefficient (ICC)

Table 3.2 Multilevel mixed-effects ordered logistic estimates for level of happiness

	Main model		Interaction model	
	[1]	[2]	[3]	[4]
Individual and household				
Women	0.150***	0.147***	0.150***	0.148***
	(0.011)	(0.011)	(0.011)	(0.011)
Age	–0.043***	–0.043***	–0.043***	–0.043***
	(0.003)	(0.003)	(0.003)	(0.003)
Age^2 (×1/100)	0.041***	0.041***	0.041***	0.041***
	(0.003)	(0.003)	(0.003)	(0.003)
Married	0.425***	0.419***	0.425***	0.419***
	(0.014)	(0.014)	(0.014)	(0.014)
Completed Primary	0.102***	0.101***	0.101***	0.099***
	(0.015)	(0.015)	(0.015)	(0.015)
Completed Junior Secondary	0.156***	0.149***	0.155***	0.147***
	(0.017)	(0.017)	(0.017)	(0.017)
Completed Senior Secondary	0.224***	0.208***	0.223***	0.207***
	(0.017)	(0.017)	(0.017)	(0.017)
Tertiary	0.455***	0.421***	0.454***	0.420***
	(0.021)	(0.021)	(0.021)	(0.021)
Currently working	–0.062***	–0.068***	–0.062***	–0.067***
	(0.013)	(0.013)	(0.013)	(0.013)
Urban	0.088***	0.074***	0.088***	0.074***
	(0.011)	(0.011)	(0.011)	(0.011)
Income: IDR 1.8–3.0 million/month	0.292***	0.286***	0.293***	0.287***
	(0.013)	(0.013)	(0.013)	(0.013)
Income: IDR 3.0–4.8 million/month	0.540***	0.524***	0.540***	0.524***
	(0.015)	(0.015)	(0.015)	(0.015)
Income: IDR 4.8+ million/month	0.876***	0.844***	0.875***	0.843***
	(0.016)	(0.016)	(0.016)	(0.016)
Giving donations *(Sedekah)*				
Any (Regular or Occasional)	0.539***		0.660***	
	(0.018)		(0.025)	
Regular		0.689***		0.809***
		(0.019)		(0.027)
Occasional		0.458***		0.558***
		(0.018)		(0.026)
Any × COVID-19 Severity			–0.036***	
			(0.005)	
Regular × COVID-19 Severity				–0.036***
				(0.006)
Occasional × COVID-19 Severity				–0.030***
				(0.006)

(continued)

Table 3.2 (continued)

	Main model		Interaction model	
	[1]	[2]	[3]	[4]
Province contextual				
Gini of Expenditure per capita	–4.386***	–4.172***	–4.291***	–4.015***
	(0.699)	(0.701)	(0.701)	(0.703)
log (GRDP per capita)	0.018	0.033	0.084	0.099
	(0.081)	(0.082)	(0.083)	(0.084)
COVID-19 Severity	–0.021***	–0.018***	0.011**	0.012**
	(0.002)	(0.002)	(0.005)	(0.005)
κ1	–3.984	–3.690	–2.697	–2.389
	(1.492)	(1.504)	(1.533)	(1.552)
κ2	–2.956	–2.662	–1.669	–1.360
	(1.492)	(1.504)	(1.533)	(1.552)
κ3	–1.565	–1.268	–0.277	0.034
	(1.492)	(1.504)	(1.533)	(1.552)
κ4	0.032	0.333	1.319	1.635
	(1.492)	(1.504)	(1.533)	(1.552)
κ5	1.331	1.635	2.619	2.937
	(1.492)	(1.504)	(1.533)	(1.552)
Variances: Province (constant)	0.127	0.130	0.131	0.135
	(0.032)	(0.032)	(0.033)	(0.034)
LR test Ordered Logit (p-score)	0.000	0.000	0.000	0.000
Intraclass Correlation (ICC)	0.037	0.038	0.038	0.039
Observations	137,958	137,958	137,958	137,958

Source: Author's calculations
Notes: statistically significant at the ** 5% level, *** 1% level

of 0.038 (results are not shown). This suggests that approximately 3.8% of the variance in the latent response is explained by variability between provinces. Despite the small magnitude of the ICC, we continue to utilize a multilevel model in this study. This decision is based on the understanding that even the smallest ICC (unless it is zero) does not necessarily indicate the absence of variation in respondents' happiness levels between provinces. The ICCs for the Main and Interaction Models in Table 3.2 are similarly small, ranging from 0.037 to 0.039 (found in the second row from the bottom).

The Likelihood Ratio (LR) test, shown in the third row from the bottom, examines whether the multilevel mixed-effects ordered logistic model provides a significantly improved fit to the data compared to the simple (single-level) ordered logistic model. A p-value of 0.000 for the LR test indicates the presence of significant between-provinces variation in happiness levels.

The line labeled "Variances: Province (constant)" in the fourth row from the bottom signifies the extent to which provinces contribute to the overall variability in happiness among individuals. The hierarchical data structure in the multilevel model considers the idea that individuals within the same province may be more similar to each other than those in different provinces due to shared contextual factors. These factors could encompass macroeconomic indicators (like the two measures controlled for in this study: the Gini coefficient of expenditures per capita and the GRDP per capita), access to local infrastructure (such as health and education), local norms and culture, and others. A higher value indicates a more significant level of diversity in self-reported happiness at the province level, suggesting that provinces have a discernible impact on individual happiness levels, potentially overshadowing the influence of individual-level factors.

3.5.1 COVID-19 Severity and Happiness Level

The estimation results from the Main Model show that, after adjusting for random effects at the provincial level, individuals residing in provinces with a higher number of COVID-19 cases per 100,000 population tended to report lower levels of happiness (Models [1]-[2]). The adverse impact of the severity of COVID-19 on overall well-being aligns with a sociological perspective that underscores how external events and crises can profoundly shape individuals' life experiences.[8]

There are many interconnected reasons for this observed decline in well-being. First, heightened exposure to COVID-19 amplifies health risks and anxiety among individuals as they cope with the fear of contracting the virus or witnessing its effects on loved ones. Such heightened apprehension and unease leads to reduced happiness (Demirbas and Kutlu 2021; van der Vegt and Kleinberg 2020). Second, regions with higher COVID-19 cases often grapple with significant economic disruptions, such as business closures, job losses, and reduced economic activity. These conditions generate financial stress, insecurity, and an overall decline in happiness (Cheng et al. 2020; Greyling et al. 2021; Kuhn et al. 2020). Third, residents in provinces experiencing greater exposure to the virus may face difficulties related to reduced social support networks, limited opportunities for social engagement, and feelings of loneliness or disconnection. These factors can substantially influence the decrease in happiness (Lepinteur et al. 2022).

Nevertheless, in the Interaction Model, the data reveals a notable shift in the relationship between COVID-19 severity and self-reported happiness when accounting for the moderating effect of making donations (Models [3]–[4]). The point estimates of COVID-19 severity are positive and statistically significant, suggesting a meaningful change in this relationship. This finding implies that individuals who

[8] We conducted a parallel analysis utilizing the total COVID-19-related deaths as an alternative measure of the pandemic's severity. The results show similar findings: the higher the total death from COVID-19 in the province where the respondent lives, the lower the level of happiness reported by the respondent. We decided not to report these estimates as it is more difficult to attribute a death to COVID-19 as the exact cause is unclear (Bittmann 2022). Some people may die directly from the disease, while others die with it such as from accompanying comorbidities.

engage in charitable actions through regular or occasional *sedekah* may experience a buffering or counterbalancing effect. Charitable behavior alleviates some of the adverse emotional and psychological impacts of a crisis like the COVID-19 pandemic, fostering resilience, a sense of community, and a renewed sense of purpose. From a sociological standpoint, this result underscores the importance of charitable actions as mechanisms for enhancing individual and collective well-being during challenging periods. It emphasizes that communities can display resilience and solidarity in specific contexts of high adversity (Kaye-Kauderer et al. 2021). People may unite to provide support, resulting in a collective sense of strength and unity and increasing self-reported happiness.

Our findings find support in international research. A study investigating the impact of the COVID-19 pandemic on people's happiness in China, Japan, South Korea, Italy, the United Kingdom, and the United States revealed that individuals living in regions with higher COVID-19 rates are more likely to report feelings of unhappiness and extreme unhappiness (Nguyen 2021). Similarly, in the Philippines, a cross-sectional study conducted over 15 months from the onset of the pandemic found that young adults who personally knew someone who had succumbed to COVID-19 experienced a significant increase in pandemic fatigue, coupled with lower subjective well-being and life satisfaction (Cleofas and Oducado 2022).

The preceding analysis addresses research question 1, which explores how variations in COVID-19 severity across regions influence the happiness of individuals in Indonesia during the pandemic.[9]

3.5.2 *Giving Sedekah and Happiness Level*

Our analytical results indicate that engaging in any form of *sedekah* is associated with a higher likelihood of reporting increased self-reported happiness compared to not making any donations (Model [1]). Similarly, both regular and occasional *sedekah* are connected to a greater probability of reporting elevated self-reported happiness when contrasted with not donating at all (Model [2]).

This phenomenon aligns with Andreoni's (1989, 1990) warm glow theory of giving, which can elucidate why individuals often report heightened happiness levels when giving donations. According to this model, making *sedekah* is not solely motivated by the desire to maximize personal gain or alleviate the suffering of others. It is deeply intertwined with the intrinsic joy and emotional fulfillment derived from helping.

The greater point estimate for regular *sedekah*, compared to occasional *sedekah*, suggests that making regular donations substantially impacts self-reported

[9] The variation in confirmed COVID-19 cases among provinces underscores significant disparities. Indonesia's capital city, DKI Jakarta, records the highest incidence of COVID-19 cases, with a rate of 5210 cases per 100,000 population. Conversely, North Sumatera reports the lowest number of cases, just 246 per 100,000 population.

happiness compared to occasional donations. The proportion of regular *sedekah* decreased between before and during the pandemic. However, the higher happiness levels observed among regular *sedekah* donors, compared to occasional *sedekah* givers, suggest that those who give regularly often experience a more profound sense of purpose, satisfaction, and emotional connection to the causes they support, ultimately contributing to their overall happiness.

The results presented above offer insights in response to research question 2, which investigates the impact of regular and occasional acts of charity on self-reported happiness. This inquiry delves into how different forms of giving can influence well-being during a global crisis.

3.5.3 The Moderating Role of Sedekah

The estimation outcomes reveal that engaging in any form of *sedekah* (Model [3]) and both regular and occasional *sedekah* (Model [4]) moderate the negative effect of COVID-19 severity on self-reported happiness.[10] By making donations, individuals proactively confront the challenges posed by the pandemic. High levels of COVID-19 severity often coincide with significant social disruptions, encompassing health-related concerns, economic challenges, and social isolation. These disruptions can overshadow the positive outcomes of charitable acts, resulting in a weakened connection between making donations and self-reported happiness.

The negative moderation indicates that the connection between COVID-19 severity and self-reported happiness is affected by making regular and occasional sedekah that weakens it or makes it less positive compared to individuals who do not donate regularly. These findings can prove that the pandemic diminishes the positive impact of both regular and occasional donations on happiness.

Figure 3.3 quantifies happiness levels by depicting predictive margins from three distinct groups of individuals, classified by their donation behaviors: non-contributors, occasional donors, and regular donors.[11] These margins were calculated using the estimates of Model [4] in Table 3.2. Among the three groups, non-givers experience the lowest happiness levels, followed by occasional *sedekah* givers, while those who regularly give *sedekah* enjoy the highest happiness levels. In greater detail, individuals who do not give *sedekah* exhibit the highest predictive margins of happiness for lower happiness levels (ranging from 0 to 2, shown as dotted lines), surpassing both regular and occasional *sedekah* givers. However, non-contributors

[10] Within the framework of our moderation analysis, a statistically significant interaction term, whether positive or negative, signifies that the impact of COVID-19 severity on self-reported happiness is conditional upon the practice of making *sedekah*. In simpler terms, the connection between COVID-19 severity and self-reported happiness is not uniform for all individuals; it hinges on whether they engage in regular or occasional *sedekah*.

[11] The term *predictive mean* refers to the predicted outcome after accounting for covariates in non-linear models, including the ordered logistic models (Mitchell 2020).

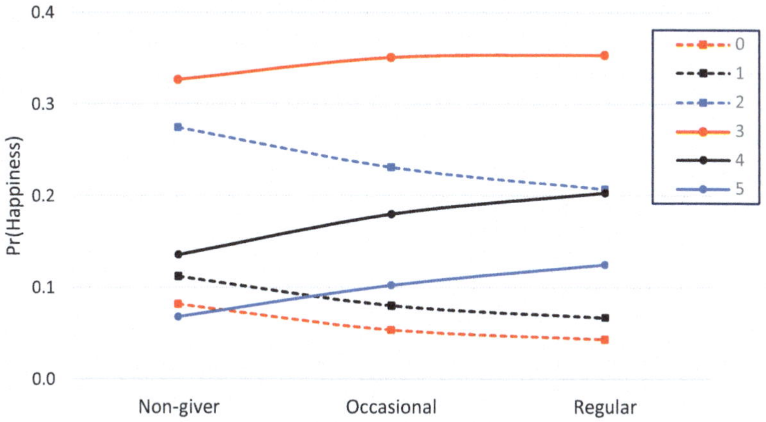

Fig. 3.3 Predictive margins of happiness levels. Notes: Calculated based on estimates of Model [4]

show the lowest predictive margins of happiness for higher happiness levels (ranging from 3 to 5, depicted as solid lines). Additionally, our findings reveal that individuals with lower happiness levels who give regular *sedekah* exhibit decreased predictive margins of happiness compared to those who give *sedekah* occasionally. Conversely, this pattern reverses for individuals with higher happiness levels.

Concerning the COVID-19 pandemic, we have yet to come across studies explicitly investigating the link between making donations and levels of happiness. Nevertheless, some studies document people's ongoing commitment to donating despite many economic challenges during the COVID-19 pandemic (Charities Aid Foundation 2022). Furthermore, a study on the practice of giving *sedekah* within the Muslim communities of Malaysia during the pandemic lockdown revealed that, despite the constraints of reduced income and limited socioeconomic activities, people remained committed to making donations (Busari et al. 2023).

The preceding discussion sheds light on our investigation of RQ3, which delves into the moderating impact of donations. The findings point to a negative form of moderation, suggesting that regular and occasional *sedekah* acts to mitigate or lessen the link between COVID-19 severity and self-reported happiness.

3.5.4 Contextual Characteristics

The significant negative coefficient for the Gini of per capita expenditures indicates that higher income inequality at the province level is consistently linked to lower self-reported happiness during the COVID-19 pandemic. The finding suggests that in provinces with greater income inequality, individuals are more likely to report reduced happiness during the crisis, likely due to the social and psychological stressors associated with income disparities. This relationship holds even when considering nuanced interactions with donation behaviors and pandemic severity.

A study conducted by Furwanti et al. (2021), utilizing cross-sectional data from all Indonesian provinces and a path analysis model, confirms that income inequality has a significant and negative impact on happiness in Indonesia. Our finding aligns with international evidence. For example, Ferrer-i-Carbonell and Ramos (2014) found a negative correlation between income inequality and happiness in Western countries, whereas the relationship in non-Western countries is mixed. Schroder (2018) noted that increasing inequality within one's country leads to lower subjective well-being. In contrast, Kelley and Evans (2017) suggested that income inequality has little impact on happiness in affluent nations but may have a neutral to positive effect in developing nations.

The province's economic prosperity, as gauged by GRDP per capita, does not display a statistically significant impact on self-reported happiness. This absence of statistical significance remains consistent even after considering interaction terms. The lack of a noteworthy relationship between GRDP per capita and self-reported happiness in this context suggests that people's well-being before and during the pandemic may have been shaped by factors beyond the economic conditions at the provincial level. However, it is important to note that the absence of statistical significance might be due to measurement complexities rather than a disregard for its sociological relevance. One plausible explanation is linked to the considerable variability in GRDP per capita observed across different districts within the province. For example, in 2021, East Java Province had an overall GRDP per capita of IDR 60.0 million. In contrast, individual GRDP per capita values ranged from IDR 20.7 million to IDR 491.3 million across its 38 *kabupaten/kota*.

Our finding aligns with a Spanish study by Cuñado and de Gracia (2012), which also did not identify a statistically significant relationship between GRDP per capita at the regional level and happiness levels. However, our results differ from those of Sujarwoto and Tampubolon (2015), who investigated happiness determinants in Indonesia at the district level and found a negative correlation between GRDP per capita and self-reported happiness.

Our analysis, which indicated a consistent connection between greater income inequality at the provincial level and reduced self-reported happiness during the COVID-19 pandemic and the limited impact of the province's economic prosperity on self-reported happiness, offers partial support for research question 4. This question delves into the effect of provincial-level macroeconomic conditions on individuals' happiness levels.

3.5.5 Individual and Household Characteristics

The point estimates for individual and household covariates indicate that holding everything else constant, respondents reported greater happiness when possessing one or more of the following attributes: being female, married, having a higher level of education, residing in urban areas, and having a higher household income, in comparison to their counterparts. Women report higher happiness levels than men, consistent with many studies, including Graham and Chattopadhyay (2012). Marriage is linked to greater happiness, as supported by Frey (2018), who notes that it can reduce loneliness and work-related stress. Higher education is associated with increased happiness, with more educated individuals experiencing greater life satisfaction, as highlighted by Chen (2012). Higher household earnings generally lead to higher happiness, aligning with research by Diener and Biswas-Diener (2002) and Lim et al. (2020). Urban residents tend to be happier than their rural counterparts, as noted by Easterlin et al. (2011), attributed to better access to material goods despite potential issues like traffic and pollution affecting urban happiness.

Conversely, currently employed respondents report lower happiness scores than those primarily dedicate their time to household responsibilities. The finding contrasts with many studies, including one encompassing twelve European countries (Di Tella et al. 2001). Several factors may contribute to this negative relationship, including job-related stress, challenges in achieving a work-life balance, job quality, concerns about job security, long commutes, adverse work environments, and potential mismatches between an individual's career aspirations and current job.

Moreover, the impact of respondent age on self-reported happiness exhibits a U-shaped pattern. Generally, happiness decreases with age until a particular point, beyond which it starts to increase. In our models, we identify this turning point at age 48. This U-shaped trend corresponds to the "midlife dip" phenomenon, as Blanchflower and Graham (2020) highlighted, where individuals often experience a dip in happiness during midlife before a subsequent upswing in later years.

3.5.6 Study Limitations

This study employs a single-question approach using a 0–10 point Likert scale to assess individual happiness. While this method offers a valuable measure, it is important to recognize that happiness is a complex concept with multiple dimensions that a single question may not fully encompass. As such, we acknowledge the necessity of considering additional aspects and subtleties to gain a more comprehensive understanding of individuals' well-being.

Furthermore, it is crucial to consider two significant data limitations when interpreting the findings. First, the SPTK datasets used in the study lack precise location information, which restricts the analysis to the provincial level and hinders a more detailed examination of the impact of COVID-19 on specific regions or communities within a province. Second, the datasets do not include information regarding the interview dates for respondents. Access to this data could have facilitated a more accurate correlation with the daily severity rate of COVID-19 at the provincial level, offering valuable insights into the temporal relationship between individuals' experiences and the evolving severity of the pandemic in their respective provinces.[12]

[12] COVID-19 pandemic severity is assessed as the total population with confirmed exposure to COVID-19 per 100,000 of the province's population. Daily data on the total affected has been accessible since March 2, 2020. Nevertheless, due to the lack of interview date information in the SPTK data, we established June 30, 2021 (the day before the commencement of SPTK face-to-face interviews) as the cutoff date for assessing the COVID-19 severity for all survey participants.

Additionally, one of the primary predictors, the act of giving *sedekah*, is influenced by explanatory variables that also play a role in determining happiness. These variables include, among other things, gender, age, marital status, education, and income. Consequently, giving *sedekah* should be regarded as an endogenous explanatory variable. Regression analyses involving endogenous variables may lead to potentially inaccurate conclusions (Wooldridge 2013). We initially attempted to employ instrumental variable estimations in our research to tackle this issue. However, our efforts to identify a robust instrument for the giving *sedekah* model at the individual and province levels proved unsuccessful, preventing us from using instrumental variable estimations in this chapter. Future research should address the endogeneity of charitable contributions, as demonstrated in studies like Ren and Ye (2017) and Ugur (2018).

3.6 Conclusion

This study investigates the interplay between generosity dynamics and individual well-being in Indonesia amidst the COVID-19 pandemic. Specifically, we aim to examine how both regular (monthly or more frequent) and occasional acts of giving, referred to as *sedekah*, affect the relationship between the severity of COVID-19 and self-reported happiness. We employ data from the Happiness Level Measurement Survey (SPTK) conducted in 2017 and 2021, which captures conditions before and during the pandemic. Our research methodology employs a Multilevel Mixed-Effects Ordered Logistic model, wherein individuals are nested within provinces for analysis.

The study formulates four research questions to elaborate on its aims. To start, research question 1 examines the impact of COVID-19 severity on self-reported happiness. The results reveal that individuals in provinces with higher COVID-19 cases reported reduced happiness, highlighting the pandemic's profound influence on well-being, including increased health risks, anxiety, economic disruptions, and reduced social support.

Second, research question 2 explores the relationship between *sedekah* and happiness. Regular and occasional *sedekah* is associated with higher self-reported happiness, aligning with the warm glow theory of giving, which emphasizes the intrinsic joy of helping. Regular donors often experience a more profound sense of purpose and connection to their causes, enhancing their happiness.

Third, research question 3, which serves as the primary research question, investigates the moderating role of *sedekah*. The negative moderation indicates that regular and occasional *sedekah* weaken the relationship between COVID-19 severity and self-reported happiness, resulting in a less notable impact than individuals who do not donate regularly. These findings prove that the pandemic diminishes the positive effect of regular and occasional donations on happiness.

Fourth, research question 4 considers contextual factors. The results indicate a connection between higher income inequality at the provincial level and reduced self-reported happiness during the COVID-19 pandemic. Economic prosperity at the provincial level has a limited impact on self-reported happiness.

This study provides a comprehensive perspective on the multi-faceted relationship between external events, acts of generosity, and contextual factors shaping individual well-being during a global crisis. These findings contribute to understanding the intricate interplay of various elements influencing individuals' happiness and overall quality of life during challenging times, such as the COVID-19 pandemic.

In light of the study's findings, we put forward recommendations for policies aimed at harnessing the potential of *sedekah* for well-being, focusing on traditional and online charitable giving. One vital policy suggestion is to prioritize and promote acts of giving *sedekah* at the individual and community levels. This could be achieved through awareness campaigns emphasizing the various benefits of regular and occasional acts of generosity, thereby nurturing a culture of giving that contributes to individual and collective well-being. Furthermore, supporting non-profit and charitable organizations engaged in disaster or pandemic relief efforts is essential. Encouraging individuals to contribute to these organizations and highlighting the substantial positive impact on donors and recipients can further bolster the spirit of generosity.

Considering the increasing availability of online platforms for making *sedekah* and its potential to magnify the impact of generosity, several recommendations can be explored (Effendi and Xuan 2021). Digital literacy programs should be implemented to ensure that individuals, especially those in remote or underserved areas, have the necessary skills and access to online platforms for *sedekah*. Public awareness campaigns can play a pivotal role in acquainting the public with these platforms and elucidating their advantages. Collaborating with religious institutions to promote online *sedekah*, underlining its alignment with faith-based values, can enhance its appeal and reach. Finally, tax deductions or incentives for individuals and businesses that donate through online platforms should be contemplated to incentivize online charitable giving. These incentives can stimulate a greater adoption of online channels for charitable giving, expanding the impact of generosity.

References

Aknin, L.B., C.P. Barrington-Leigh, E.W. Dunn, J.F. Helliwell, J. Burns, R. Biswas-Diener, I. Kemeza, P. Nyende, C.E. Ashton-James, and M.I. Norton. 2013. Prosocial spending and well-being: Cross-cultural evidence for a psychological universal. *Journal of Personality and Social Psychology* 104 (4): 635–652. https://doi.org/10.1037/a0031578.

Aknin, L.B., A.V. Whillans, M.I. Norton, and E.W. Dunn. 2019. Happiness and prosocial behavior: An evaluation of the evidence. In *World happiness report*, ed. J.F. Helliwell, R. Layard, J.D. Sachs, and J.-E. De Neve, 67–88. New York: Sustainable Development Solutions Network.

Andrade, C. 2020. The limitations of online surveys. *Indian Journal of Psychological Medicine* 42 (6): 575–576. https://doi.org/10.1177/0253717620957496.

Andreoni, J. 1989. Giving with impure altruism: Applications to charity and Ricardian equivalence. *Journal of Political Economy* 97 (6): 1447–1458.

———. 1990. Impure altruism and donations to public goods: A theory of warm-glow giving. *The Economic Journal* 100: 464–477.

Badan Pusat Statistik. 2017. *Indeks kebahagiaan 2017 [Happiness index 2017]*. Jakarta, Indonesia: Badan Pusat Statistik.

———. 2021. *Indeks kebahagiaan 2021 [Happiness index 2021]*. Jakarta, Indonesia: Badan Pusat Statistik.

Bittmann, F. 2022. Is there a dose-response relationship? Investigating the functional form between COVID-19 incidence rates and life satisfaction in a multilevel framework. *Journal of Happiness Studies*. https://doi.org/10.1007/s10902-022-00542-1.

Blanchflower, D., and C. Graham. 2020. *The mid-life dip in well-being: Economists (who find it) versus psychologists (who don't)!* Cambridge, MA: National Bureau of Economic Research. https://doi.org/10.3386/w26888.

Boenigk, S., and M.L. Mayr. 2016. The happiness of giving: Evidence from the German Socioeconomic Panel that happier people are more generous. *Journal of Happiness Studies* 17 (5): 1825–1846. https://doi.org/10.1007/s10902-015-9672.

Borualogo, I.S., and F. Casas. 2022. Subjective well-being of children and adolescents during the COVID-19 pandemic in Indonesia: two data collections. *Current Psychology*. https://doi.org/10.1007/s12144-022-03346-x.

Brodeur, A., D. Gray, A. Islam, and S. Bhuiyan. 2021. A literature review of the economics of COVID-19. *Journal of Economic Surveys* 35 (4): 1007–1044. https://doi.org/10.1111/joes.12423.

Busari, S.A., M.B. Sitiris, and J.A. Adebiyi. 2023. Ṣadaqah (Charity) attitudes of Muslims during COVID-19 pandemic lockdown: An interpretative phenomenology. *International Journal of Fiqh and Usul al-Fiqh Studies* 7 (1): 78–87.

Charities Aid Foundation. 2022. *World giving index 2022: A global view of giving trends*. London, UK: Charities Aid Foundation.

Chen, W.-C. 2012. How education enhances happiness: Comparison of mediating factors in four east Asian countries. *Social Indicators Research* 106 (1): 117–131. https://doi.org/10.1007/s11205-011-9798-5.

Cheng, T.C., S. Kim, and K. Koh. 2020. *The impact of COVID-19 on subjective well-being: Evidence from Singapore*. Bonn: IZA–Institute of Labor Economics.

Cleofas, J.V., and R.M.F. Oducado. 2022. COVID-19 death occurrences, pandemic fatigue, and well-being. *Journal of Loss and Trauma* 27 (7): 679–682. https://doi.org/10.1080/15325024.2021.1971423.

Cuñado, J., and F.P. de Gracia. 2012. Environment and happiness: New evidence for Spain. *Social Indicators Research* 112 (3): 549–567. https://doi.org/10.1007/s11205-012-0038-4.

Demirbas, N., and R. Kutlu. 2021. Effects of COVID-19 fear on society's quality of life. *International Journal of Mental Health and Addiction* 20: 2813–2822. https://doi.org/10.1007/s11469-021-00550-x.

Diener, E., and R. Biswas-Diener. 2002. Will money increase subjective well-being? A literature review and guide to needed research. *Social Indicators Research* 57 (2): 119–169. https://doi.org/10.1023/a:1014411319119.

Di Tella, R., R.J. MacCulloch, and A. Oswald. 2001. Preferences over inflation and unemployment: Evidence from surveys of happiness. *The American Economic Review* 91 (1): 335–341.

Dwidienawati, D., D. Tjahjana, D. Gandasari, and M. Faisal. 2021. Happiness and satisfaction after 1 year of the COVID-19 pandemic. *Journal of Southwest Jiaotong University* 56 (2): 111–123. https://doi.org/10.35741/issn.0258-2724.56.2.10.

Easterlin, R.A., L. Angelescu, and J.S. Zweig. 2011. The impact of modern economic growth on urban-rural differences in subjective well-being. *World Development* 39 (12): 2187–2198. https://doi.org/10.1016/j.worlddev.2011.04.015.

Effendi, T.D., and N.T. Xuan. 2021. Online donation for Covid-19 as connective action in Indonesia and Vietnam. *Journal of Social and Political Sciences* 4 (2): 192–204. https://doi.org/10.31014/aior.1991.04.02.288.

Faghih, N., and A. Forouharfar, eds. 2022. *Socioeconomic dynamics of the COVID-19 crisis: Global, regional, and local perspectives*. 1st ed. Cham: Springer Nature.

Ferrer-i-Carbonell, A., and X. Ramos. 2014. Inequality and happiness. *Journal of Economic Surveys* 28 (5): 1016–1027. https://doi.org/10.1111/joes.12049.

Filantropi Indonesia. 2021, June 15. *Indonesia returns as the most generous country in the world*. https://filantropi.or.id/en/indonesia-returns-as-the-most-generous-country-in-the-world/. Accessed 1 June 2023.

Frey, B.S. 2018. *Economics of happiness*. 1st ed. Cham: Springer.

Furwanti, R., D.M. Lestari, M. Muflikha, and M.B. Wibowo. 2021. Determinant of macroeconomics: Does income inequality influence happiness? Evidence from Indonesia. *JEJAK* 14 (1): 146–156. https://doi.org/10.15294/jejak.v14i1.28278.

Geertz, C. 1985. *Local knowledge: Further essays in interpretive anthropology*. New York: Basic Books.

Graham, C., and S. Chattopadhyay. 2012. Gender and well-being around the world: Some insights from the economics of happiness. *Working papers*. http://ideas.repec.org/p/hka/wpaper/2012-010.html.

Greyling, T., S. Rossouw, and T. Adhikari. 2021. The good, the bad and the ugly of lockdowns during Covid-19. *PLoS One* 16 (1): e0245546. https://doi.org/10.1371/journal.pone.0245546.

Hai-Anh, H., and L.D. Toan. 2022. Does the COVID-19 pandemic disproportionately affect the poor? Evidence from a six-country survey. *TSE working papers*. https://ideas.repec.org/p/tse/wpaper/127425.html.

Halimatussadiah, A., C.H. Siregar, H. Bintara, J.F. Rezki, L.A.M. Putri, M.R. Aufari, N.K. Sholihah, R.R. Fadilla, and W. Al Kautsar. 2021. *Buku statistik survei dampak pandemi COVID 19 [Statistical book of survey of the impact of the COVID-19 pandemic]*. Institute for Economic and Social Research, Faculty of Economics and Business, Universitas Indonesia (LPEM-FEB UI). https://www.lpem.org/wp-content/uploads/2021/12/BUKU_STATISTIK_v8_opt.pdf. Accessed 19 Nov 2022.

Helliwell, J.F., R. Layard, J.D. Sachs, and J.-E. De Neve, eds. 2020. *World happiness report 2020*. New York: Sustainable Development Solutions Network.

Helliwell, J.F., R. Layard, J.D. Sachs, J.-E. De Neve, L.B. Aknin, and S. Wang, eds. 2022. *World happiness report 2022*. New York: Sustainable Development Solutions Network.

———, eds. 2023. *World happiness report 2023*. New York: Sustainable Development Solutions Network.

Hyman, L. 2013. Happiness and memory: Some sociological reflections. *Sociological Research Online* 19 (2): 1–9. https://doi.org/10.5153/sro.3268.

Indrawati, S.M., S. Nazara, T. Anas, C.F. Ananda, and K. Verico, eds. 2022. *Keeping Indonesia safe from the covid-19 pandemic: Lessons learnt from the national economic recovery programme*. Singapore and Jakarta, Indonesia: ISEAS Publishing and Ministry of Finance of the Republic of Indonesia.

Iskandarsyah, A., W. Yudiana, A. Shabrina, and J. Passchier. 2022. Perception of information about COVID-19 and protective behaviours in relation to feelings of anxiety and happiness. *International Journal of Public Health Science* 11 (1): 8–19. https://doi.org/10.11591/ijphs.v11i1.21018.

Jun, H.J., M. Kang, D.K. Yoon, S.A. Lee, and H. Park. 2022. The effects of charitable giving on life satisfaction of older Korean adults: The moderating role of relationship satisfaction and social trust. *Research on Aging* 44 (7–8): 600–610. https://doi.org/10.1177/01640275211065441.

Kaye-Kauderer, H., J.H. Feingold, and A, Feder, S. Southwick, and D. Charney. 2021. Resilience in the age of COVID-19. *BJPsych Advances* 27 (3): 166–178. https://doi.org/10.1192/bja.2021.5.

Kelley, J., and M.D.R. Evans. 2017. The new income inequality and well-being paradigm: Inequality has no effect on happiness in rich nations and normal times, varied effects in extraordinary circumstances, increases happiness in poor nations, and interacts with individuals' perceptions, attitudes, politics, and expectations for the future. *Social Science Research* 62: 39–74. https://doi.org/10.1016/j.ssresearch.2016.12.007.

Kuah, K.E., G. Guiheux, and F.K.G. Lim, eds. 2023. *COVID-19 responses of local communities around the world: Exploring trust in the context of risk and fear*. New York: Routledge.

Kuhn, U., H.S. Klaas, E. Antal, N. Dasoki, F. Lebert, O. Lipps, G.-A. Monsch, J.-E. Refle, V.-A. Ryser, R. Tillmann, and M. Voorpostel. 2020. Who is most affected by the Corona crisis? An analysis of changes in stress and well-being in Switzerland. *European Societies* 23 (sup1): S942–S956. https://doi.org/10.1080/14616696.2020.1839671.

Lepinteur, A., A.E. Clark, A. Ferrer-i-Carbonell, A. Piper, C. Schröder, and C. D'Ambrosio. 2022. Gender, loneliness and happiness during COVID-19. *Journal of Behavioral and Experimental Economics* 101: 101952. https://doi.org/10.1016/j.socec.2022.101952.

Lim, H.-E., D. Shaw, P.-S. Liao, and H. Duan. 2020. The effects of income on happiness in east and south Asia: Societal values matter? *Journal of Happiness Studies* 21 (2): 391–415. https://doi.org/10.1007/s10902-019-00088-9.

Mehmetoglu, M., and T.G. Jakobsen. 2017. *Applied statistics using Stata: A guide for the social sciences*. Singapore: Sage.

Mitchell, M.N. 2020. *Interpreting and visualizing regression models using Stata*. 2nd ed. College Station, TX: Stata Press.

Morgan, P.J. 2021. *Impacts of COVID-19 on households in ASEAN countries and their implications for human capital development*. Asian Development Bank 1226. https://www.adb.org/publications/impacts-covid-19-households-asean-countries. Accessed 3 Nov 2022.

Nguyen, C.V. 2021. *Does the COVID-19 pandemic cause people to be unhappy? Evidence from a six-country survey*. Global Labor Organization (GLO). http://hdl.handle.net/10419/228738. Accessed 15 Feb 2023.

Pattinasarany, I.R.I. 2018. Happiness and life satisfaction among East and Southeast Asian countries. *Paper presented at the fourth conference of International Consortium for Social Well-Being Studies*. Seoul National University.

Pholphirul, P. 2015. Happiness from giving: Quantitative investigation of Thai Buddhists. *Applied Research in Quality of Life* 10 (4): 703–720. https://doi.org/10.1007/s11482-014-9349-8.

Rabe-Hesketh, S., and A. Skrondal. 2022. *Multilevel and longitudinal modeling using Stata*. 4th ed. College Station, TX: Stata Press.

Rahmanita, M., Nurbaeti, F. Asmaniati, T.R. Dewi, and N. Widyastuti. 2021. COVID-19 pandemic: Happiness revisited through work and leisure during the stay at home period. *Journal of Hunan University Natural Sciences* 48 (4): 100–107.

Ren, Q., and M. Ye. 2017. Donations make people happier: Evidence from the Wenchuan earthquake. *Social Indicators Research* 132 (1): 517–536. https://doi.org/10.1007/s11205-016-1233-5.

Schroder, M. 2018. Income inequality and life satisfaction: Unrelated between countries, associated within countries over time. *Journal of Happiness Studies* 19: 1021–1043. https://doi.org/10.1007/s10902-017-9860-3.

Snijders, T.A., and R.J. Bosker. 2012. *Multilevel analysis: an introduction to basic and advanced multilevel modeling*. 2nd ed. Singapore: Sage.

Song, J., C. Gu, and B. Zuo. 2019. Effect of charitable behavior on life satisfaction: A parallel multivariable mediation model. *Social Behavior and Personality* 47 (3): 1–8. https://doi.org/10.2224/sbp.7701.

StataCorp. 2021. *Stata multilevel mixed-effects reference manual release 17*. College Station, TX: Stata Press.

Sujarwoto, S., and G. Tampubolon. 2015. Decentralisation and citizen happiness: A multilevel analysis of self-rated happiness in Indonesia. *Journal of Happiness Studies* 16: 455–475. https://doi.org/10.1007/s10902-014-9518-3.

Tadic, M., H. Braam, K. Van Vliet, and R. Veenhoven. 2014. Memory-experience gap in early adolescents' happiness reports. *Child Indicators Research* 7: 21–40. https://doi.org/10.1007/s12187-013-9194-6.

Tiefenbach, T., and F. Kohlbacher. 2014. Happiness in Japan in times of upheaval: Empirical evidence from the national survey on lifestyle preferences. *Journal of Happiness Studies* 16 (2): 333–366. https://doi.org/10.1007/s10902-014-9512-9.

Tjahjana, D., D. Dwidienawati, A.H. Manurung, and D. Gandasari. 2021. Does people's well-being get impacted by COVID-19 pandemic measure in Indonesia? *Studies of Applied Economics* 39 (4). https://doi.org/10.25115/eea.v39i4.4873.

Ugur, Z.B. 2018. Donate more, be happier! Evidence from the Netherlands. *Applied Research in Quality of Life* 13 (1): 157–177. https://doi.org/10.1007/s11482-017-9512-0.
Utama, R.Y., H. Palani, and A.Z. Rabbani. 2021. Giving more enhances your happiness: Evidence from Indonesia. *Communication in Humanity and Social Science* 1 (1): 24–34. https://doi.org/10.21924/chss.1.1.2021.8.
van der Vegt, I., and B. Kleinberg. 2020. Women worry about family, men about the economy: Gender differences in emotional responses to COVID-19. *Lecture Notes in Computer Science* 12467: 397–409. https://doi.org/10.1007/978-3-030-60975-7_29.
Winzer, L., B. Samutachak, and R.S. Gray. 2018. Religiosity, spirituality, and happiness in Thailand from the perspective of Buddhism. *Journal of Population and Social Studies* 26 (4): 332–343. https://doi.org/10.25133/jpssv26n4.023.
Wooldridge, J.M. 2013. *Introductory econometrics: A modern approach*. 5th ed. Mason, OH: South-Western, Cengage Learning.
Worldometer. 2023. Countries where Coronavirus has spread—Worldometer. https://www.worldometers.info/coronavirus/countries-where-coronavirus-has-spread/. Accessed 23 Feb 2023.
Wu, Y.-Y., Y.-T. Yu, Y.-D. Yao, M.-H. Su, W.-C. Zhang, S.-M. Ti, X.-Y. Lin, S. Zhang, S.-Q. Zhang, and H.-L. Yang. 2021. Share rose, get fun: The influence of donation on happiness. *Frontiers in Sociology* 6: 675968. https://doi.org/10.3389/fsoc.2021.675968.
Zheng, X., J. Chen, and J., and Y. Li. 2021. The association between charitable giving and happiness: Evidence from the Chinese General Social Survey. *Quality & Quantity* 55: 2103–2138. https://doi.org/10.1007/s11135-021-01104-y.

Indera Ratna Irawati Pattinasarany holds the position of Associate Professor in the Department of Sociology at Universitas Indonesia. She obtained her master's degree in sociology from Michigan State University, USA, and completed her Ph.D. in sociology at Universitas Indonesia. Her research focuses on social stratification and mobility, social inequality, social well-being, and sociology of education. Actively involved in both international and national sociological associations, Indera is a current member of the International Sociological Association, contributing to RC28 (Social Stratification), RC55 (Social Indicators), and RC04 (Sociology of Education). Additionally, she plays a crucial role in fostering international cooperation within the Indonesian Sociological Association.

Chapter 4
The Well-Being of Young People in Europe During the Pandemic: The Social Ties, Labor Market Integration, and the Social Inequalities

Dragan Stanojević, Bojan Todosijević, and Anja Gvozdanović

4.1 Introduction

Throughout the COVID-19 pandemic, spanning from spring 2020 to spring 2023, European countries encountered significant social, economic, and political repercussions due to the implementation of policies designed to curb the spread of the virus and address its consequences. Physical distancing, social isolation, curfews, movement restrictions, limitations on public space interactions, institutional closures (especially educational institutions), transition to remote work, and employee layoffs, have served as policy instruments employed to varying extents across European nations for over 2 years. The adverse implications on the well-being of the youth have been well-documented, prompting an increasing discourse regarding the "COVID generation," characterized by a significant deterioration in mental health, substantial disruptions in education, heightened vulnerability in the labor market, and hindrances to prospective career trajectories (UNICEF 2020).

Young people[1] were more frequently subject to job loss, cessation of job-seeking efforts, and encountered challenges in making ends meet (Palmer and Small 2021).

[1] In the field of youth studies, conceptualizations of the youth through age range vary considerably, often delimited at 25, 30, or 35 years. For the purpose of our analysis, we propose categorizing youth as individuals aged 15–35 years. This broader spectrum pertains to distinct developmental stages, starting from puberty and concluding when physiological and emotional maturity is attained, often encompassing an extended duration (Furlong 2012).

D. Stanojević (✉)
Faculty of Philosophy, University of Belgrade, Belgrade, Serbia
e-mail: dstanoje@f.bg.ac.rs

B. Todosijević
Institute of Social Sciences, Belgrade, Serbia

A. Gvozdanović
Institute for Social Research in Zagreb, Zagreb, Croatia

C. Suter et al. (eds.), *Well-being During the Pandemic*, Social Indicators Research Series 90, https://doi.org/10.1007/978-3-031-63440-6_4

Pre-existing involvement in precarious employment structures, notably temporary and part-time contracts, rendered them more susceptible to challenges associated with financial instability and housing insecurity, both exacerbated during the pandemic. Countries have adopted diverse and often inadequately transparent and sustained approaches towards the pandemic, implementing, modifying, and retracting various policy measures. These actions have further heightened the sense of insecurity and distrust. Furthermore, imposing restrictions on gatherings and suspending a significant portion of political activities (including the prohibition of protests, collective actions, election postponements, etc.) has compounded the youth's perception of diminished connectedness and reduced readiness for collective action.

During the COVID-19 crisis, the trajectory of youth life satisfaction exhibited notable fluctuations, correlating with the imposition and alleviation of isolation measures. Despite the apparent rise in life satisfaction during the spring and summer of 2020, coinciding with the relaxation of restrictions, the enforcement of more rigorous measures in 2021 precipitated the nadir of youth life satisfaction (Eurofound 2021).

The subject of this chapter is the relationship between life satisfaction, as an indicator of the well-being of young individuals, and various forms of integration—social, economic, and political—during the pandemic. Common sense suggests that higher level of social integration often corresponds to increased access to resources, heightened resilience, and consequently, a greater level of life satisfaction. This assumption becomes particularly compelling when examining these relationships amid the COVID-19 crisis, which has resulted in social isolation and the atomization of individuals (Baarck et al. 2021). However, our pivotal research question that we aim to address is whether young people who are more effectively integrated are more satisfied or if certain forms of integration are associated with greater dissatisfaction and frustration. Alternatively, it is of interest to ascertain whether dissatisfaction might, in fact, foster a greater propensity to connect with others and engage in collective actions. This inquiry gives rise to several specific questions. In what manner have informal contacts, social interactions, and connections with others functioned as factors of resilience? Are different forms of political integration (participation) associated with life satisfaction? How is labor market integration related to life satisfaction, and in what manner, if at all? Do societies characterized by greater equality and solidarity contribute to a more positive self-perception among young individuals?

We will first focus on the theoretical background of the relationship between life satisfaction and the three dimensions of integration: social ties, participation in the labor market, and political participation. Namely, we will discuss the findings of current research regarding the link between life satisfaction of youth and social integration (including informal contacts and experiences of discrimination), labor market integration and political participation in Europe. Following this, in the methodological section, we will delineate the indicators used and the methodology applied. In the subsequent section, we will present the analyses, and in the discussion, we will endeavor to connect the findings with theoretical frameworks and contextual characteristics.

4.2 Theoretical Background

4.2.1 Social Integration

Primary Social Ties and Social Capital In this study, we examine the role of horizontal social ties, primarily friendships and familial connections. Social capital, consisting of trust-based connections, represents both a societal and individual resource in everyday life. This is especially true for strong ties (Granovetter 1973), characterized not only by reciprocity, trust, and shared norms but also by emotional intensity and frequent contact. Friendships, classified as bonding social capital by Putnam (2000), provide young people with a sense of security and belonging, generating practical knowledge and skills related to the challenges of growing up and facing life's inevitable limitations (Boeck 2007). Close friendships also offer social support during times of crisis and stress, addressing current material, emotional, and other needs (Amichai-Hamburger et al. 2013). Active friendships and networks, or awareness of their "safety-net" function, contribute to life satisfaction and subjective well-being, regardless of age (Crocetti and Meeus 2014; Delhey and Dragolov 2016).

During the COVID-19 pandemic, public health policies in most European Union countries focused on reducing the number of COVID-19 cases and minimizing the risk of virus spread. This involved some form of lockdown and restrictions on movement, discouraging social interactions. Such circumstances posed a significant challenge, necessitating adaptation to a crisis with an uncertain endpoint. During the pandemic, two notable phenomena among young people were detected: the increase in feelings of social isolation (Baarck et al. 2021) and the shift of social interactions, especially during school closures, towards the virtual realm facilitated by digital technologies (Drouin et al. 2020; Fernandes et al. 2020). At the same time, both social isolation and intensified online communication are not mutually exclusive but can be complementary.

Social isolation refers to an inadequate or insufficient number and poor quality of interactions with others, influenced by various individual and social factors (Clair et al. 2021). During the early stages of the COVID-19 outbreak, a significant proportion of individuals in the European Union experienced frequent feelings of loneliness, more than doubling the rate found in a comparable survey from pre-pandemic 2016. Notably, the impact of isolation and lockdown measures was particularly pronounced among the youth. In the period from April to July 2020, young people experienced a surge in loneliness to four times the rate reported 4 years earlier (Baarck et al. 2021).

Recent psychological studies indicate a correlation between higher levels of social isolation and lower levels of life satisfaction and subjective well-being (Birditt et al. 2021; Clair et al. 2021). Conversely, a sense of belonging and social support associated with intense social interactions is positively correlated with higher well-being and life satisfaction across all age cohorts (Ahmadiani et al. 2022; Ciziceno

2022; Crowley and Walsh 2018, 2021; Helliwell 2006; Onal et al. 2022; Putnam 2000; Sarmiento Prieto et al. 2023). Therefore, the widespread feeling of social isolation is likely to impact the level of well-being or life satisfaction among young people. Given the growing prevalence of the "online life" of young people, it raises the question of whether the importance of online social interactions for well-being and life satisfaction is equivalent to that in the real world. Happiness and feelings of loneliness among young people during the COVID-19 pandemic were not correlated with the intensity of their virtual interactions (Towner et al. 2022). If we extrapolate this finding to the relationship between social capital and life satisfaction, we can cautiously conclude that their connection is effectively built when relationships of trust and reciprocity are established and maintained through regular face-to-face contact.

Hypothesis 1: Young people with higher levels of bonding social capital express significantly higher levels of life satisfaction.

Ethnic Discrimination Research dedicated to the pandemic period and social inequalities almost unanimously concludes that the pandemic has exacerbated and underscored existing gender, racial, economic, and ethnic inequalities. In addition, ethnic minorities across European countries generally reported lower life satisfaction than members of the ethnic majority even before the pandemic (Kööts-Ausmees and Realo 2016). Therefore, minority groups, already facing an unfavorable social position, experienced even greater challenges during the pandemic, with significant differences in access to healthcare, employment, housing solutions, and income (Gould and Wilson 2020). A global review and meta-analysis of ethnic inequalities during the pandemic confirmed that the disparities in health outcomes were primarily due to varying levels of risks, with institutional racism and racial discrimination recognized as underlying causes (Irizar et al. 2023). The health and economic burden of the crisis were unevenly distributed across social categories in most Western societies (Ahmed et al. 2023; Fouskas et al. 2022; Irizar et al. 2023; Katikireddi et al. 2021; Platt 2021). For instance, data on COVID-19 mortality in the UK showed that nearly all ethnic minority groups faced greater mortality risks compared to the White British majority within the same age cohort (Platt and Warwick 2020). Given this context, it is expected that groups more exposed to various stressors related to life security during the pandemic are at a greater risk of compromised mental health and, consequently, reduced life satisfaction (Lenoir and Wong 2023).

The crisis, uncertainty, and unpredictable daily life create fertile ground for the rise of xenophobia, racism, and nationalism in the public and political spheres. In times of crisis, widespread feelings of insecurity, personal threat, and social instability contribute to an increase in authoritarian tendencies, known as the authoritarian reflex (Inglehart 2018). Some citizens develop a tendency to rally around authoritative figures, displaying a strong sense of unity and conformity within their group, strict adherence to the group's standards, and a dismissal of those not part of the group (Inglehart 2018). Elias et al. (2021) argue that the COVID-19 pandemic is linked to racism and xenophobia in two fundamental ways. First, there is an increase in racist sentiment towards minority groups during periods of widespread existential threat. In the past, ethnic or racial minorities were often targeted with dehumanizing narratives by the majority, blaming them for various societal misfortunes (Elias et al. 2021), and the COVID-19 pandemic is no exception. The second way in which the pandemic and racism are connected is the social moment in the Western world when the pandemic began, characterized by the rise in exclusive nationalism that then intensified xenophobic racism. With an ongoing anti-migrant narrative in the political life of some European societies, the pandemic era further complicated the integration process for immigrants, asylum seekers, and refugees (Fouskas et al. 2022). Additionally, individuals of Asian descent experienced anti-Asian discrimination (Litam and Oh 2021; Wang et al. 2021), contributing to the mental health deterioration of this ethnic group. For example, experiences of COVID-19-related racial discrimination among American Chinese were identified as a strong predictor of depression (Litam and Oh 2021). In Canada, individuals born in the country expressed significantly higher levels of life satisfaction than Asian immigrants before the pandemic (Helliwell et al. 2020). Regarding the mental health of young people, a German study found that the state of mental health before and during the early stages of the pandemic remained relatively consistent among ethnic Germans and various minority groups. However, the stress associated with the pandemic posed threats to the mental health of young people, particularly due to increased experiences of discrimination and health concerns among Asian minorities and health concerns within Turkish, Middle Eastern, and African minority communities (Plenty et al. 2021).

Hypothesis 2: Young people who belong to an ethnic minority express significantly lower levels of life satisfaction than those who belong to an ethnic majority.

4.2.2 Labor Market Integration

Employment constitutes a significant aspect of the transition to adulthood, serving as a crucial prerequisite for financial autonomy (Arnett 2014; Furlong et al. 2017). The work transitions of young people in European countries commonly start with a series of temporary and insecure jobs, and those with lower educational backgrounds often experience extended periods of unemployment. Consequently, their life trajectories are exposed to various risks and uncertainties (Beck 1992; Furlong and Cartmel 1997). Furlong et al. (2017, 18) characterize this position as liminal, as it does not enable young individuals to become "fully adult." In a society marked by job insecurity, planning becomes challenging, constraining the agency of young people and leading to discomfort and anxiety (Chesters and Cuervo 2019). Therefore, the relationship between labor market integration and the well-being of young individuals exhibits robust associations.

When employed and adequately rewarded for their efforts, young individuals express higher satisfaction levels than those who are unemployed and inactive.

Moreover, those engaged in more secure employment with permanent contracts report greater satisfaction than their counterparts involved in temporary and less stable contractual arrangements (Vancea and Utzet 2017). Furthermore, young individuals classified as Not in Education, Employment, or Training (NEET) report lower life satisfaction compared to their peers who are employed or undergoing education (Jongbloed and Giret 2022).

While these associations are generally present, the mechanism through which one's position in the labor market leads to (dis)satisfaction is complex and contextually conditioned.[2] Employed individuals generate income, affording them a level of control to manage their lives and the ability to organize their future, making improvements in various life domains such as housing, relationships, and family (Furlong et al. 2017). Although income is commonly recognized as the primary reason for increased life satisfaction, a job can also serve as the foundation for identity (Ezzy 1993), self-esteem, a sense of purpose, but also a way to structure daily activities, to generate social capital, and more (Jahoda 1981; Voßemer and Eunicke 2015).

Getting and losing a job can have varying effects on life satisfaction depending on the situation and the significance individuals attribute to these events. As Frey and Stutzer (2002, 101) point out "individuals tend to evaluate their own situation relative to other persons. For most persons, unemployment lowers their happiness less if they are not alone with this particular fate. When unemployment is seen to hit many persons, one knows or hears of, both the psychic and the social effects are mitigated." Furthermore, the flexibility of contracts and working hours may be desirable in some instances and imposed options in others, contingent upon the social context and the individual's circumstances. For example, during academic studies, temporary employment may be preferable as it allows flexibility, but a similar arrangement may be challenging for a young parent responsible for bills and child-rearing. Flexible work arrangements, such as remote work, ordinarily provide greater autonomy and control over the work process and the potential for better work-life balance (Gajendran and Harrison 2007). Data during the COVID-19 crisis indicate that such arrangements presented new challenges as boundaries between private and work life were disrupted, especially when most household members were intensely present within the household. Nevertheless, remote work remained associated with higher satisfaction compared to in-office work (Kondratowicz et al. 2022; Susilo 2020).

Analyses of the labor market situation during the COVID-19 crisis reveal that young individuals were particularly vulnerable to risks, given that, even before the pandemic, this age group had the highest proportion engaged in non-standard and precarious employment (MacDonald 2017). Temporary jobs are the first to be affected in times of crisis, leading young people in such positions to be among the

[2] In the literature, various theoretical frameworks are used to explain this relationship. These include functionalist and deprivation approach (Jahoda 1981), vitamin model (Warr 1987), agency theory (Fryer 1986), and sociological approach via identity theory (Ezzy 1993), all of which serve as foundational concepts that are subsequently critiqued and developed further. Voßemer and Eunicke (2015) provide an extensive overview of the literature and research on the relationship between employment and the well-being of young people.

first to lose their jobs, consequently elevating the unemployment rate. At the EU level, within just 1 year of the crisis's inception, youth employment dropped 2.8 percentage points (European Union 2022). Prior to the onset of the pandemic, youth in European countries were disproportionately employed in sectors particularly vulnerable to the crisis, namely accommodation and food services, wholesale and retail, and health and social work.

From August 2019 to August 2020, the share of unemployed individuals in the EU increased from 15 to 18.5%. The NEET category increased by approximately 1.5 percentage points between 2019 and 2020 (Konle-Seidl and Picarella 2021). These data only partially reveal the depth of the problem, as a significant number of young individuals (an additional 2.4 percentage points) lost their jobs, became temporarily inactive, or ceased their job search, leading to a substantial rise in the inactivity rates among the youth (Anderton et al. 2020; Konle-Seidl and Picarella 2021). The situation in non-EU European countries was similar, with minor variations.

Hypothesis 3: Young people who are employed are more satisfied compared to those who are unemployed.

Hypothesis 4: Young people who work from home are more satisfied compared to those who worked in offices during the COVID-19 crisis

4.2.3 Political Participation and Life Satisfaction

Political integration is an essential aspect of general social integration, especially for the young people in democracies as they are entering adulthood and the world of political rights and duties. Political integration is a complex phenomenon that could be expressed in various ways. Arguably, political *participation* is among its most direct indicators. Taking part in political activities such as voting in elections, contacting politicians, joining a political party, or participating in demonstrations are signs of being integrated into the political domain of the social world.

Political participation[3] is an obvious candidate variable for helping understand youth well-being in society. The COVID-19 era is perhaps a particularly relevant context, as it was a period of increased politicization in many countries (e.g., Rothgerber et al. 2020). However, it is not immediately and intuitively clear why political participation should be associated with life satisfaction. Political activity is rarely accompanied by immediate reward (utility in economists' terminology) but is often accompanied by frustration. Pacheco and Lange (2010, 688), therefore, rhetorically ask: "Given political participation as a seemingly futile activity to realize individual preferences, why would we expect a positive relationship between

[3] According to Verba and Nie (1972, 9), "Political participation is the means by which the interests, desires and demands of the ordinary citizen are communicated (...) all those activities by private citizens that are more or less directly aimed at influencing the selection of governmental personnel and/or decisions they make."

participation and enhanced utility?" Indeed, while political participation is a rather popular research topic, the relationship with life satisfaction only recently gained momentum, while research focused on youth political participation is still relatively rare (cf., Weiss 2020).

Participating in politics is, in fact, found to be associated with the feeling of well-being in different countries in various ways (e.g., Dorn et al. 2008; Frey and Stutzer 2000b; He et al. 2022; Laurence 2021; Lindholm 2020; Owen et al. 2008; Pacheco and Lange 2010; Vega-Tinoco et al. 2022). The involved mechanism may be based on the feeling of accomplishment, a sense of efficacy, self-appreciation for taking part in an activity aimed to contribute to the welfare of the society ("procedural utility," Frey and Stutzer 2000b), and so on. Laurence (2021, 322), for instance, concludes "that participation's impact needs to be understood through both social- and psychological-resource models, with positive indirect effects observed via structural/cognitive elements of social capital as well as perceived control/social efficacy."

At the same time, researchers argued that it is the experience of well-being that affects political participation (e.g., Barnes et al. 1979; Flavin and Keane 2012; Lindholm 2020; Weitz-Shapiro and Winters 2011). For instance, Weitz-Shapiro and Winters (2011, 118) conclude that "our data are more consistent with the claim that happiness causes people to participate." The causality is explained by interpreting subjective well-being as a "psychological resource for the purpose of political participation due to its positive influence on self-efficacy and motivation to invest time and effort into political activities" (Lindholm 2020, 472). Also, the influence may be exerted through identification with the socio-political system and broader social integration. In line with these ambiguities, Lorenzini (2015, 383) observed that "Several researchers have used subjective well-being to explain political participation [...]. Others have analysed it as resulting from political institutions and participation," however, he prefers the "satisfaction influences participation" causal direction rather than vice versa.

Not only could causal direction go both ways, but the direction of association has also been found to be positive, negative, and non-existent. For instance, feelings of not-well-being may be a strong motive for political participation as a generator of the desire to change (something in) society. Indeed, it was reported that life *dissatisfaction* may foster youth propensity for political protest (e.g., Barnes et al. 1979; Lorenzini 2015; Marsh 1977). Conversely, Flavin and Keane (2012) concluded that life satisfaction does not contribute to protest activities. To make matters more complex and difficult for a simple résumé, Lorenzini (2015, 382–3) found an interesting interaction of political participation with unemployment in Switzerland, concluding that life satisfaction (LS) "fosters unemployed youth protest activities. In addition, [...] LS hinders employed youth contacting activities."

One reason contributing to the diversity of research findings is the complexity of the phenomenon of political participation. It has been noted long ago that political participation is not a simple and unitary phenomenon easy to define (e.g., Barnes et al. 1979; Fox 2014; Sabucedo and Arce 1991; Van Deth 2014; Weiss 2020). To better understand it and derive more useful research hypotheses, separating various forms or modes of political participation proved helpful. Lindholm (2020), for instance, differentiates formal and protest-oriented political participation. Similar, and perhaps the best known, is the division between conventional and unconventional modes of participation (Barnes et al. 1979).

Conventional modes of political participation are those that are, so to say, prescribed by the actual political system and widely regarded as common and legitimate modes of participation. Examples are voting at elections, political party activism, or writing letters to representatives. Given the system-supporting and institutionalized nature of the conventional political participation, it is unsurprising that a positive association with well-being is often found with indicators of this form of political participation (e.g., Flavin and Keane 2012). *Unconventional* modes of political participation would be those that are less commonly practiced and often not explicitly codified (non-institutionalized) or even allowed by the political system (Pitti 2018). Here, the examples would be online engagement, participation in demonstrations and protests, signing petitions, boycotting products, and similar.

This distinction seems particularly useful for the study of association with life satisfaction. Conventional participation might be seen as stemming more from the perceived legitimacy of the system, trust in the rules of the democratic process, and so on. With the sense of performing the duty of basic political participation (e.g., voting), this would lead to an enhanced feeling of well-being. Yet, another dynamic is also conceivable. For instance, high political polarization, i.e., strong negative attitudes towards political opponents, may stimulate both conventional participation and decrease feelings of well-being.

The unconventional forms of participation often reflect a negative attitude concerning some issues that are strong enough to motivate one for some unconventional activities. This is relevant since those activities are often seen as resource-demanding (in terms of time, money, and risks). Hence, these political participation forms seem likely to be associated with lower life satisfaction. In fact, such findings (e.g., negative association of life satisfaction with protest activity) have been reported in the literature (e.g., Barnes et al. 1979; Lorenzini 2015; Marsh 1977), although not universally (e.g., Flavin and Keane 2012). This is not necessarily surprising. Unconventional activism, such as pro-government demonstrations, can also be system-supportive and, therefore, positively or not associated with life satisfaction.

While we follow the literature in separating the two outlined forms of political participation, we treat voting at elections as a separate entity, the third form of political participation. While it is perhaps the most conventional of all forms, it is also unique. It is the most widespread form of participation in democracies—every citizen has the right to participate in elections, and many do. In fact, in some countries, voting in national elections is compulsory. All other forms of conventional participation (those represented in our data, at least) are far less often practiced. Hence, the motivation behind voting and other forms of conventional participation might differ. Voting is a more explicit and direct expression of the system's acceptance, so we expect it to be most positively associated with life satisfaction. While this could apply to the general population, it seems to be especially relevant for the youth because it appears that those more conventional ones are more likely to take part in voting earlier (youth initially shows lower levels of participation, which then increases with age, cf. Quintelier 2007).[4]

It is time to turn to the issue of what should be expected to be specific for youth political participation under the extraordinary conditions of the COVID-19 pandemic. Unsurprisingly, the expectations are not clear because the individual ESS (European Social Survey) studies analyzed here were not conducted simultaneously, which means they were conducted during different phases of the pandemic. Also, different countries implemented different policies (e.g., restrictions on free movement), making deriving specific predictions unfeasible. Still, in general terms, participation might have been increasingly motivated by negative feelings, i.e., general dissatisfaction, given that governments were often blamed for not performing well in that context. Higher life satisfaction/well-being under such conditions could be accompanied by a more passive political outlook, especially because avoiding unnecessary social contacts would also mean avoiding some forms of political activism. So, overall, we would expect life satisfaction to be *negatively* associated with unconventional political participation and positively with conventional political participation, especially voting. The voting variable is specific in several regards. The ESS (European Social Survey) question asks about voting at "the last election," which in some cases means before the pandemic, and in others during a pandemic phase with fewer restrictions. In both cases, we may expect the association to be more akin to the usual findings of the positive association of voting with life satisfaction.

The derived expectations do not seem particularly specific for young people, partly because the background literature reports general findings, not specifically for age categories.[5] Research on youth political attitudes and behavior outlined certain specificities, well summarized by Quintelier (2007, 165), who concluded that "young people are less concerned with politics, less politically knowledgeable, do not participate in social or political activities, are more apathetic, and have low levels of political interest." However, these findings mainly deal with the level of certain variables but not so much with the relationships between variables, which is the concern of the present paper.

---

[4] For example, while the latter half of the twentieth century witnessed a decrease in overall electoral participation, this decline was particularly notable among young people (Fieldhouse et al. 2007). Conversely, some scholars argue that over the past few decades, voter turnout has remained steady and relatively high among young people in Europe (Pilkington and Pollock 2015).

[5] For a recent literature review on youth political participation, see Weiss (2020). In her words, "In conclusion, it can be said that the definition of youth political participation is currently nothing more than general political participation." (Weiss 2020, 9). The main difference is in the level of political engagement, and in different conception of the "political" among the younger generations. No generalizations seem to have been made about different relationships between political participation and other major variables in this context, including life satisfaction.

Hypotheses 5, 6, 7: life satisfaction is positively associated with (5) voting and (6) conventional participation, and (7) negatively with unconventional political participation.

4.3 Contextual Variations

In comparative research, it is important to consider the potential role of contextual variables, whether as background variables to control for the role of some cross-country differences or as variables that have direct and interactive effects. In this paper, we focus on two contextual variables dealing with inequalities between and within countries: GDP (Gross Domestic Product) per capita and the GINI inequality coefficient.

The relationship between *income inequality* (GINI) and life satisfaction is not unequivocal. National and cross-country research shows mixed effects, indicating a positive (Cheung 2018; Berg and Veenhoven 2010), or a negative (Alesina et al. 2004; Graafland and Lous 2018; Schröder 2016; Verme 2011) association between. These discrepancies result from various methodological approaches, employed variables, statistical techniques, and contextual specificities (Verme 2011). In the sociology, the most prominent theory that explains the relationship between inequality and satisfaction is the theory of *relative deprivation* (Runciman 1966). This approach highlights the significance of reference groups with whom individuals compare themselves and the importance of the perception of the fairness of distribution, suggesting that higher levels of inequality lead to lower life satisfaction. The perception of inequality and actual social disparities often lead to dissatisfaction, but also societies marked by inequality tend to experience related issues such as social isolation, poverty, crime, and socio-political instability, which further influence overall satisfaction levels. Comparative analyses of European societies generally indicate a *negative* association between life satisfaction and income inequalities (Alesina et al. 2004; Hajdu and Hajdu 2014). Europeans generally exhibit lower life satisfaction in countries characterized by significant income disparities. Research specifically focusing on young individuals in this regard is lacking, and our assumption is that greater income inequalities among European countries will lead to lower life satisfaction among the youth.

GDP Per Capita Although the debate on the manner and extent of the relationship between wealth and satisfaction is ongoing, the majority of studies investigating cross-country differences indicate a positive association between GDP per capita and life satisfaction. Research in Europe also demonstrates clear connections between these two variables (Degutis et al. 2010), and Pittau et al. (2010, 358) provide explanations for the content of this relationship "in Europe GDP per capita is highly correlated with levels and quality of basic facilities and services, such as transportation and communications systems, and with levels and quality of public institutions like schools and hospitals, as well as with low levels of crime and corruption," leading to a higher degree of comfort, predictability, and consequently, satisfaction.

4.4 Method

4.4.1 Data

To examine the relationship between life satisfaction, different forms of social integration, and characteristics of the social context, we used data from the tenth cycle of the European Social Survey[6] (ESS10-2023), conducted across 31 countries during the years 2020–2022. The ESS data collection was performed during the COVID-19 crisis and was marked by several disruptions due to national-level health measures that prevented in-person interviews. Sub-populations comprising individuals aged 15–35 years were extracted for this analysis.[7] The ESS instrument encompasses a set of indicators that measure social, economic, and political integration. We used two standard indicators of contextual variations—GINI and GDP per capita. For the GDP per capita (expressed in current US dollars) data, we used the World Data Bank database (World Bank 2022). The source for the GINI coefficient was the EUROSTAT database (Eurostat 2021).

4.4.2 Research Design and Analytical Methods

Dependent Variable
Outcome variable—*life satisfaction* was assessed using the following question: "All things considered, how satisfied are you with your life as a whole nowadays?" Responses were recorded on an 11-point scale, where a rating of 0 indicates extreme dissatisfaction, and a rating of 10 represents extreme satisfaction.

Independent Variables
Social Integration. To better understand the role of social integration in shaping well-being, we employed two indicators: the frequency of social contacts and the experience of ethnic discrimination. For the first indicator, "Frequency of Social Contacts," posed a fundamental question: "How often do you socially meet with friends, relatives, or colleagues?" Respondents were given a scale of 1 to 7, from "Never" to "Every day," allowing us to capture the regularity of social interactions. The second indicator delved into the experience of ethnic discrimination as a pertinent factor that can influence an individual's sense of belonging and overall well-being.

---

[6] European Social Survey European Research Infrastructure (ESS ERIC). (2023). ESS10 integrated file, edition 3.2 [Data set]. Sikt—Norwegian Agency for Shared Services in Education and Research. https://doi.org/10.21338/ess10e03_2.

[7] While this data, when isolated, is not representative for the youth population on a per-country basis, it nevertheless provides adequate information to explore associations between the variables of interest.

Political Participation. Political integration is an important aspect of general social integration, especially for young people in democracies. We treat political integration as commensurable to political participation. Our investigation was guided by three distinct indicators: conventional participation, unconventional participation, and voting. Conventional participation encompassed activities such as wearing campaign badges, contacting politicians, and active involvement in political parties or action groups. Voting was measured by whether respondents participated in the most recent election. Unconventional participation included diverse activities, from online engagement to participation in demonstrations, signing petitions, engagement with civic organizations, and making purchase decisions for political reasons. These are fairly standard measures used to operationalize political participation.

Labor Market Integration. This facet was assessed through three indicators: employment status, work location (office or home), and the impact of the COVID-19 pandemic on the labour market. Employment status classified individuals into either employed or unemployed/inactive categories. Work location is considered the place of work, distinguishing between office-based and remote work, which took on a new dimension of relevance during the pandemic. Additionally, the study investigated the "Force Majeure" indicator, which assessed whether respondents experienced various labor market disruptions since the onset of the COVID-19 pandemic, including job losses, reductions in income, decreased working hours, furloughs, and forced unpaid leave or holiday.

Social Context Indicators. We examined social context variables that capture the disparities between countries, shedding light on the economic and income inequalities that can significantly influence well-being. Two primary indicators were used to assess these inequalities: GDP per capita and the GINI coefficient. GDP per capita provides insights into the average income or wealth possessed by the population in a given nation and serves as a measure of wealth differences between countries. The GINI coefficient measures the distribution of income among a population, with a higher GINI coefficient indicating greater income inequality.

Control Variables. To ensure the robustness of our analysis, we also incorporated several control variables, including gender, age, education level, urban or rural residence, and marital or union status.

We employed a random intercept multilevel linear regression analysis as our analytical method, encompassing a sample of 31 countries. MLM (multilevel modelling) offers the capacity to discern the effects of individual characteristics of young respondents as well as the social context within which they reside. In this manner, it becomes possible to ascertain the extent to which personal attributes, social context, and their interactions impact the level of life satisfaction. We present two tables, each featuring ten models. To weight the data, we used the weights that take into account the survey's design, population characteristics, and the relative numerical relationship between countries (*anweight*).

4.5 Results

The initial model presented in Table 4.1 is a random variance component model without independent variables. In the first model, all independent predictors at Level I are included. The second model introduces an additional contextual variable (the GINI coefficient and GDP per capita, respectively) as the indicators at Level II. In all subsequent models, interactions between the indicators at Level II and the Level I analysis are incorporated.

Social Ties Young people who have a greater number of friends and contacts with whom they socialize more frequently tend to experience higher levels of life satisfaction. All models consistently demonstrate this positive association, thus affirming the significance of social connections for the well-being of young people. Those who reported experiencing ethnic discrimination exhibit a lower level of satisfaction compared to their counterparts without that experience.

Labor Market Young individuals who are employed tend to experience higher levels of satisfaction compared to those who are unemployed or inactive. Unemployment among young people during COVID-19 signifies the absence of income and the ability to plan and manage their lives in times of crisis. Additionally, being absent from the labor market in a context of already reduced social interactions has further confined young individuals to narrow social relationships, making their lives even more isolated. Those who have encountered some issues in their workplace during the COVID-19 crisis report lower levels of satisfaction compared to their peers with stable working arrangements. The reduction in earnings, job loss, or the experience of being furloughed has introduced additional layers of uncertainty and insecurity into the transitional life paths of young individuals through the labor market. Each incremental rise in risk has correspondingly led to diminished satisfaction among the youth, underscoring the significance of stability and certainty as pivotal sources of contentment. The finding that young individuals who worked in an office reported lower levels of satisfaction compared to those who predominantly worked from home is interesting. It appears that better work-life balance, as well as privacy and security during the crisis period, were more significant sources of satisfaction than every day in-person interactions with colleagues.

Political Participation All three measures of political participation are significantly associated with life satisfaction. The associations are virtually unaffected by adding the macro-level variables, thus making the results in the two tables practically indistinguishable. Both conventional and unconventional modes of political participation are *negatively* associated with life satisfaction. This means that higher levels of both modalities of political participation/integration are accompanied by, on average, *lower* levels of life satisfaction. The results for voting at elections are different, however: the coefficient is positive in this case. This means that, on average, voting at elections is accompanied by a relatively higher life satisfaction.

Table 4.1 MLM—Life satisfaction, young people aged 15–35, Europe, ESS round 10 (2020–2021)

Predictors	Model 0	Model 1	Model 2	Model 3	Model 4	Model 5	Model 6	Model 7	Model 8
(Intercept)	0.00	0.00	–0.02	0.02	0.05	0.00	0.02	–0.01	0.02
Female		–0.02	–0.02	–0.02	–0.02	–0.02	–0.02	–0.03	–0.02
Age		–0.01**	–0.01**	–0.01**	–0.01**	–0.01**	–0.01**	–0.01**	–0.01**
Higher ed.		0.12***	0.12***	0.12***	0.12***	0.12***	0.12***	0.12***	0.12***
In education		0.10***	0.09***	0.09***	0.09***	0.09***	0.09***	0.09**	0.09***
Urban		–0.01	–0.02	–0.02	–0.02	–0.02	–0.02	–0.02	–0.02
Married/in partnership		0.34***	0.34***	0.34***	0.34***	0.34***	0.34***	0.34***	0.34***
How often socially meet with friends ...		0.18***	0.19***	0.17***	0.18***	0.18***	0.18***	0.18***	0.18***
Conventional		–0.11***	–0.10***	–0.10***	–0.10***	–0.10***	–0.10***	–0.10***	–0.10***
Vote		0.17***	0.16***	0.16***	0.11*	0.17***	0.17***	0.16***	0.16***
Unconventional		–0.10***	–0.10***	–0.10***	–0.10***	–0.08**	–0.11***	–0.10***	–0.10***
Employed		0.28***	0.29***	0.28***	0.29***	0.29***	0.28***	0.24***	0.28***
At office		–0.13***	–0.13***	–0.13***	–0.13**	–0.13***	–0.09**	–0.13***	–0.13***
Force Majeure		–0.03**	–0.03**	–0.03**	–0.03**	–0.03**	–0.03**	–0.03**	–0.03**
Discrimination (ethnic)		–0.25***	–0.25***	–0.26***	–0.25***	–0.25***	–0.25***	–0.24***	–0.25**
Gini			–0.09*	–0.09*	–0.12	–0.09*	–0.10*	–0.08	–0.09*
Gini × How often socially meet				0.04**					
Gini × Vote					0.04				
Gini × Unconventional						–0.01			
Gini × At office							–0.07		
Gini × Employed								0.06	
Gini × Discrimination (ethnic)									–0.14

(continued)

Table 4.1 (continued)

Predictors	Model 0	Model 1	Model 2	Model 3	Model 4	Model 5	Model 6	Model 7	Model 8
Random effects									
σ^2	0.78	0.65	0.65	0.65	0.65	0.65	0.65	0.65	0.65
τ_{00}	$0.08_{country}$	$0.07_{country}$	$0.06_{country}$	$0.06_{country}$	$0.11_{country}$	$0.06_{country}$	$0.07_{country}$	$0.06_{country}$	$0.06_{country}$
τ_{11}				$0.00_{country.}$ *socially meet	$0.03_{country.}$ *vote	$0.01_{country.}$ *unconventional	$0.01_{country.}$ *at office	$0.03_{country.}$ *employed	$0.11_{country.}$ *dscrimintaion
ρ_{01}				$-0.66_{country}$	$-0.79_{country}$	$0.10_{country}$	$-0.81_{country}$	$0.07_{country}$	$0.26_{country}$
ICC	0.10	0.10	0.09	0.09	0.09	0.09	0.09	0.09	0.09
N - country	31	31	31	31	31	31	31	31	31
Observations	14,435	11,079	11,079	11,079	11,079	11,079	11,079	11,079	11,079

*<0.5, **<0.01, ***<0.001

Contextual Variables When it comes to differences between social contexts or countries, the results are as follows. Firstly, the impact of contextual variables is not very high, and they only marginally improve the models (the Intraclass Correlation Coefficient (ICC) decreases slightly). However, income inequality, expressed through the GINI coefficient, exhibits negative associations with the level of satisfaction among young individuals. If they reside in a country with pronounced income inequalities, on average, they will be less satisfied compared to young people living in societies with lower levels of inequality (Ahn et al. 2016). The results of interactions between GINI and social contacts are intriguing. As income inequality increases, the significance of social contacts becomes greater for satisfaction. If young individuals live in a country with pronounced income inequalities, having more contacts will lead to higher satisfaction compared to young people in countries with lower levels of inequality. This is an interesting finding because it suggests that personal informal networks compensate for structural inequalities.

In Table 4.2, the first two models are identical to the previous ones. In the third model, an indicator of GDP per capita is introduced, showing positive associations with life satisfaction. As society becomes wealthier, young individuals are, on average, more satisfied with their lives. Neither social contacts nor labor market integration are statistically significantly associated with GDP per capita. This implies that the effects of labor market integration, political integration, and the level of social interactions do not exhibit interactive impacts with the aggregate wealth on life satisfaction. Irrespective of a nation's economic wealth, political participation, labor market integration, and the level of social interactions have similar effects on life satisfaction.

However, there is a positive interaction between GDP per capita, discrimination, and satisfaction. Young individuals who report experiencing ethnic discrimination have a higher level of satisfaction if they live in wealthier countries compared to young people who have experienced the same discrimination in countries with lower GDP per capita.

Table 4.2 MLM—Life satisfaction, young people aged 15–35, Europe, ESS round 10 (2020–2021)

Predictors	Model 0	Model 1	Model 2	Model 3	Model 4	Model 5	Model 6	Model 7	Model 8
(Intercept)	0.00	0.00	0.00	0.01	0.05	–0.01	0.01	–0.00	0.01
Female		–0.02	–0.02	–0.02	–0.02	–0.02	–0.02	–0.02	–0.02
Age		–0.01**	–0.01**	–0.01**	–0.01**	–0.01**	–0.01**	–0.01**	–0.01**
Higher ed.		0.12***	0.12***	0.12***	0.12***	0.12***	0.12***	0.12***	0.12***
In education		0.10***	0.10***	0.10***	0.10***	0.10***	0.10***	0.09**	0.10***
Urban		–0.01	–0.01	–0.01	–0.02	–0.01	–0.02	–0.02	–0.02
Married/in partnership		0.34***	0.34***	0.34***	0.34***	0.34***	0.34***	0.34***	0.34***
How often socially meet with friends ...		0.18***	0.18***	0.18***	0.18***	0.18***	0.18***	0.19***	0.18***
Conventional		–0.11***	–0.11***	–0.11***	–0.11***	–0.11***	–0.11***	–0.11***	–0.11***
Vote		0.17***	0.17***	0.17***	0.11*	0.17***	0.17***	0.17***	0.17***
Unconventional		–0.10***	–0.10***	–0.10***	–0.10***	–0.08**	–0.11***	–0.11***	–0.10***
Employed		0.28***	0.28***	0.28***	0.28***	0.28***	0.28***	0.23***	0.28***
At office		–0.13***	–0.13***	–0.13***	–0.13***	–0.14***	–0.08*	–0.13***	–0.13***
Force Majeure		–0.03**	–0.03**	–0.03**	–0.03**	–0.03**	–0.03**	–0.03**	–0.03**
Discrimination (ethnic)		–0.25***	–0.25***	–0.26***	–0.25***	–0.26***	–0.26***	–0.25***	–0.31***
GDP/c			0.09*	0.10*	0.11	0.06	0.10*	0.09*	0.09*
GDP/c × How often socially meet				–0.01					
GDP/c × Vote					–0.02				
GDP/c × Unconventional						0.06			
GDP/c × At office							–0.01		
GDP/c × Employed								0.01	
GDP/c × Discrimination (ethnic)									0.27**

Random effects									
σ^2	0.78	0.65	0.65	0.65	0.65	0.65	0.65	0.65	0.65
τ_{00}	$0.07_{country}$	$0.06_{country}$	$0.06_{country}$	$0.06_{country}$	$0.11_{country}$	$0.06_{country}$	$0.07_{country}$	$0.06_{country}$	$0.06_{country}$
τ_{11}				$0.01_{country.*socially\ meet}$	$0.03_{country.*vote}$	$0.01_{country.*unconventional}$	$0.02_{country.*at\ office}$	$0.04_{country.*employed}$	$0.04_{country.*discrimination}$
ρ_{01}				$-0.74_{country}$	$-0.81_{country}$	$-0.12_{country}$	$-0.84_{country}$	$0.17_{country}$	$-0.03_{country}$
ICC	0.10	0.08	0.09	0.09	0.09	0.09	0.09	0.09	0.09
N - country	31	31	31	31	31	31	31	31	31
Observations	14,435	11,079	11,079	11,079	11,079	11,079	11,079	11,079	11,079

*<0.5, **<0.01, ***<0.001

4.6 Discussion

This analysis confirms the positive associations between social capital and the life satisfaction among young people during the pandemic, aligning with a series of other similar studies (Ahmadiani et al. 2022; Ciziceno 2022; Crowley and Walsh 2018, 2021; Helliwell 2006; Onal et al. 2022; Putnam 2000; Sarmiento Prieto et al. 2023). It means that the sense of belonging, trust, reciprocity, and security arising from strong connections, or bonding social capital, is an important predictor of life satisfaction. Moreover, it is shown that in uncertain and unstable times, social capital is precisely one of the crucial resources for young people to build their own resilience, reflected in a higher degree of life satisfaction. This understanding is particularly important in the context of the increasingly prevalent sense of social isolation or the weakening of quality interpersonal relationships in real life. Simultaneously, due to epidemiological reasons, many activities have shifted to digital platforms, and contacts have largely been reduced to digitally mediated relationships. Despite the intensification of online connections, judging by our results and those of other studies (Towner et al. 2022), it can be assumed that the virtual world has not adequately replaced or substituted for face-to-face relationships and the personal benefits they bring. This analysis has also shown that such contacts have the potential to create quality relationships and, consequently, emotional and other resources that lead to life satisfaction.

Belonging to an ethnic minority is a significant predictor of reduced life satisfaction. The social position of ethnic minorities in European societies, even in the pre-pandemic era, was, on average, less favorable, and their life satisfaction was lower compared to the ethnic majority. The combination of an average unfavorable position in social structure and smoldering xenophobia and nationalism constituted the social context in which members of ethnic and racial minorities faced the pandemic, which, according to some studies, further exacerbated existing social inequalities and made them more visible (Ahmadiani et al. 2022; Ciziceno 2022; Onal et al. 2022; Sarmiento Prieto et al. 2023). We can assume that all of this contributed to lower level of life satisfaction among young members of ethnic minorities.

These results indicate that for life satisfaction, affiliation with a close circle of people with whom a young person can establish a quality relationship is important. Additionally, a higher degree of inclusiveness in society towards minority cultural identities also contributes to higher life satisfaction.

Labor market integration emerges as a highly significant determinant of life satisfaction. Young individuals who are employed and have not experienced disruptions in the labor market during the crisis exhibit greater satisfaction compared to those who are unemployed and have faced job loss and/or income reduction. Part of this (dis)satisfaction may stem from the sense of security provided by employment and income, while another aspect is derived from a sense of belonging and the ability to maintain social connections with colleagues. During the crisis, remote work proved to be a more significant source of satisfaction for the youth than in-office work. In addition to the classic reasons such as reduced commute times, fewer workplace distractions, a more comfortable work environment, lower health risks, fewer social conflicts, and a safer social environment should be added.

The reported results confirm our expectations that the three indicators of political participation are associated with life satisfaction. The fact that the associations are virtually unaffected by adding the macro-level variables supports the solidity of the determined relationships. However, the hypotheses about the *direction* of the associations are not entirely confirmed, making the findings particularly interesting. The results concerning voting are in line with Hypothesis 5 and with the bulk of the literature: Young European voters tend to express higher levels of life satisfaction, on average, compared to the abstainers.

However, although voting is perhaps the most conventional political behavior (next to voter abstinence), other forms of political activities that we categorized as conventional are negatively associated with life satisfaction. Those youngsters who engage in activities such as wearing a campaign badge, contacting a politician, or being active in a political party or action group tend to be somewhat *dissatisfied*. This is contrary to our Hypothesis 6 and to numerous findings reported in the literature (e.g., Frey and Stutzer 2000a, b; He et al. 2022; Laurence 2021; Owen et al. 2008; Pacheco and Lange 2010; Vega-Tinoco et al. 2022; Weitz-Shapiro and Winters 2011). Unlike Vega-Tinoco et al. (2022), who also used ESS data, for instance, we found that it is voting that is positively associated, while the other forms of (civic in their terminology) participation are *negatively* associated with life satisfaction. Perhaps this reflects the generation differences—they dealt with older adults (aged 50+), while our study is focused on the youth, and we use a newer wave of the ESS data (ESS10 from 2020 to 2021). Plus, our data were collected during the COVID-19 era.

Tentatively expected is the negative association between life satisfaction and *unconventional* modes of political activity (such as online engagement, participation in demonstrations, and signing petitions). This kind of activism has often been associated with lower life satisfaction (e.g., Barnes et al. 1979; Lorenzini 2015; Marsh 1977), so our results confirm Hypothesis 7 and support this stream of findings. After finding that voting is positively associated with life satisfaction in Latin America, Weitz-Shapiro and Winters (2011, 119) speculated: "Although happier people may be more likely to vote, perhaps those less satisfied with their lives are more likely to contact their elected representatives or participate in protests." We provide evidence from Europe supporting this speculation.

Nonetheless, we infer that the general hypothesis—that political integration is indeed a correlate (if not causally related to) of life satisfaction, is supported. Voting is certainly the most conventional aspect among the specific modes of participation covered by the included ESS variables. Not only is it the most widespread, but it also represents the acceptance of the political system and involvement, or integration, into formal political life. Voting does not require any additional motivation (although it may include) except the feeling of duty and acceptance of the basic rules of political life in a democracy (procedural utility); hence, the positive association with life satisfaction. The other activities listed here under both conventional and unconventional categories require additional motivation, which often might be the belief that voting is insufficient or ineffective. Thus, while some of the unconventional activities, such as taking part in demonstrations, might sometimes involve crossing the borders of legality, the remaining activities are not that radically different from those categorized as conventional ones.[8] It seems as if taking any political activity besides voting requires special motivation, which is somehow associated with lower life satisfaction. It may be that dissatisfaction with some political issue and the perception that perhaps voting does not change things is caused by lower life satisfaction. Likewise, lower life satisfaction, which may be caused by political dissatisfaction, may lead to political activism, both more or less conventional. In any case, the reciprocal causal direction may work here (Ding et al. 2015; Laurence 2021).

The literature is inconsistent regarding the hypothesized causal direction (e.g., Pirralha 2017, 2018; Weitz-Shapiro and Winters 2011), and in the present study, we cannot disentangle it because we do not have adequate data. Here, we focus on the existence of the associations under the assumption that well-being is the dependent variable (as specified in the statistical models presented above). However, some studies tried disentangling the causal direction conundrum (e.g., Laurence 2021; Pirralha 2017, 2018). Relying on a 3-wave panel using the German Socio-Economic Panel (SOEP) data, Pirralha (2018, 803) concluded that "our findings offer no support for the idea of a causal relationship between political participation and LS."[9] To make things more interesting, Ding et al. (2015, 252) found in Australia that "increasing informal social connectedness in one year most strongly predicts better mental health the next year, followed by civic engagement; while increased political participation in one year predicts *worse* mental health the next year" (emphasis in original).

The association of youth activism with reduced satisfaction levels may also be specific to periods of crisis, such as the COVID-19 pandemic. But, a more reliable answer will have to wait for future research with more adequate datasets. In any case, the diverse relationship with different indicators of political participation shows the value of differentiating modes of participation, especially the separation of voting from the rest of the conventional modes.

[8] For instance, the unconventional category includes activity named "online engagement". However, authors such as Morozov (2009) find online participation as an illusion of participation. In his words, "'Slacktivism' is an apt term to describe feel-good online activism that has zero political or social impact." (Morozov 2009).

[9] Similar is another Pirralha's study, using Dutch LISS panel data. Again, "our results do not offer support for a link between political participation and individual wellbeing" (Pirralha 2017, 338).

4.7 Conclusion

The overall results support the hypothesis about the positive association of the three domains of social integration—social relationships, labor market integration, and some forms of political participation—with greater life satisfaction. We conclude that even in uncertain and unstable times, social capital is one of the crucial resources for young people to build their own resilience, as reflected in a higher degree of life satisfaction.

The lack of integration into a broader society, as reflected in belonging to a discriminated ethnic minority, is also a significant predictor of reduced life satisfaction. Perhaps the context of the pandemic, when various minorities in Europe had harder-than-average time, only enhanced this negative association. Overall, regarding social integration, the results show that affiliation with a close circle of people with whom a young person can establish a quality relationship and living in a society where a young person feels included both contribute to higher life satisfaction.

Interestingly, however, social contacts that come with in-office work do not seem to count as contributing to life satisfaction. It may be due to the pandemic's context, but remote work proved to be a significant source of satisfaction for the youth rather than in-office work. Apart from that, labor market integration, as indicated by being in the labor force (employed), emerged as a highly significant determinant of life satisfaction.

The results also confirmed some of the hypotheses about the contribution of political participation to life satisfaction. Corroborating numerous previous findings, young European voters tend to express higher levels of life satisfaction, on average, compared to the abstainers.

However, other forms of political activism—both those activities classified as conventional (wearing a campaign badge, contacting a politician, or being active in a political party or action group) and unconventional ones (e.g., participation in protests and demonstrations)—are negatively associated with life satisfaction. The negative association of life satisfaction with unconventional participation is not uncommon in literature, perhaps showing that dissatisfaction is an important motivator of political activism. It is less commonly observed that conventional forms of participation are also associated with reduced life satisfaction.

Future research endeavors should be focused on longitudinal research for a comprehensive understanding of the evolution of the correlations identified in the present study, particularly in the context of a post-pandemic world. This strategic focus would enable us to discern whether the observed role of social integration is a reflection of the health crisis period, or indicative of a "new reality," signifying more enduring transformations in the behaviors and attitudes of the youth demographic.

References

Ahmadiani, M., S. Ferreira, and J. Kessler. 2022. What makes people happy? Evidence from International Data. *Journal of Happiness Studies* 23 (5): 2083–2111. https://doi.org/10.1007/s10902-021-00478-y.

Ahmed, A., M. Lundahl, and E. Wadensjö. 2023. Ethnic discrimination during the Covid-19 pandemic. In *Migration and integration in a post-pandemic world: Socioeconomic opportunities and challenges*, ed. L. Lerpold, Ö. Sjöberg, and K. Wennberg, 291–314. Cham: Springer.

Ahn, H., S.J. Roll, W. Zeng, J.J. Frey, S. Reiman, and J. Ko. 2016. Impact of income inequality on workers' life satisfaction in the US: A multilevel analysis. *Social Indicators Research* 128: 1347–1363.

Alesina, A., R. Di Tella, and R. MacCulloch. 2004. Inequality and happiness: are Europeans and Americans different? *Journal of Public Economics* 88 (9–10): 2009–2042. https://doi.org/10.1016/j.jpubeco.2003.07.006.

Amichai-Hamburger, Y., M. Kingsbury, and B.H. Schneider. 2013. Friendship: An old concept with a new meaning? *Computers in Human Behavior* 29 (1): 33–39.

Anderton, R., V. Botelho, A. Consolo, A. Dias da Silva, C. Foroni, M. Mohr, and L. Vivian. 2020. The impact of the COVID-19 pandemic on the euro area labour market. *Economic Bulletin*, issue 8, ECB. https://ideas.repec.org/a/ecb/ecbart/202100082.html.

Arnett, J.J. 2014. *Emerging adulthood: The winding road from the late teens through the twenties*. 2nd ed. Oxford: Oxford University Press. https://doi.org/10.1093/acprof:oso/9780199929382.001.0001.

Baarck, J., A. Balahur-Dobrescu, L.G. Cassio, B. D'hombres, Z. Pasztor, and G. Tintori. 2021. *Loneliness in the EU. Insights from surveys and online media data*. Luxembourg: Publications Office of the European Union. https://doi.org/10.2760/46553. JRC125873.

Barnes, S.H., M. Kaase, K.R. Allerback, B. Farah, F. Heunks, and R. Inglehart. 1979. *Political action: Mass participation in five Western democracies*. Beverly Hills, CA: Sage.

Beck, U. 1992. *Risk society*. London: Sage.

Berg, M., and R. Veenhoven. 2010. Income inequality and happiness in 119 nations, Chapter 11. In *Social policy and happiness in Europe*, ed. Bent Greve, 174–194. Cheltenham, UK: Edgar Elgar.

Birditt, K.S., A. Turkelson, K.L. Fingerman, C. Polenick, and A. Oya. 2021. Age differences in stress, life changes, and social ties during the COVID-19 pandemic: Implications for psychological well-being. *The Gerontologist* 61 (2): 205–216.

Boeck, T. 2007. Young people, social capital and the navigation of life transitions. *Paper for the DfES Youth Strategy Review*. Leicester: DfES. https://dora.dmu.ac.uk/bitstream/handle/2086/4975/BoeckPhD.pdf. Accessed 22 Dec 2023.

Chesters, J., and H. Cuervo. 2019. Adjusting to new employment landscapes: Consequences of precarious employment for young Australians. *The Economic and Labour Relations Review* 30 (2): 222–240. https://doi.org/10.1177/1035304619832740.

Cheung, F. 2018. Income redistribution predicts greater life satisfaction across individual, national, and cultural characteristics. *Journal of Personality and Social Psychology* 115 (5): 867–882. https://doi.org/10.1037/pspp0000164.

Ciziceno, M. 2022. The conceptions of quality of life, wellness and well-being: A literature review. In *Sport and quality of life: Practices, habits and lifestyles*, Social indicators research series, ed. P. Corvo and F. Massimo Lo Verde, vol. 84, 11–27. Cham: Springer. https://doi.org/10.1007/978-3-030-93092-9_2.

Clair, R., M. Gordon, M. Kroon, and C. Reilly. 2021. The effects of social isolation on well-being and life satisfaction during pandemic. *Humanities and Social Sciences Communications* 8 (1): 1–6. https://doi.org/10.1057/s41599-021-00710-3.

Crocetti, E., and W. Meeus. 2014. "Family comes first!" Relationships with family and friends in Italian emerging adults. *Journal of Adolescence* 37 (8): 1463–1473.

Crowley, F., and E. Walsh. 2018. How important are personal ties, trust and tolerance for life satisfaction in Europe? *SRERC working paper series, no. SRERCWP2018-1*. Cork: University College Cork, Spatial and Regional Economic Research Centre (SRERC). http://hdl.handle.net/10419/195053.

———. 2021. Tolerance, social capital, and life satisfaction: A multilevel model from transition countries in the European Union. *Review of Social Economy* 82 (1): 23–50. https://doi.org/10.1080/00346764.2021.1957994.

Degutis, M., S. Urbonavičius, and A. Gaižutis. 2010. Relation between GDP and life satisfaction in the European Union. *Ekonomika* 89 (1): 9–21.

Delhey, J., and G. Dragolov. 2016. Happier together. Social cohesion and subjective well-being in Europe. *International Journal of Psychology* 51 (3): 163–176.

Ding, N., H.L. Berry, and L.V. O'Brien. 2015. One-year reciprocal relationship between community participation and mental well-being in Australia: A panel analysis. *Social Science & Medicine* 128: 246–254. https://doi.org/10.1016/j.socscimed.2015.01.022.

Dorn, D., Fischer, J. A., Kirchgässner, G., & Sousa-Poza, A. (2008). Direct democracy and life satisfaction revisited: new evidence for Switzerland. *Journal of Happiness Studies*, 9, 227–255. https://doi.org/10.1007/s10902-007-9050-9.

Drouin, M., B.T. McDaniel, J. Pater, and T. Toscos. 2020. How parents and their children used social media and technology at the beginning of the COVID-19 pandemic and associations with anxiety. *Cyberpsychology, Behavior, and Social Networking* 23 (11): 727–736.

Elias, A., J. Ben, F. Mansouri, and Y. Paradies. 2021. Racism and nationalism during and beyond the COVID-19 pandemic. *Ethnic and Racial Studies* 44 (5): 783–793.

Eurofound. 2021. *Living, working and COVID-19 (Update April 2021)—Mental health and trust decline across EU as pandemic enters another year*. Luxembourg: Publications Office of the European Union. https://www.eurofound.europa.eu/system/files/2021-11/ef21064en.pdf. Accessed 2 Jan 2024. https://doi.org/10.2806/76802.

European Union. 2022. The effects of COVID-19 on youth employment. European Youth Portal. https://youth.europa.eu/news/effects-of-covid-19-youth-employment_en. Accessed 24 Dec 2023.

Eurostat. 2021. *Gini coefficient of equivalised disposable income—EU-SILC survey*. Luxembourg: European Commission in Luxembourg City. https://ec.europa.eu/eurostat/databrowser/view/tessi190/default/table.

Ezzy, D. 1993. Unemployment and mental health. A critical review. *Social Science and Medicine* 37: 41–52.

Fernandes, B., U.N. Biswas, R.T. Mansukhani, A.V. Casarín, and C.A. Essau. 2020. The impact of COVID-19 lockdown on internet use and escapism in adolescents. *Revista de psicología clínica con niños y adolescentes* 7 (3): 59–65.

Fieldhouse, E., M. Tranmer, and A. Russell. 2007. Something about young people or something about elections? Electoral participation of young people in Europe: Evidence from a multilevel analysis of the European Social Survey. *European Journal of Political Research* 46 (6): 797–822. https://doi.org/10.1111/j.1475-6765.2007.00713.x.

Flavin, P., and M. Keane. 2012. Life satisfaction and political participation: Evidence from the United States. *Journal of Happiness Studies* 13 (1): 63–78. https://doi.org/10.1007/s10902-011-9250-1.

Fouskas, T., G. Koulierakis, F.M. Mine, A. Theofilopoulos, S. Konstantopoulou, F. Ortega-de-Mora, D. Georgiadis, and G. Pantazi. 2022. Racial and ethnic inequalities, health disparities and racism in times of COVID-19 pandemic populism in the EU: Unveiling anti-migrant attitudes, precarious living conditions and barriers to integration in Greece. *Societies* 12 (6): 1–22. https://doi.org/10.3390/soc12060189.

Fox, S. 2014. Is it time to update the definition of political participation? *Parliamentary Affairs* 67 (2): 495–505. https://doi.org/10.1093/pa/gss094.

Frey, B., and A. Stutzer. 2000a. Happiness, economy and institutions. *The Economic Journal* 110 (466): 918–938. https://doi.org/10.1111/1468-0297.00570.

———. 2000b. Happiness prospers in democracy. *Journal of Happiness Studies* 1 (1): 79–102. https://doi.org/10.1023/A:1010028211269.

———. 2002. *Happiness and economics: How the economy and institutions affect human well-being*. Princeton, NJ: Princeton University Press.

Fryer, D. 1986. Employment deprivation and personal agency during unemployment: A critical discussion of Jahoda's explanation of the psychological effects of unemployment. *Social Behaviour* 1 (1): 3–23.

Furlong, A. 2012. *Youth studies: An introduction*. London: Routledge.

Furlong, A., and F. Cartmel. 1997. *Young people and social change: Individualization and risk in late modernity*. Buckingham: Open University Press.

Furlong, A., J. Goodwin, H. O'Connor, S. Hadfield, S. Hall, K. Lowden, and R. Plugor. 2017. *Young people in the labour market: Past, present, future. Series: Youth, young adulthood and society*. London: Routledge.

Gajendran, R.S., and D.A. Harrison. 2007. The good, the bad, and the unknown about telecommuting: Meta-analysis of psychological mediators and individual consequences. *Journal of Applied Psychology* 92: 1524–1541. https://doi.org/10.1037/0021-9010.92.6.1524.

Gould, E., and V. Wilson. 2020. *Black workers face two of the most lethal preexisting conditions for coronavirus—racism and economic inequality*. Washington, DC: Economic Policy Institute. https://www.epi.org/publication/black-workers-covid/. Accessed 12 Dec 2023.

Graafland, J., and B. Lous. 2018. Economic freedom, income inequality and life satisfaction in OECD countries. *Journal of Happiness Studies* 19: 2071–2093. https://doi.org/10.1007/s10902-017-9905-7.

Granovetter, M.S. 1973. The strength of weak ties. *American Journal of Sociology* 78 (6): 1360–1380.

Hajdu, T., and G. Hajdu. 2014. Reduction of income inequality and subjective well-being in Europe. *Economics* 8 (1): 20140035. https://doi.org/10.5018/economics-ejournal.ja.2014-35.

He, L., K. Wang, T. Liu, T. Li, and B. Zhu. 2022. Does political participation help improve the life satisfaction of urban residents: Empirical evidence from China. *PLoS One* 17 (10): 1–23. https://doi.org/10.1371/journal.pone.0273525.

Helliwell, J. F., 2006. Well-being, social capital and public policy: what's new?. *The economic journal*, 116(510): C34–C45. doi: https://doi.org/10.1111/j.1468-0297.2006.01074.x.

Helliwell, J. F., G. Schellenberg, and J. Fonberg. 2020. *Life satisfaction in Canada before and during the COVID-19 pandemic*. Analytical Studies Branch Research Paper Series, Statistics Canada Catalogue no. 11F0019M—No. 457. https://www150.statcan.gc.ca/n1/en/pub/11f0019m/11f0019m2020020-eng.pdf. Accessed 21 Dec 2023.

Inglehart, R.F. 2018. The silent revolution in reverse: The rise of Trump and the authoritarian populist parties. In *Cultural evolution, people's motivations are changing, and reshaping the world*, 173–199. Cambridge: Cambridge University Press. https://doi.org/10.1017/9781108613880.

Irizar, P., D. Pan, D. Kapadia, L. Bécares, S. Sze, H. Taylor, S. Amele, E. Kibuchi, P. Divall, L.J. Gray, L.B. Nellums, S.V. Katikireddi, and M. Pareek. 2023. Ethnic inequalities in COVID-19 infection, hospitalisation, intensive care admission, and death: A global systematic review and meta-analysis of over 200 million study participants. *EClinicalMedicine* 57: 1–24. https://doi.org/10.1016/j.eclinm.2023.101877.

Jahoda, M. 1981. Work, employment, and unemployment: Values, theories, and approaches in social research. *American Psychologist* 36 (2): 184–191. https://doi.org/10.1037/0003-066X.36.2.184.

Jongbloed, J., and J.F. Giret. 2022. Quality of life of NEET youth in comparative perspective: Subjective well-being during the transition to adulthood. *Journal of Youth Studies* 25 (3): 321–343. https://doi.org/10.1080/13676261.2020.1869196.

Katikireddi, S.V., S. Lal, E.D. Carrol, C.L. Niedzwiedz, K. Khunti, R. Dundas, and B. Barr. 2021. Unequal impact of the COVID-19 crisis on minority ethnic groups: A framework for understanding and addressing inequalities. *Journal of Epidemiology and Community Health* 75 (10): 970–974. https://doi.org/10.1136/jech-2020-216061.

Kondratowicz, B., D. Godlewska-Werner, P. Połomski, and M. Khosla. 2022. Satisfaction with job and life and remote work in the COVID-19 pandemic: The role of perceived stress, self-efficacy and self-esteem. *Current Issues in Personality Psychology* 10 (1): 49–60. https://doi.org/10.5114/cipp.2021.108097.

Konle-Seidl, R., and F. Picarella. 2021. *Youth in Europe: Effects of COVID-19 on their economic and social situation.* Luxembourg: Policy Department for Economic, Scientific and Quality of Life Policies Directorate-General for Internal Policies, European Parliament. https://www.europarl.europa.eu/RegData/etudes/STUD/2021/662942/IPOL_STU(2021)662942_EN.pdf.

Kööts-Ausmees, L., and A. Realo. 2016. Life satisfaction among ethnic minorities in Europe. *Journal of Cross-Cultural Psychology* 47 (3): 457–478.

Laurence, J. 2021. The impact of youth engagement on life satisfaction: A quasi-experimental field study of a UK national youth engagement scheme. *European Sociological Review* 37 (2): 305–329. https://doi.org/10.1093/esr/jcaa059.

Lenoir, R., and K.K.Y. Wong. 2023. Impact of the COVID-19 pandemic on young people from black and mixed ethnic groups' mental health in West London: A qualitative study. *BMJ Open* 13 (5): 1–10. https://doi.org/10.1136/bmjopen-2023-071903.

Lindholm, A. 2020. Does subjective well-being affect political participation? *Swiss Journal of Sociology* 46 (3): 467–488. https://doi.org/10.2478/sjs-2020-0023.

Litam, S.D.A., and S. Oh. 2021. Effects of COVID-19-related racial discrimination on depression and life satisfaction among young, middle, and older Chinese Americans. *Adultspan Journal* 20 (2): 70–84. https://doi.org/10.1002/adsp.12111.

Lorenzini, J. 2015. Subjective well-being and political participation: A comparison of unemployed and employed youth. *Journal of Happiness Studies* 16 (2): 381–404. https://doi.org/10.1007/s10902-014-9514-7.

MacDonald, R. 2017. Precarious work: The growing precarité of youth. In *Routledge handbook of youth and young adulthood*, ed. A. Furlong, 2nd ed., 156–163. London: Routledge.

Marsh, A. 1977. *Protest and political consciousness*, Vol. 49, Sage library of social research. Beverly Hills, CA: Sage.

Morozov, E. 2009. The brave new world of slacktivism. *Foreign Policy* 19 (5) https://tinyurl.com/y7tl6xqz. Accessed 10 Sept 2018.

Onal, O., F.Y. Evcil, E. Dogan, M. Develi, E. Uskun, and A.N. Kisioglu. 2022. The effect of loneliness and perceived social support among older adults on their life satisfaction and quality of life during the COVID-19 pandemic. *Educational Gerontology* 48 (7): 331–343.

Owen, A.L., J. Videras, and C. Willemsen. 2008. Democracy, participation, and life satisfaction. *Social Science Quarterly* 89 (4): 987–1005. https://doi.org/10.1111/j.1540-6237.2008.00595.x.

Pacheco, G., and T. Lange. 2010. Political participation and life satisfaction: A cross-European analysis. *International Journal of Social Economics* 37 (9): 686–702. https://doi.org/10.1108/03068291011062489.

Palmer, A.N., and E. Small. 2021. COVID-19 and disconnected youth: Lessons and opportunities from OECD countries. *Scandinavian Journal of Public Health* 49 (7): 779–789. https://doi.org/10.1177/14034948211017017.

Pilkington, H., and G. Pollock. 2015. "Politics are bollocks": Youth, politics and activism in contemporary Europe. *The Sociological Review* 63 (2_suppl): 1–35. https://doi.org/10.1111/1467-954x.12260.

Pirralha, A. 2017. Political participation and well-being in the Netherlands: Exploring the causal links. *Applied Research in Quality of Life* 12 (2): 327–341. https://doi.org/10.1007/s11482-016-9463-x.

———. 2018. The link between political participation and life satisfaction: A three wave causal analysis of the German SOEP household panel. *Social Indicators Research* 138 (2): 793–807.

Pittau, M.G., R. Zelli, and A. Gelman. 2010. Economic disparities and life satisfaction in European regions. *Social Indicators Research* 96 (2): 339–361. https://EconPapers.repec.org/RePEc:spr:soinre:v:96:y:2010:i:2:p:339-361.

Pitti, I. 2018. Unconventional political participation: An overview. In *Youth and unconventional political engagement*, ed. I. Pitti, 7–21. Cham: Palgrave Macmillan. https://doi.org/10.1007/978-3-319-75591-5_2.

Platt, L. 2021. COVID-19 and ethnic inequalities in England. *LSE Public Policy Review* 2021/1 (4): 1–14. https://doi.org/10.31389/lseppr.33.

Platt, L., and R. Warwick. 2020. *Are some ethnic groups more vulnerable to COVID-19 than others*. The Institute for Fiscal Studies, Nuffield Foundation. ISBN 978-1-912805-75-4. https://blcf.org.uk/assets/dei/EthnicVulnerabilityCovid.pdf. Accessed 3 Jan 2024.

Plenty, S., C. Bracegirdle, J. Dollmann, and O. Spiegler. 2021. Changes in young adults' mental well-being before and during the early stage of the COVID-19 pandemic: Disparities between ethnic groups in Germany. *Child and Adolescent Psychiatry and Mental Health* 15 (1): 1–14.

Putnam, R.D. 2000. *Bowling alone: The collapse and revival of American community*. New York: Simon and Schuster.

Quintelier, E. 2007. Differences in political participation between young and old people. *Contemporary Politics* 13 (2): 165–180. https://doi.org/10.1080/13569770701562658.

Rothgerber, H., T. Wilson, D. Whaley, D.L. Rosenfeld, M. Humphrey, A.L. Moore, and A. Bihl. 2020. Politicizing the COVID-19 pandemic: Ideological differences in adherence to social distancing [Preprint]. *PsyArXiv*. https://doi.org/10.31234/osf.io/k23cv. Accessed 3 Jan 2024.

Runciman, W.G. 1966. *Relative deprivation and social justice: A study of attitudes to social inequality in twentieth-century England*. Berkeley, CA: University of California Press.

Sabucedo, J.M., and C. Arce. 1991. Types of political participation: A multidimensional analysis. *European Journal of Political Research* 20 (1): 93–102. https://doi.org/10.1111/j.1475-6765.1991.tb00257.x.

Sarmiento Prieto, J.P., C.P. Castro-Correa, A. Arrieta, M. Jerath, and S. Arensburg. 2023. Relevance of social capital in preserving subjective well-being in the face of the COVID-19 pandemic. *Risk, Hazards & Crisis in Public Policy* 14 (2): 159–178.

Schröder, M. 2016. How income inequality influences life satisfaction: Hybrid effects evidence from the German SOEP. *European Sociological Review* 32 (2): 307–320.

Susilo, D. 2020. Revealing the effect of work-from home on job performance during the COVID-19 crisis: Empirical evidence from Indonesia. *Journal of Contemporary Issues in Business & Government* 26: 23–40. https://doi.org/10.47750/cibg.2020.26.01.002.

Towner, E., L. Tomova, D. Ladensack, K. Chu, and B. Callaghan. 2022. Virtual social interaction and loneliness among emerging adults amid the COVID-19 pandemic. *Current Research in Ecological and Social Psychology* 3: 100058. https://doi.org/10.1016/j.cresp.2022.100058.

UNICEF. 2020. *Averting a lost COVID generation: A six point plan to respond, recover and reimagine a post-pandemic world for every child*. United Nations Children's Fund (UNICEF), November 2020. New York: UNICEF. https://www.unicef.org/media/86881/file/Averting-a-lost-covid-generation-world-childrens-day-data-and-advocacy-brief-2020.pdf. Accessed 3 Jan 2024.

Vancea, M., and M. Utzet. 2017. How unemployment and precarious employment affect the health of young people: A scoping study on social determinants. *Scand J Public Health* 45 (1): 73–84. https://doi.org/10.1177/1403494816679555.

Van Deth, J.W. 2014. A conceptual map of political participation. *Acta politica* 49 (3): 349–367. https://doi.org/10.1057/ap.2014.6.

Vega-Tinoco, A., A.I. Gil-Lacruz, and M. Gil-Lacruz. 2022. Civic participation as a promoter of well-being: Comparative analysis among European countries. *Social Indicators Research* 164 (1): 217–237. https://doi.org/10.1007/s11205-022-02947-0.

Verba, S., and N.H. Nie. 1972. *Participation in America*. New York: Harper and Row.

Verme, P. 2011. Life satisfaction and income inequality. *Review of Income and Wealth* 57: 111–127.

Voßemer, J., and N. Eunicke. 2015. The impact of labor market exclusion and job insecurity on health and well-being among youth—a literature review. *EXCEPT working papers, WP no 2*. Talinn: Tallinn University. http://www.exceptproject.eu/working-papers/.

Wang, S., C. Xiabing, L. Yong, L. Chloé, Y. Ran, and F. Madrisotti. 2021. "I'm more afraid of racism than of the virus!": Racism awareness and resistance among Chinese migrants and their descendants in France during the Covid-19 pandemic. *European Societies* 23 (S1): S721–S742.
Warr, P.B. 1987. *Work, unemployment, and mental health*. Oxford: Oxford University Press.
Weiss, J. 2020. What is youth political participation? Literature review on youth political participation and political attitudes. *Frontiers in Political Science* 2: 1. https://doi.org/10.3389/fpos.2020.00001.
Weitz-Shapiro, R., and M.S. Winters. 2011. The link between voting and life satisfaction in Latin America. *Latin American Politics and Society* 53 (4): 101–126.
World Bank. 2022. *GDP per capita, PPP (current international $)*. World Bank Data. https://data.worldbank.org/indicator/NY.GDP.PCAP.PP.CD.

Dragan Stanojević is an Assistant Professor at the University of Belgrade Faculty of Philosophy, Department of Sociology. His research is focused on family relations, youth and children, political participation, social inequalities, social inclusion, and life course patterns. He served as the NC of the European Social Survey in Serbia during its IX and X rounds. He is actively involved in various research activities across Europe, contributing as a senior researcher within the Pool of European Youth Researchers (PEYR) and the European Platform for Learning Mobility (EPLM).

Bojan Todosijević is a Principal research fellow at the Centre for Political Studies and Public Opinion Research, Institute of Social Sciences (IDN), Belgrade, Serbia. His research covers topics such as the structure of social attitudes, the influence of ideological orientations on political attitudes and behavior, nationalist attitudes, political intolerance, and populist ideology. More recently, his focus turned towards electoral behavior in Serbia. A comparative approach and quantitative methodology characterize his research and publications. He is an expert on statistical data analysis and public opinion research methodology.

Anja Gvozdanović is a Senior Research Associate in the field of sociology, affiliated with the Centre for Youth and Gender Studies at the Institute for Social Research in Zagreb, Croatia. Her research interests include youth sociology, political culture, social capital, values and social trust, reconciliation and peacebuilding in Croatia and Western Balkans.

Part II
The Impact of COVID-19 on Employment and Workers' Well-being

Chapter 5
Employment Vulnerabilities of Female and Young Adults in Arab Countries: Trends Since the Onset of COVID-19

Shireen AlAzzawi and Vladimir Hlasny

5.1 Introduction

Across much of the world, the COVID pandemic became synonymous with lock-down measures that greatly reduced economic activity and often affected the most vulnerable workers hardest because of the nature of their jobs and provisions of their contracts. Workers in Arab countries already faced precarious working conditions pre-pandemic. For years the regional labor markets failed to create enough decent employment opportunities to absorb the bulk of fresh graduates. Public employment has been on a decline due to economic reform programs in place since the turn of the century. Meanwhile, formal private job openings failed to fill the gap, particularly for marginal workers such as women and youths (Assaad et al. 2020), in part due to competition from the large informal economy. Economic growth over the past decade, relatively strong in a few cases, did not translate into growth in formal employment (Prince et al. 2018).

Over 60% of all workers in the region are informally employed, while young adults face even more vulnerability in employment on account of their missing job experience, their skills that do not match firms' needs, and their sheer number (Tzannatos 2021). Over 85% of young adults have been estimated to hold informal jobs (ILO 2020a, b). Vulnerability of employment can thus be said to be one of the most critical conditions facing Arab young adults (Fehling et al. 2015), given that their jobs lack security and stability, paid leaves, social and health insurance coverage, and in many cases physical safety. Such vulnerability almost always stays with them throughout

S. AlAzzawi (✉)
Santa Clara University, Santa Clara, CA, USA
e-mail: salazzawi@scu.edu

V. Hlasny
Ewha Womans University, Seoul, Korea

United Nations Economic and Social Commission for Western Asia (UN ESCWA), Beirut, Lebanon

C. Suter et al. (eds.), *Well-being During the Pandemic*, Social Indicators Research Series 90, https://doi.org/10.1007/978-3-031-63440-6_5

their careers as studies have found that transitions to better job opportunities are rare for those who start out in vulnerable positions (AlAzzawi and Hlasny 2022). Moreover, regional youth unemployment was already the highest in the world pre-pandemic, at over 30% for men and 40% for women, and the pandemic was expected to further aggravate young adults' plight in terms of both unemployment and informality. Employers' drive toward cost-cutting, irregularization, and gig and platform employment will particularly affect young adults and other at-risk groups.

In response to the onset of COVID, Arab countries' governments implemented a widening range of measures to alleviate the health impacts. Egypt put in place relatively lenient policy responses to the pandemic in the first half of 2020, and maintained the measures at a consistent level longer, reducing them gradually only in mid-2021—refer to Fig. 5.1. As a result, Egypt retained positive economic growth throughout the span of the pandemic, albeit at less than half the pre-2020 projected rates (Assaad et al. 2022).

Jordan started out with a very stringent regulatory regime in the spring of 2020, but did not keep it up very long. It was hit with resurgent waves of the pandemic in the second half of 2020 and early 2021, requiring further mitigation measures throughout the first half of 2021. These were rolled back only in the second half of the year. Jordan thus faced lingering socio-economic impacts of the pandemic throughout 2021.

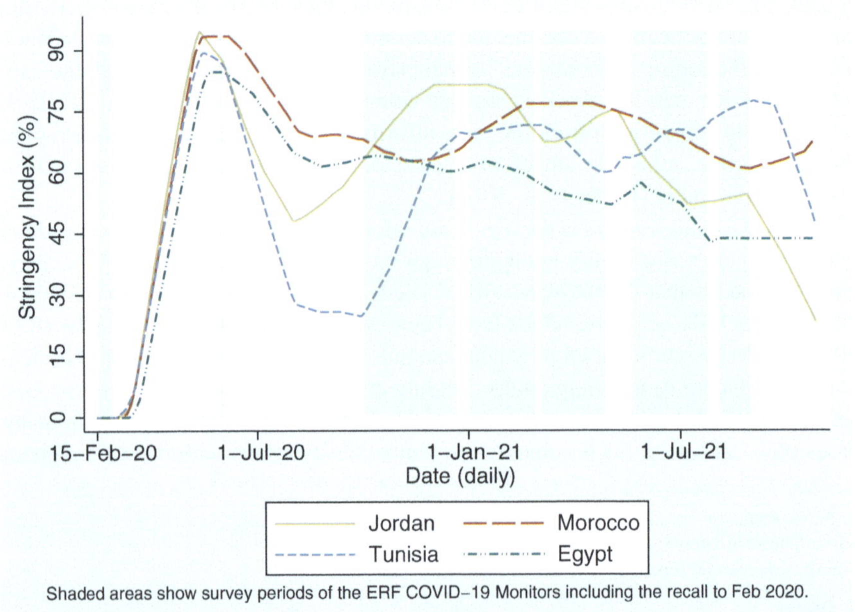

Fig. 5.1 Stringency index, 30-day moving average, by country and date. Note: shaded areas show survey periods. Round 0 occurred during end-Feb 2020; round 1 during June 2020 and during October–November 2020; round 2 during January–February 2021; round 3 during March–April 2021; round 4 during May–July 2021; round 5 during August–September 2021

Morocco similarly relied on harsh closure policies in the second quarter of 2020, but kept them for a longer spell of time. It endured a large negative effect on economic growth, but labor market indicators finally started to recover in the first two quarters of 2021. Following a resurgence of cases, the stringent closure regime was brought back in the second quarter of 2021 and was only slowly rolled back later in the year.

In Tunisia, government responses failed to contain the pandemic because of their volatile intensity throughout the year 2020. The closure regime was fairly strong in the first half of the year, then was relaxed significantly in the second half, before being tightened again throughout the year 2021. Tunisia ended up suffering the largest negative impact on its economy in 2020, which lingered well into the following year.

Amid the social distancing and market shutdowns implemented across the region to tackle the pandemic, workers without solid attachments to well established employers faced particularly adverse prospects in terms of employability, job stability, and decent working conditions. Shutdowns exerted a heavy toll on all labor market sectors in Arab countries including manufacturing and industry, but it was particularly the service sector—where most of the recent secondary and tertiary school graduates and women seek work—that took the greatest pummeling (ILO 2020c). Employers demoted, furloughed or laid off workers, and those in the informal sector were likely to be the hardest hit given the lack of job protection, and the lack of personal cushions such as savings, access to credit, and family connections. The International Labour Organization (ILO) estimates that women lost between 20 and 30% more working hours than men throughout the years 2020 and 2021.

Economic recovery in the second half of the year 2021 did not provide the needed relief. Throughout 2021–2023, the world has continued suffering supply chain bottlenecks, which have led to inflationary pressures. Central banks' delayed responses to these challenges ended up slowing down growth, even before the Ukraine-Russian Federation war and other regional conflicts have started further compounding the ongoing effects of the pandemic.

Tracking the employment status of vulnerable groups across the distinct stages of the pandemic is critical to understanding the cyclicality and trajectory of the region's chronic employment problem, and the path to recovery from crises. This study thus contributes to answering questions such as: Which worker groups are particularly hurt by health epidemics in the short term? How do the workers' outcomes change with the progress of the pandemic and the regulatory efforts to contain it, and how long do the impacts of such shocks last? What are some effective ways to help different groups of workers, and when are the most critical points for intervention?

This study evaluates the employment outcomes and job-transition prospects of workers, separately for women and men, and for young and older workers, across various phases of the COVID pandemic. Young workers are defined as those 17–29 years of age, while those 30–59 years old are classified as older workers. Respondents older than 59 are omitted as not of the prime working age, and as candidates for early or regular retirement. We rely on five rounds of high-frequency panel surveys carried out over the period of June 2020 through September 2021, with a pre-COVID recall module to February 2020, for four developing Arab countries already facing severe labor market challenges. We focus on workers' experience of losing hours or being laid off, and their employment status, because these outcomes represent the main aspirations of labor market entrants in Arab countries, and are crucial for workers' career progress, lifetime outcomes, and well-being.

The rest of the chapter is structured as follows. Section 5.2 provides some background regarding employment vulnerability of workers in Arab countries and worldwide to the pandemic. Section 5.3 lays out our analytical approach and data sources. Section 5.4 presents the main results, and Sect. 5.5 summarizes our key findings and their significance for the process of recovery from the pandemic.

5.2 Early Assessments of the Pandemic Impacts

Studies since the onset of COVID have shown that particular groups of workers have been affected particularly gravely by lockdowns and the associated economic downturn (AlAzzawi 2023; Delaporte and Peña 2020; Dingel and Nieman 2020; Hatayama et al. 2020; Saltiel 2020; ILO 2020d). The crisis has particularly hit workers in sectors with a risk of downturns due to the lockdowns and social distancing rules; informally employed workers; and workers with limited opportunities for teleworking, due to poor access to reliable technology, or the nature of their jobs. The impact is also projected to be stronger in countries with limited public-sector employment and with fiscal constraints preventing their governments from intervening more robustly in the economy.

International agencies[1] and national statistical agencies have shared early results of rapid assessments of the pandemic's impact on countries' labor markets and various social indicators. For example, the World Bank rapid survey in Yemen, undertaken between March and April 2020, found that 18% of households could not reach their jobs due to COVID-imposed mobility restrictions and 31% were either not receiving salaries or receiving less than before the pandemic. The share of households citing low wages and a loss of employment as the most difficult challenges facing them increased from 45 to 49%, relative to before the outbreak. The assessment for Iraq focused on poverty and concluded that introducing a full curfew would have had a severe impact on poverty due to changes in workers' labor income, increasing the poverty headcount for the country as a whole by 10 percentage points

[1] The World Bank (2020) listed the results of rapid phone surveys assessing the impact of the pandemic on households. UNDP (2020) provided detailed summaries and references to rapid assessments conducted to examine the impact of the pandemic on key issues such as health, poverty, labor markets, migrant workers, small and medium enterprises and women. UN ESCWA assessed that in the first year of the pandemic, the distribution of incomes and wealth in the region substantially widened, and poverty headcount in the 14 middle and low-income Arab countries rose from 29.2 to 32.4% of the population.

and increasing the poverty gap by 3 points. In Djibouti, findings from a rapid phone survey also confirmed a strong impact of the crisis on the labor market with almost 20% of breadwinners losing their jobs since the onset of the pandemic. This impact was particularly pronounced for households in the bottom income quintile. Among those who lost their jobs, 68% identified COVID-related reasons as the cause of their current economic inactivity. Among those who kept their pre-pandemic employment type, 42% were working less or not at all, with a simultaneous reduction in income: 45% of those working less than previously received no income at all, while 36% received only partial wage payments.

Assessments conducted in the following months continued reporting similarly troubling trends. In Tunisia as of October 2020, labor force participation rate stagnated at 41% of the working age population, and unemployment rate increased from 13 to 22% (ILO and ERF 2021). In Jordan, rapid assessment in mid-2021 (UN Women, Arab States 2021) indicated that 13% of women and one-fifth of men who had been employed before the pandemic lost their jobs by the summer of 2021. Of these, 85% were informal-sector workers and 15% were formal. Young adults specifically were prone to be unemployed, as 81% of them had been unemployed even prior to March 2020, and 71% of those employed were subsequently laid off by the summer of 2021. As many as 45% of respondents said that someone in their household had become unemployed during the pandemic.

5.3 Analytical Approach

In light of the existing evidence from across Arab countries, we aim to evaluate the impacts of the pandemic on young adults and women statically as well as dynamically, accounting for the severity of government responses to the pandemic and for workers' pre-COVID circumstances. We start by analyzing the labor market experiences of February-2020 wage workers across different phases of the pandemic—being laid off, working fewer hours, or no longer being wage workers—differentiating between those employed in the public or formal private sector, and those employed informally inside or outside establishments. Next we evaluate workers' transitions from their initial February-2020 status to their new statuses at different points in time.

To assess the factors behind workers' employment outcomes, and the sources of the young/non-young gaps, we turn to multinomial logit models of workers' experience of having lost pay or hours, or been laid off, and of their employment status. This approach has been successfully used with employment types in numerous studies (AlAzzawi and Hlasny 2022; Assaad and Krafft 2014; Aygun et al. 2022). Multinomial logit estimates the probability that a worker will attain a specific employment type relative to the probability of the baseline option—remaining inactive. First, we estimate a multinomial logit model of the workers' probability of experiencing a loss of hours or pay, being temporarily suspended, or being permanently terminated. Next, we estimate a multinomial model of workers' labor market status—employed, unemployed and inactive—and a more detailed model of workers' employment type emphasizing several degrees of job vulnerability—formal, informal within establishments, informal outside establishments, self-employed or unpaid, and non-employed—and disregarding the difference between those unemployed and inactive. This is valuable, as workers' transitions between different types of informal employment hold different implications than the retention of formal employment, or the transitions between unemployment and economic inactivity. This model gives insights into the "cascading" impacts of the pandemic on workers: some formal workers may have lost their job amenities (and landed in informality), among these some were temporarily suspended (became irregular), or consigned to work externally without a contract or without pay (became self-employed/unpaid family workers), and some were laid off permanently (unemployed/inactive).

These multinomial logit models control for workers' predispositions for individual employment types, by controlling either for workers' pre-pandemic February-2020 status (in the models of workers' experiencing of employment shocks), or for the fitted time-invariant probabilities of workers' attaining the alternative employment statuses (in the models of employment outcomes; refer to AlAzzawi and Hlasny 2023). Accounting for the pre-pandemic/predisposed status alleviates potential bias due to latent worker-level heterogeneity, as well as inefficiency due to error autocorrelation. Moreover, it changes the interpretation of estimates as the drivers of the short-term changes in workers' status (rather than of workers' cumulative up-to-date career outcomes).

Workers' propensity to transition between employment types is made a function of tightness of the pandemic regulation, which proxies for the fluctuating labor market conditions in regard to all workers. This and other key covariates are interacted with the female or youth indicator to allow distinct effects across the respective sex and age groups. Hence, the specific vulnerability of young and female workers to the stringency regime is assessed using the *young* × *stringency* and *female* × *stringency* interaction terms. We conjecture that the coefficients on *stringency*, *young*, *young* × *stringency*, *female* and *female* × *stringency* are positive for the more adverse labor market outcomes such as informality, loss of hours and pay, layoff, and inactivity. Similarly, their coefficients are expected to be negative for favorable outcomes such as no adverse shocks, remaining employed, and retaining a formal position.

For control variables, we use workers' school completion level, potential work experience (age less 16 for young workers, age less 29 for those older), and proximity to various geographic labor markets—residence in a cluster of administrative regions, and a *rural/urban* indicator. The regressions are estimated on pooled rounds of the Economic Research Forum (ERF) COVID-19 Monitors, but separately for each country, in order to pick up different labor market dynamics across the four countries. For reporting the results, we present the average marginal effects (AMEs) of the unit increases in the explanatory variables on the probability of experiencing a particular labor-market shock or attaining a particular employment type. To assess the relevance of explanatory variables in the multinomial model, we test the individual and joint significance of the estimated AMEs across all categories of the dependent variables ($AME_{xj=1}, \ldots, AME_{xj=J}$ for each variable x). Errors in regressions are clustered at the worker level to alleviate the effect of their autocorrelation on the measures of model fit. Coefficient standard errors are also corrected for heteroskedasticity and autocorrelation of unknown forms. All data analysis is performed using Stata 14 software (StataCorp 2015).

Data

Data for the analysis come from the ERF COVID-19 Monitor surveys (OAMDI 2021), which are moderate-size rapid telephone surveys conducted by the ILO and ERF between June 2020 and September 2021. ERF COVID-19 Monitors are unbalanced panel surveys with a limited module of recall questions to February 2020 ("round 0"), allowing us to track the same workers and their employment outcomes over the span of up to 19 months, from February 2020 to September 2021. For the purpose of this study, we use three rounds for Egypt (June 2020, January–February 2021, and June–July 2021) and Jordan (January–February, June–July 2021, and August–September 2021), and four rounds for Morocco and Tunisia (October–November 2020, January–February 2021, March–April 2021, and June–July 2021). Sudan is excluded from this analysis because of the country's different setting, and the different distribution of key survey variables.

Each survey round covers just over 2000 individuals (2500 in Jordan), giving approximately 9400 panel observations for 4500 workers in Egypt (including refresher samples and "round 0"), 8400 observations for 3400 workers in Jordan, 11,300 observations for 4600 workers in Morocco, and 9600 observations for 3000 workers in Tunisia. The surveys contain individual-level expansion weights facilitating representativeness within a certain sample-frame of respondents contactable by telephone. The surveys include information on workers' employment type, employment shocks, hours worked, income, and the status of self-employed workers' enterprise. For the alternative dependent variables in the main model specifications, workers' labor market experiences in rounds 1–5, and their employment status in rounds 0–5 are used. For explanatory variables, we account for workers' education, family status and dependents by age, residence and other demographics.

Individual-level survey data are supplemented with country-level information on the strictness of governments' day-to-day COVID responses (Hale et al. 2023). A 30-day moving average of the stringency index in each country is constructed and matched to survey respondents according to their actual individual survey dates.

5.4 Main Results

This section presents our main results regarding workers' job status transitions and experiences amid COVID, and the socioeconomic factors playing a role in them. We then discuss some broad commonalities and differences between the demographic groups of interest and the four countries.

Figure 5.2 reports the labor market experiences at different phases of the pandemic of individuals who were wage workers as of February 2020, distinguishing men and women, and young and older adults. Across all four countries, public sector employees were least likely to be affected by temporary or permanent layoffs, or experienced decreased hours over the past 60 days, regardless of their age cohort and sex. If they encountered any shocks, the most prominent shock was in the form of decreased hours. Regardless of age, women were more likely to "no longer be a wage worker" (henceforth, WW). Figure 5.3 investigates this dimension of transitions into lower employment statuses further.

As shown in Fig. 5.2a–c, young adults were often more likely to experience a reduction in hours or a temporary layoff, especially in Egypt and Tunisia. Informal workers across all four countries were more likely to be affected by these shocks than formal private sector workers, and especially informal workers outside of establishments, who were likely to experience temporary layoffs. Within that group, high shares of young men in particular faced the risk of temporary layoffs. By June 2021 (Fig. 5.2d) the situation seemed to have improved somewhat in Jordan and Morocco, relative to Egypt and Tunisia where many workers continued to face

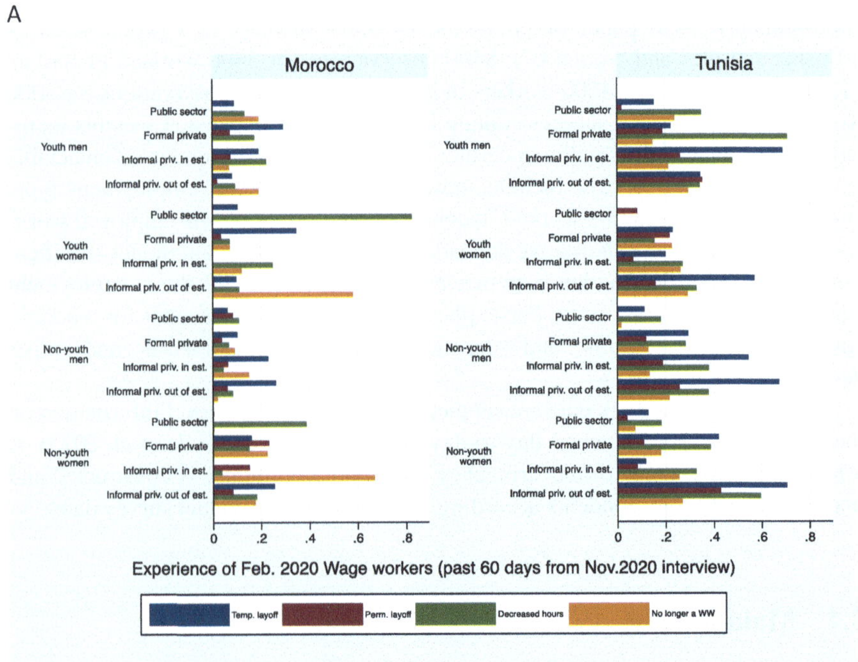

Fig. 5.2 (**a**) Experience of Feb. 2020 wage workers in past 60 days from Nov. 2020, by age and sex. (**b**) Experience of Feb. 2020 wage workers in past 60 days from Feb. 2021 by age and sex. (**c**) Experience of Feb. 2020 wage workers in past 60 days from Apr. 2021. (**d**) Experience of Feb. 2020 wage workers in past 60 days from June 2021 by age and sex. (**e**) Experience of Feb. 2020 wage workers in past 60 days from Aug. 2021, overall and by age and sex

B

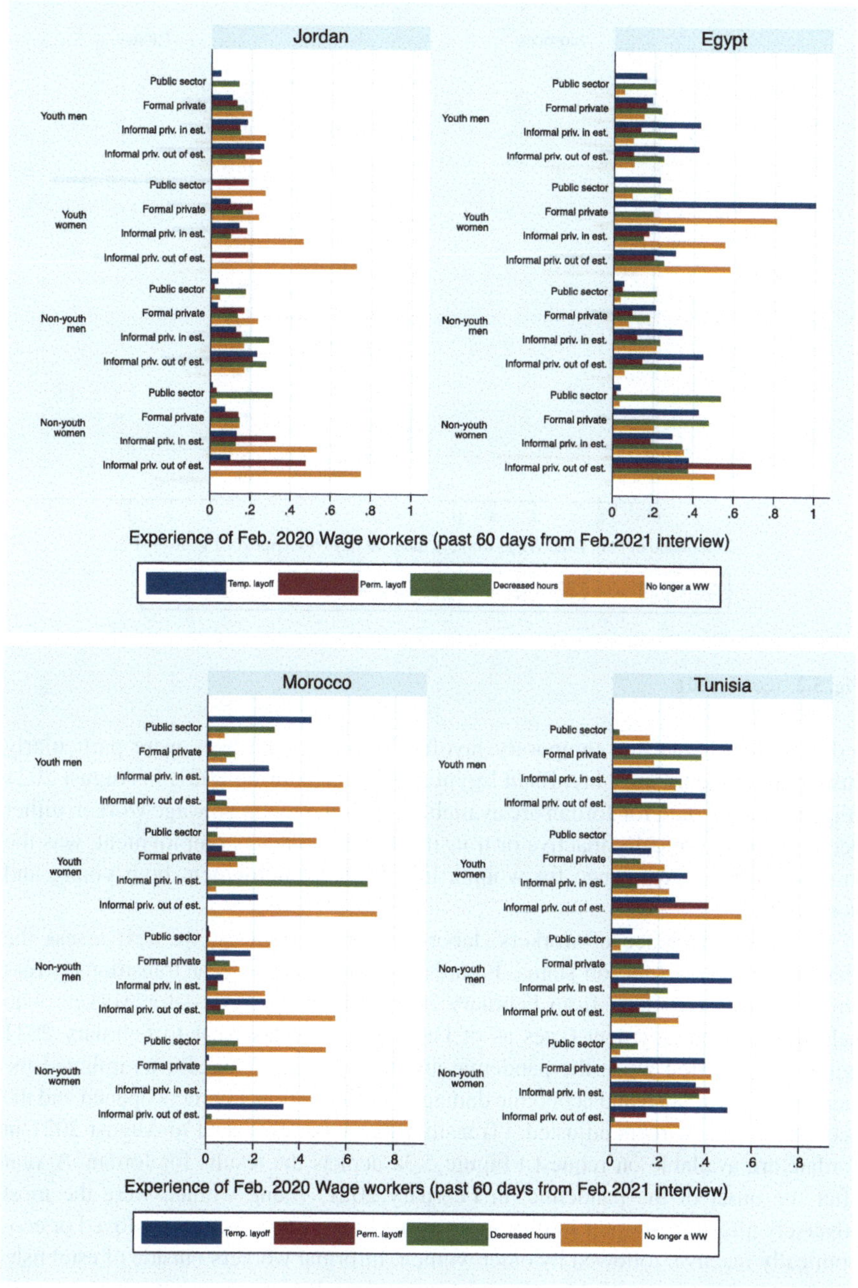

Fig. 5.2 (continued)

c

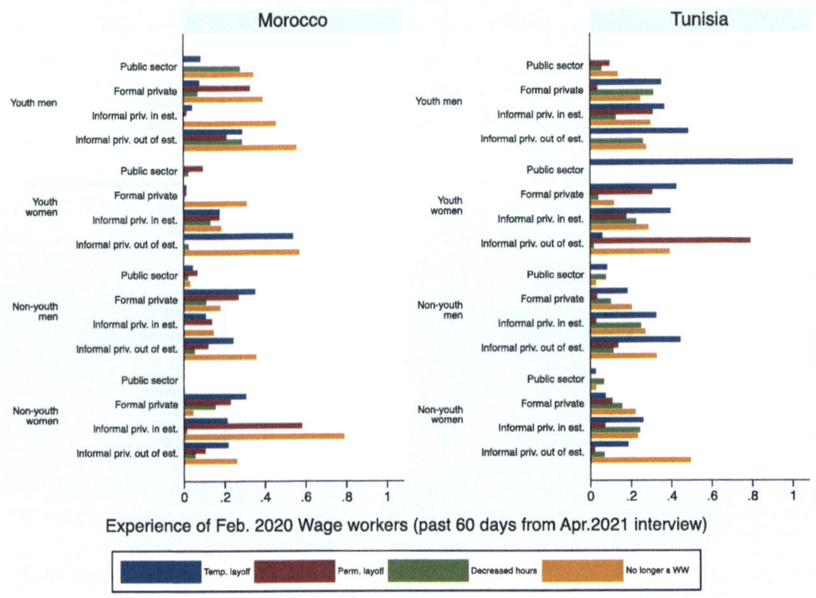

Fig. 5.2 (continued)

reductions in hours and temporary layoffs. Women of all ages were particularly susceptible to temporary layoffs in Egypt and Tunisia during 2021. In August 2021 (Fig. 5.2e; only data for Jordan are available), no longer being a wage worker, either becoming economically inactive or transitioning to nonwage employment, was the most prominent experience for women in informal employment both young and non-young.

Given this evidence of workers' labor market experiences, we next assess the changes in their actual job status. Figure 5.3 shows year-to-year transitions across employment categories—from February 2020 to February 2021—for workers who held different employment types as of February 2020. The year to February 2021 represents a period when the pandemic and the associated lockdowns inflicted the clearest health-related and economic damages, before national borders opened and the economies and workers adjusted. (Transitions to June 2021, and to August 2021 in Jordan, are available on request.) Figure 5.3a depicts the results for Jordan. A year after the onset of the pandemic, in February 2021, young women were the most adversely affected group in Jordan, more prone to become either unemployed or economically inactive, followed by older women. Informal workers outside of establishments were also more likely to become unemployed or inactive, but young women were again hit the hardest in that category. By June and August 2021 (available on request) somewhat of a recovery occurred, with fewer women becoming unemployed or inactive, but for young men who had been informally employed in February 2020, larger shares ended up unemployed in February 2021 than a year earlier.

D

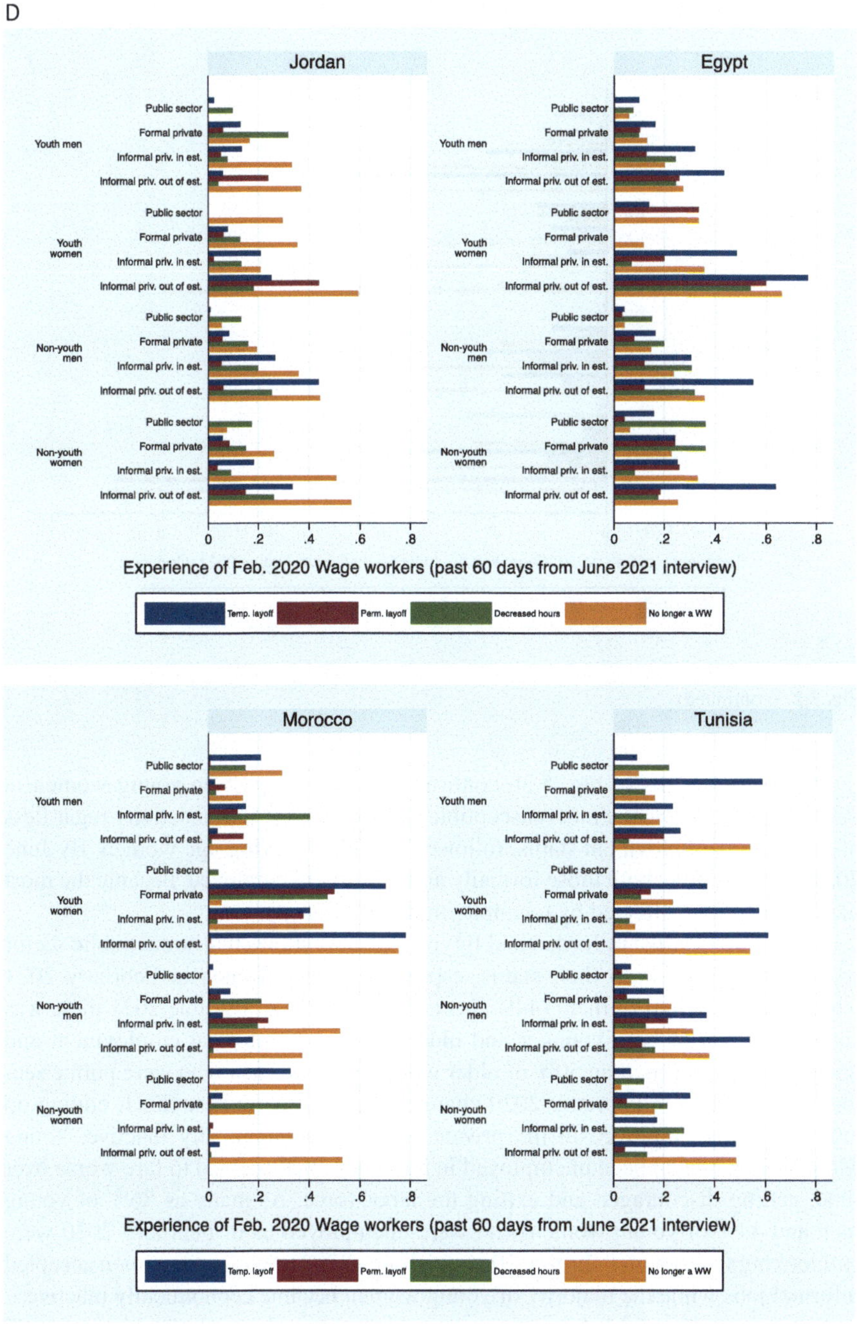

Fig. 5.2 (continued)

E

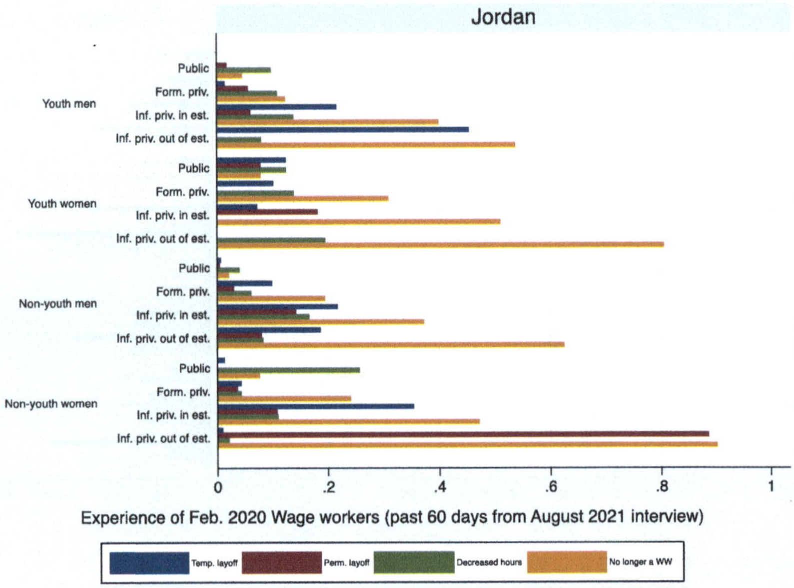

Fig. 5.2 (continued)

For Egypt, results in Fig. 5.3b confirm the strong impact on young women in February 2021, being the most susceptible to unemployment or inactivity regardless of their initial employment status, followed by older working-age women. By June 2021, older women, both those formally and informally employed, became the most likely group to be affected by unemployment or inactivity.

In Morocco, unlike in Jordan and Egypt, Fig. 5.3c shows that some public sector workers could not keep their status, especially young women in February 2021 when nearly one half of them (44%) became unemployed. By June 2021 there was some transition of both younger and older workers to informal employment and unemployment. More than 50% of older working-age women who were public sector wage workers in February 2020 changed their status by June 2021, ending up either formally employed in the private sector or economically inactive. Young Moroccans who had been unemployed in February 2020 seemed to fare worse over time, getting discouraged and exiting the labor force. As many as 86% of young men and 44% of young women who were unemployed as of February 2020 were still looking for a job in February 2021. By June of 2021, many young men accepted informal jobs while the majority of young women became economically inactive.

For Tunisia, Fig. 5.3d shows that a large share of workers who had been formal wage workers in the private sector in February 2020 transitioned to informality, and in the case of women to unemployment or inactivity. Moreover, large shares of women, especially older adults, who had changed their status, became

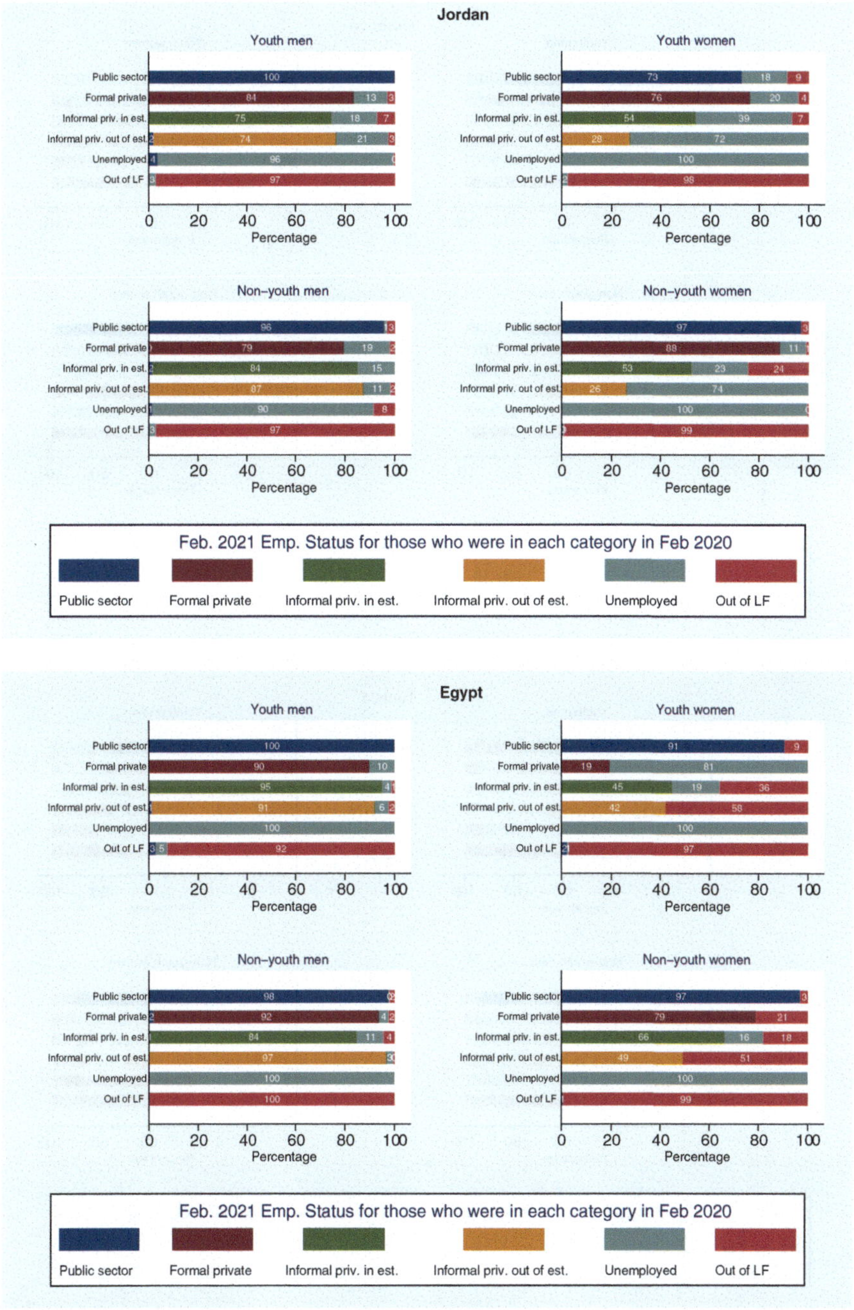

Fig. 5.3 (**a**) Employment status transitions from Feb 2020 to Feb 2021, Jordan, by age and sex. (**b**) Employment status transitions from Feb 2020 to Feb 2021, Egypt, by age and sex. (**c**) Employment status transitions from Feb 2020 to Feb 2021, Morocco, by age and sex. (**d**) Employment status transitions from Feb 2020 to Feb 2021, Tunisia, by age and sex

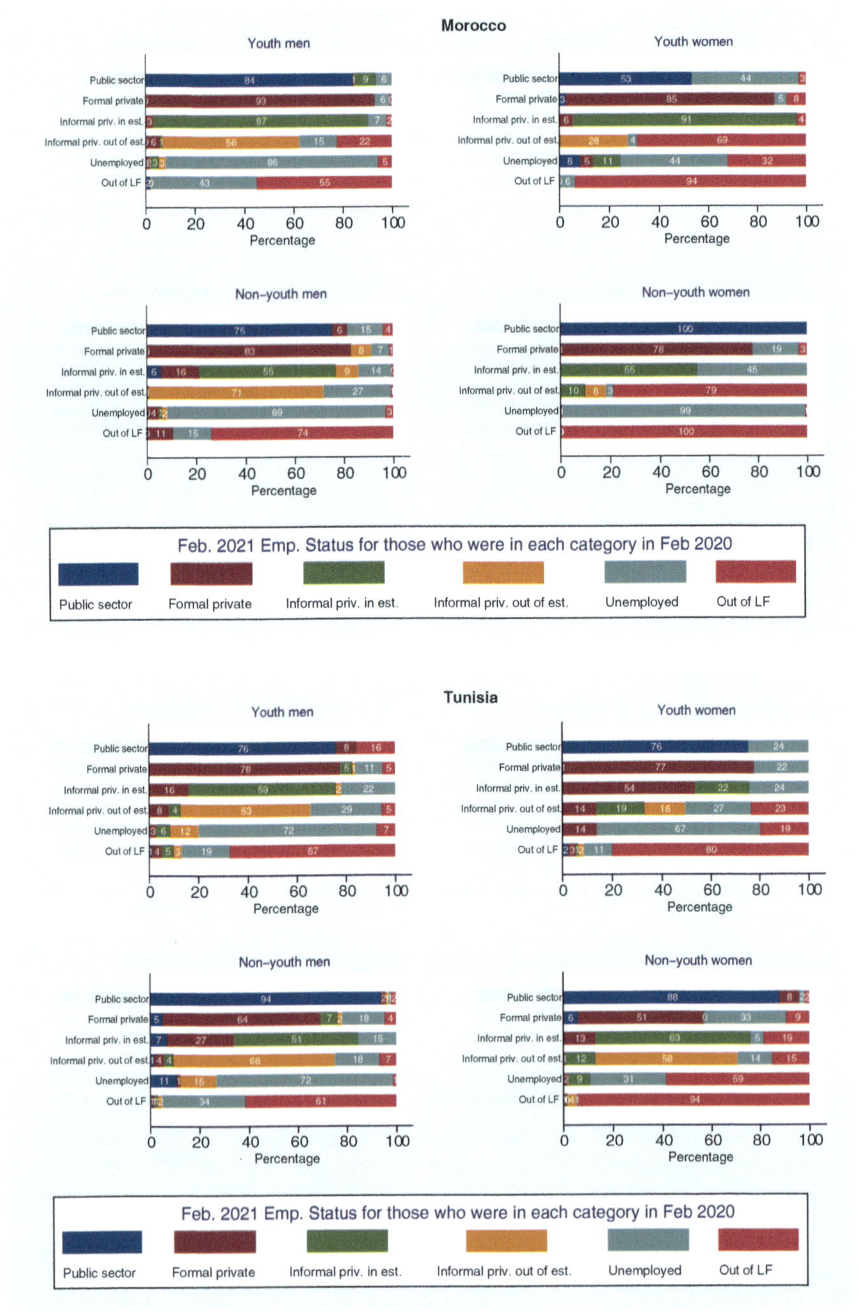

Fig. 5.3 (continued)

economically inactive by February 2021, confirming the lingering effect of the pandemic on female workers.

Factors Contributing to Workers' Adverse Outcomes
In light of the employment shocks and transitions observed across different groups and countries, we next assess the factors affecting them. Table 5.1 reports the results of multinomial logistic models of labor-market experiences, controlling for lagged pre-pandemic status. Groups of columns per country—columns 1–3 for Egypt, 4–6 for Jordan, 7–9 for Morocco, and 10–12 for Tunisia—report on the multinomial logits of workers' experience of no impact, lost pay/hours, or a layoff, respectively. The results confirm that the stringency regime had the expected negative effect on workers' experiencing "no adverse impact" and an aggravating effect on those experiencing lost hours/pay or a layoff. Young adults were more prone to losing hours/pay or being laid off even under less stringent COVID regimes (except in Morocco), but the effect changed signs when their youth status is interacted with the stringency regime, an indication of collinearity of the two variables and the difficulty of estimating their effects separately. Women's prospects did not differ from men's, but their prospect of experiencing no adverse impact fell compared to men under stringent COVID regimes. Mothers with pre-school children were less likely to not see any adverse impacts, and more likely to lose their jobs (in all countries but Morocco). The effect of having school-age children is inconclusive.

Other covariates provide interesting, for the most part expected, results: higher levels of education and of job experience appear to protect workers from the most adverse impacts including layoffs (except in Jordan for the case of work experience). Being married apparently does not affect workers' prospects. Workers' pre-existing vulnerability is related negatively with their odds of escaping adverse impacts, and positively with their odds of being laid off.

Table 5.2 reports the results of multinomial logistic models of workers' employment outcomes: employed, unemployed and searching, and economically inactive. COVID regime *stringency* is confirmed to have a negative effect on workers' employment chances, and a positive effect on their odds of staying unemployed (with the prospects of remaining inactive being inconclusive). Young adults have a lower risk of being employed, and a higher risk of remaining unemployed and searching, regardless of the degree of COVID regime stringency, but the effects disappear or are overturned under tighter COVID stringency. Women have lower odds of being employed than men, but this effect disappears when accounting for tighter stringency regimes. Workers' education is associated positively with employment prospects and negatively with the prospect of becoming inactive (except in Tunisia). Workers' potential work experience is associated positively with becoming inactive, and negatively with the prospect of remaining unemployed and job-searching. This is consistent with younger workers of both sexes striving to remain active, while older workers, particularly females, becoming discouraged.

Tables 5.3 and 5.4 report on similar specifications using five values for the categorical dependent variable: Formal; informal in establishments; informal out

Table 5.1 Multinomial logit regressions of labor market experience over the past 60 days, controlling for workers' pre-COVID vulnerability

	Egypt			Jordan			Morocco			Tunisia		
	(1) No impact	(2) Lost pay/hrs	(3) Laid off	(4) No impact	(5) Lost pay/hrs	(6) Laid off	(7) No impact	(8) Lost pay/hrs	(9) Laid off	(10) No impact	(11) Lost pay/hrs	(12) Laid off
Stringency	–0.094	0.148	–0.054	–0.567***	0.316*	0.251	–8.224**	2.006	6.218*	–0.296	0.246	0.050
	(0.276)	(0.240)	(0.245)	(0.197)	(0.183)	(0.174)	(3.535)	(3.264)	(3.259)	(0.258)	(0.261)	(0.211)
Young	–0.673**	0.527**	0.146	–0.338*	0.381**	–0.042	0.505	–0.394	–0.112	–0.984***	0.515	0.469
	(0.330)	(0.248)	(0.241)	(0.173)	(0.159)	(0.121)	(0.612)	(0.474)	(0.514)	(0.314)	(0.354)	(0.297)
Young × stringency	1.163**	–0.956**	–0.208	0.456	–0.599**	0.143	–0.919	0.720	0.199	1.337***	–0.711	–0.626
	(0.573)	(0.429)	(0.420)	(0.289)	(0.268)	(0.202)	(0.859)	(0.678)	(0.729)	(0.474)	(0.558)	(0.476)
Female	0.351	–0.726**	0.375	0.181	–0.218	0.037	–0.784	0.377	0.408	0.019	0.156	–0.176
	(0.372)	(0.291)	(0.301)	(0.199)	(0.180)	(0.133)	(0.652)	(0.481)	(0.553)	(0.260)	(0.309)	(0.265)
Female × stringency	–0.739	1.311***	–0.572	–0.364	0.359	0.006	1.043	–0.459	–0.583	–0.084	–0.237	0.320
	(0.649)	(0.495)	(0.517)	(0.323)	(0.288)	(0.222)	(0.918)	(0.666)	(0.786)	(0.396)	(0.467)	(0.403)
Basic educ. complet.	–0.084	0.055	0.029	0.167**	–0.098	–0.069	0.120**	–0.052	–0.067*	–0.004	0.049	–0.044
	(0.061)	(0.051)	(0.057)	(0.077)	(0.074)	(0.061)	(0.047)	(0.040)	(0.039)	(0.051)	(0.047)	(0.047)
Secondary education	0.020	0.070*	–0.091**	0.192**	–0.070	–0.122**	0.129***	–0.035	–0.094**	0.047	0.024	–0.071*
	(0.051)	(0.037)	(0.044)	(0.077)	(0.076)	(0.060)	(0.049)	(0.040)	(0.041)	(0.046)	(0.038)	(0.042)
Higher education	0.088	0.083**	–0.171***	0.150*	0.001	–0.150**	0.212***	–0.039	–0.173***	0.109**	0.120***	–0.229***
	(0.055)	(0.040)	(0.047)	(0.077)	(0.077)	(0.061)	(0.061)	(0.053)	(0.047)	(0.054)	(0.044)	(0.040)
Age-16 (-29 adults)	0.003	0.001	–0.004**	–0.002	–0.001	0.003**	0.010***	–0.005**	–0.006**	0.002	0.004**	–0.006***
	(0.002)	(0.002)	(0.002)	(0.002)	(0.002)	(0.001)	(0.003)	(0.002)	(0.002)	(0.003)	(0.002)	(0.002)
Married	0.012	0.017	–0.029	–0.021	0.042	–0.022	–0.033	0.024	0.009	–0.038	0.023	0.016
	(0.045)	(0.039)	(0.033)	(0.037)	(0.032)	(0.022)	(0.051)	(0.041)	(0.039)	(0.046)	(0.039)	(0.039)
Female × kids <6 yo	–0.129***	0.057*	0.072**	–0.006	–0.018	0.023	0.016	–0.057	0.040	–0.023	–0.033	0.056*
	(0.050)	(0.034)	(0.034)	(0.032)	(0.029)	(0.017)	(0.069)	(0.053)	(0.046)	(0.043)	(0.040)	(0.030)

Female × kids at schl.	–0.020	0.023	–0.002	–0.047*	0.055**	–0.008	–0.036	–0.009	0.045	0.018	0.006	–0.024
	(0.037)	(0.027)	(0.029)	(0.025)	(0.022)	(0.015)	(0.035)	(0.027)	(0.034)	(0.029)	(0.028)	(0.023)
Rural				–0.009	0.062	–0.053	0.091	–0.018	–0.073	0.334**	–0.353**	0.019
				(0.072)	(0.057)	(0.060)	(0.088)	(0.085)	(0.089)	(0.156)	(0.159)	(0.084)
Informal, in-estab, Feb '20	–0.209***	–0.025	0.234***	–0.239***	0.079**	0.161***	–0.068	0.024	0.044	–0.193***	–0.003	0.196***
	(0.045)	(0.032)	(0.037)	(0.043)	(0.036)	(0.032)	(0.065)	(0.055)	(0.050)	(0.056)	(0.056)	(0.051)
Informal, out-of-estab, Feb '20	–0.274***	–0.073**	0.347***	–0.264***	0.053	0.211***	–0.042	–0.010	0.051	–0.203***	–0.106**	0.309***
	(0.044)	(0.035)	(0.042)	(0.062)	(0.055)	(0.050)	(0.047)	(0.038)	(0.037)	(0.051)	(0.044)	(0.043)
Obs. (indv. clusters)		1662 (1399)			2222 (1531)			2196 (1865)			2872 (1421)	
Chi-squared (dg.fr.)		243.4*** (42)			235.6*** (38)			120.8*** (58)			290.8*** (54)	
Pseudo R-squared		0.116			0.104			0.091			0.131	

Notes: Authors' calculations based on ERF COVID-19 Household Monitor, rounds 1–5, among those who were wage workers in Feb-2020. AMEs shown. Governorate fixed effects controlled for. The baseline group is the 30-year old, non-married, urban males with unfinished basic education holding formal jobs as of February 2020. Samples weighted by individual-level weights. Heteroskedasticity and autocorrelation-robust standard errors clustered at worker level in parentheses, * $p < 0.1$, ** $p < 0.05$, *** $p < 0.01$

Table 5.2 Multinomial logit regressions of labor market status, controlling for workers' time-constant risk of vulnerability

	Egypt			Jordan			Morocco			Tunisia		
	(1) Employed	(2) Unemployed	(3) Inactive	(4) Employed	(5) Unemployed	(6) Inactive	(7) Employed	(8) Unemployed	(9) Inactive	(10) Employed	(11) Unemployed	(12) Inactive
Stringency	−0.127***	0.149***	−0.022	−0.268***	0.124**	0.145***	−0.173***	0.008	0.165***	−0.031	0.148***	−0.117***
	(0.016)	(0.021)	(0.022)	(0.030)	(0.049)	(0.049)	(0.039)	(0.036)	(0.049)	(0.036)	(0.041)	(0.044)
Young	−0.071**	0.046*	0.024	−0.072**	0.099***	−0.027	−0.106**	0.040	0.067*	0.025	0.031	−0.056
	(0.031)	(0.024)	(0.028)	(0.028)	(0.031)	(0.025)	(0.047)	(0.042)	(0.040)	(0.054)	(0.044)	(0.049)
Young × stringency	0.078***	−0.067***	−0.011	0.070*	−0.163***	0.093**	−0.048	0.079	−0.031	−0.022	−0.117**	0.140***
	(0.020)	(0.020)	(0.023)	(0.038)	(0.047)	(0.042)	(0.056)	(0.050)	(0.050)	(0.054)	(0.055)	(0.048)
Female	−0.010	−0.162	0.172	−0.361**	−0.338**	0.700***	−0.393	0.186	0.207	0.468***	−0.426***	−0.043
	(0.101)	(0.101)	(0.108)	(0.168)	(0.152)	(0.168)	(0.243)	(0.263)	(0.221)	(0.161)	(0.132)	(0.132)
Female × stringency	0.055***	0.020	−0.075***	0.151***	0.292***	−0.443***	0.076	0.124**	−0.200***	−0.010	0.168***	−0.158***
	(0.018)	(0.023)	(0.025)	(0.036)	(0.051)	(0.050)	(0.060)	(0.059)	(0.054)	(0.047)	(0.051)	(0.045)
Basic educ. complet.	0.012	0.031*	−0.043*	0.049	−0.043	−0.006	0.111***	−0.060	−0.051	−0.051	0.001	0.050
	(0.026)	(0.016)	(0.026)	(0.046)	(0.034)	(0.039)	(0.042)	(0.047)	(0.041)	(0.035)	(0.026)	(0.032)
Secondary education	0.052*	0.026*	−0.078***	0.081	−0.043	−0.037	0.262***	−0.164***	−0.098	−0.131**	0.091*	0.040
	(0.027)	(0.016)	(0.026)	(0.053)	(0.038)	(0.043)	(0.067)	(0.057)	(0.066)	(0.056)	(0.050)	(0.041)
Higher education	0.082	0.084*	−0.167***	0.187**	0.065	−0.252***	0.429***	−0.228***	−0.201**	−0.353***	0.312***	0.040
	(0.058)	(0.051)	(0.055)	(0.077)	(0.063)	(0.058)	(0.086)	(0.061)	(0.088)	(0.095)	(0.117)	(0.084)
Age-16 (-29 adults)	0.002	−0.003**	0.001	−0.005**	−0.005**	0.009***	0.002	−0.006**	0.004**	−0.002	−0.001	0.003*
	(0.002)	(0.001)	(0.001)	(0.002)	(0.002)	(0.002)	(0.003)	(0.002)	(0.002)	(0.002)	(0.002)	(0.002)
Married	−0.014	0.051**	−0.036	−0.071**	−0.037*	0.109***	−0.009	−0.126***	0.135***	−0.100**	0.020	0.080**
	(0.026)	(0.020)	(0.023)	(0.028)	(0.023)	(0.024)	(0.032)	(0.030)	(0.025)	(0.044)	(0.032)	(0.036)
Female × kids <6 yo	0.010	−0.013	0.003	−0.017	−0.010	0.027***	0.011	−0.014	0.002	−0.047*	0.028*	0.020
	(0.014)	(0.010)	(0.011)	(0.015)	(0.012)	(0.010)	(0.029)	(0.024)	(0.018)	(0.024)	(0.017)	(0.016)

Female × kids at schl.	–0.016*	0.017**	–0.000	0.008	–0.008	–0.000	–0.020	–0.001	0.021*	–0.018	0.022	–0.003
	(0.010)	(0.007)	(0.008)	(0.010)	(0.009)	(0.008)	(0.017)	(0.013)	(0.011)	(0.015)	(0.014)	(0.010)
Prob(Informal in-estab)	–0.022	0.151	–0.129	–1.438***	0.390	1.047**	–1.023	–0.425	1.448*	–0.627	1.285**	–0.658
	(0.138)	(0.109)	(0.138)	(0.472)	(0.354)	(0.510)	(0.867)	(0.689)	(0.784)	(0.771)	(0.636)	(0.737)
Prob(Infrm,out-of-estab)	0.728***	0.089	–0.817***	1.690***	–0.375	–1.315**	1.159**	–1.173***	0.015	–0.396	0.295	0.101
	(0.250)	(0.177)	(0.303)	(0.615)	(0.569)	(0.645)	(0.464)	(0.394)	(0.441)	(0.345)	(0.265)	(0.311)
Prob(Self-emp/unpaid)	–0.032	0.404**	–0.372	–0.541	0.161	0.380	0.630***	–0.202	–0.428**	–0.724**	0.696**	0.027
	(0.225)	(0.189)	(0.291)	(0.378)	(0.344)	(0.405)	(0.244)	(0.229)	(0.188)	(0.322)	(0.291)	(0.278)
Prob(non-empl)	–0.542***	0.434**	0.108	–0.317	0.555**	–0.238	0.500	–0.793	0.292	–1.920***	1.126***	0.795***
	(0.182)	(0.174)	(0.183)	(0.253)	(0.228)	(0.235)	(0.542)	(0.595)	(0.460)	(0.376)	(0.314)	(0.271)
Obs. (indv. clusters)	9372 (4438)			8336 (3384)			11,267 (4606)			9586 (3007)		
Chi-squared (dg. fr.)	1373*** (46)			981.1*** (42)			672.5*** (58)			830.4*** (54)		
Pseudo R-squared		0.329			0.276			0.211			0.235	

Notes: Authors' calculations based on ERF COVID-19 Household Monitor, Rounds 0–5. AMEs shown. Governorate, and rural residence fixed effects controlled for. The baseline group is the 30-year old, non-married, urban males with unfinished basic education. Samples weighted by individual-level weights. Heteroskedasticity and autocorrelation-robust standard errors clustered at worker level in parentheses, * $p < 0.1$, ** $p < 0.05$, *** $p < 0.01$

Table 5.3 Multinomial logit regressions of vulnerable status, controlling for workers' time-constant risk of vulnerability: Egypt and Jordan

	Egypt					Jordan				
	(1) Formal	(2) Informal: In estab.	(3) Informal: Out of estab	(4) Self-emp/ unpaid	(5) Non-employed	(6) Formal	(7) Informal: In estab.	(8) Informal: Out of estab	(9) Self-emp/ unpaid	(10 Non-employed
Stringency	–0.138***	–0.176***	–0.063***	0.035	0.341***	–0.270***	–0.052**	–0.042***	–0.000	0.365***
	(0.034)	(0.038)	(0.023)	(0.025)	(0.035)	(0.036)	(0.022)	(0.015)	(0.017)	(0.042)
Young	–0.142***	0.015	0.038	–0.016	0.105***	–0.047	0.045***	–0.010	–0.042	0.054*
	(0.047)	(0.034)	(0.028)	(0.039)	(0.032)	(0.032)	(0.016)	(0.012)	(0.026)	(0.030)
Young × stringency	–0.012	0.039	–0.003	0.048	–0.071	0.001	–0.012	0.039*	0.040	–0.069
	(0.069)	(0.054)	(0.040)	(0.043)	(0.049)	(0.053)	(0.028)	(0.021)	(0.032)	(0.053)
Female	0.171	–0.508***	0.021	–0.006	0.321***	0.115	0.150	–0.215**	–0.525***	0.474**
	(0.135)	(0.142)	(0.116)	(0.149)	(0.109)	(0.192)	(0.098)	(0.105)	(0.166)	(0.200)
Female × stringency	0.075	0.190**	–0.048	–0.042	–0.175***	0.068	0.025	–0.055	0.237***	–0.274***
	(0.076)	(0.084)	(0.067)	(0.070)	(0.050)	(0.059)	(0.034)	(0.043)	(0.059)	(0.055)
Basic educ. complet.	0.067***	–0.036	0.013	–0.020	–0.025	0.130***	0.004	–0.001	–0.035	–0.098**
	(0.024)	(0.022)	(0.016)	(0.030)	(0.028)	(0.039)	(0.023)	(0.023)	(0.043)	(0.046)
Secondary education	0.134***	–0.001	–0.006	–0.044	–0.083***	0.190***	0.006	–0.012	–0.053	–0.132**
	(0.030)	(0.026)	(0.021)	(0.037)	(0.028)	(0.052)	(0.031)	(0.028)	(0.051)	(0.054)
Higher education	0.284***	0.031	–0.014	–0.099*	–0.202***	0.273***	–0.018	0.024	–0.022	–0.257***
	(0.089)	(0.065)	(0.041)	(0.057)	(0.060)	(0.095)	(0.039)	(0.057)	(0.078)	(0.080)
Age-16 (-29 adults)	0.009***	–0.004**	–0.000	–0.002	–0.002	–0.003	–0.001	–0.002	–0.000	0.006***
	(0.002)	(0.002)	(0.001)	(0.002)	(0.002)	(0.003)	(0.001)	(0.001)	(0.002)	(0.002)
Married	0.063**	–0.135***	0.076***	–0.004	0.000	0.007	–0.039**	–0.017	–0.008	0.057*
	(0.029)	(0.030)	(0.027)	(0.030)	(0.027)	(0.035)	(0.017)	(0.012)	(0.026)	(0.031)
Female × kids <6 yo	0.039*	–0.047*	0.009	–0.010	0.008	–0.006	–0.011	–0.040*	0.013	0.043***
	(0.022)	(0.025)	(0.020)	(0.023)	(0.015)	(0.021)	(0.009)	(0.023)	(0.016)	(0.016)

Female × kids at schl.	–0.018	0.022	–0.022*	–0.003	0.022**	–0.004	–0.006	0.000	0.008	0.001
	(0.014)	(0.013)	(0.013)	(0.016)	(0.010)	(0.014)	(0.007)	(0.008)	(0.014)	(0.011)
Rural						0.091	0.004	–0.070*	–0.139**	0.113*
						(0.057)	(0.033)	(0.039)	(0.059)	(0.061)
Prob(Informal in-estab)	0.222	–0.131	0.125	–0.168	–0.048	–0.938*	–0.113	–0.292	–0.249	1.592***
	(0.192)	(0.149)	(0.123)	(0.153)	(0.144)	(0.511)	(0.223)	(0.183)	(0.393)	(0.489)
Prob(Infrm,out-of-estab)	0.357	0.144	0.051	0.028	–0.579**	1.379*	0.154	0.254	–0.242	–1.544**
	(0.293)	(0.230)	(0.147)	(0.221)	(0.232)	(0.750)	(0.284)	(0.280)	(0.409)	(0.668)
Prob(Self-emp/unpaid)	–0.324	0.576***	0.292**	–0.080	–0.464**	–0.025	0.375*	–0.134	–0.298	0.083
	(0.240)	(0.195)	(0.137)	(0.192)	(0.234)	(0.415)	(0.196)	(0.197)	(0.280)	(0.393)
Prob(non-empl)	–0.413	0.638***	–0.014	–0.169	–0.042	–0.577*	–0.224	0.278*	0.419*	0.104
	(0.259)	(0.246)	(0.206)	(0.251)	(0.194)	(0.318)	(0.160)	(0.148)	(0.235)	(0.312)
Obs. (indv. clusters)		5521 (4438)					5947 (3384)			
Chi-squared (dg. fr.)		1911*** (92)					1229*** (84)			
Pseudo R-squared			0.298					0.255		

Notes: Authors' calculations based on ERF COVID-19 Household Monitor, rounds 0–5. AMEs shown. Governorate fixed effects controlled for. Samples weighted by individual-level weights. Heteroskedasticity and autocorrelation-robust standard errors clustered at worker level in parentheses, * $p < 0.1$, ** $p < 0.05$, *** $p < 0.01$

Table 5.4 Multinomial logit regressions of vulnerable status, controlling for workers' time-constant risk of vulnerability: Morocco and Tunisia

	Morocco					Tunisia				
	(1) Formal	(2) Informal: In estab.	(3) Informal: Out of estab	(4) Self-emp/ unpaid	(5) Non-employed	(6) Formal	(7) Informal: In estab.	(8) Informal: Out of estab	(9) Self-emp/ unpaid	(10) Non-employed
Stringency	–0.160***	–0.002	–0.021	–0.083***	0.265***	–0.113***	–0.001	–0.027	–0.046**	0.187***
	(0.030)	(0.014)	(0.026)	(0.032)	(0.038)	(0.028)	(0.015)	(0.017)	(0.023)	(0.038)
Young	–0.075**	0.013	0.071*	–0.077	0.069	0.007	0.060**	0.019	–0.008	–0.077
	(0.038)	(0.015)	(0.042)	(0.048)	(0.045)	(0.052)	(0.026)	(0.029)	(0.039)	(0.058)
Young × stringency	0.044	–0.014	–0.109**	0.128**	–0.049	–0.015	–0.032*	0.006	–0.016	0.058
	(0.048)	(0.019)	(0.046)	(0.060)	(0.059)	(0.052)	(0.019)	(0.036)	(0.045)	(0.059)
Female	–0.237	0.051	0.152	–0.417*	0.451*	0.415**	0.022	–0.256	–0.018	–0.163
	(0.153)	(0.103)	(0.195)	(0.253)	(0.250)	(0.167)	(0.075)	(0.156)	(0.150)	(0.182)
Female × stringency	0.049	0.002	–0.092*	0.082	–0.041	0.118**	0.041*	0.006	–0.040	–0.125**
	(0.049)	(0.025)	(0.053)	(0.068)	(0.057)	(0.047)	(0.021)	(0.037)	(0.050)	(0.049)
Basic educ. complet.	0.095**	–0.006	–0.019	0.021	–0.091**	–0.019	–0.031	0.007	0.023	0.020
	(0.041)	(0.016)	(0.029)	(0.051)	(0.046)	(0.035)	(0.025)	(0.021)	(0.035)	(0.035)
Secondary education	0.426***	0.013	–0.014	–0.144**	–0.281***	–0.054	–0.044	0.069	–0.046	0.075
	(0.115)	(0.049)	(0.058)	(0.068)	(0.073)	(0.058)	(0.033)	(0.059)	(0.056)	(0.058)
Higher education	0.787***	–0.004	–0.069	–0.224***	–0.490***	–0.126	–0.056	0.046	–0.115**	0.252**
	(0.111)	(0.062)	(0.063)	(0.040)	(0.071)	(0.079)	(0.039)	(0.114)	(0.058)	(0.117)
Age-16 (-29 adults)	0.005**	–0.001	–0.003	0.001	–0.002	0.001	–0.003***	–0.001	0.000	0.003
	(0.002)	(0.001)	(0.002)	(0.003)	(0.003)	(0.002)	(0.001)	(0.001)	(0.002)	(0.002)
Married	0.035	–0.015	–0.013	–0.015	0.007	–0.051	–0.001	0.031	–0.031	0.052
	(0.024)	(0.011)	(0.022)	(0.029)	(0.031)	(0.039)	(0.014)	(0.031)	(0.030)	(0.045)
Female × kids <6 yo	0.053*	–0.004	–0.047*	0.008	–0.009	–0.001	–0.021	0.024	–0.034	0.032
	(0.027)	(0.009)	(0.024)	(0.043)	(0.028)	(0.029)	(0.013)	(0.020)	(0.027)	(0.025)

Female × kids at schl.	–0.049***	0.001	0.030*	0.012	0.006	–0.013	–0.003	–0.017	0.012	0.021
	(0.017)	(0.008)	(0.017)	(0.020)	(0.017)	(0.016)	(0.006)	(0.014)	(0.016)	(0.015)
Rural	0.023	–0.051*	–0.091	0.081	0.037	0.093	–0.005	–0.071	0.065	–0.082
	(0.067)	(0.030)	(0.061)	(0.079)	(0.087)	(0.087)	(0.030)	(0.050)	(0.070)	(0.087)
Prob(Informal in-estab)	–0.979	0.090	–0.749	0.966*	0.672	–0.979	0.090	–0.749	0.966*	0.672
	(0.875)	(0.263)	(0.550)	(0.504)	(0.886)	(0.875)	(0.263)	(0.550)	(0.504)	(0.886)
Prob(Infrm,out-of-estab)	–0.568*	–0.284**	0.778***	–0.686**	0.759**	–0.568*	–0.284**	0.778***	–0.686**	0.759**
	(0.334)	(0.125)	(0.259)	(0.307)	(0.339)	(0.334)	(0.125)	(0.259)	(0.307)	(0.339)
Prob(Self-emp/unpaid)	–0.678**	0.014	0.034	–0.174	0.804***	–0.678**	0.014	0.034	–0.174	0.804***
	(0.285)	(0.097)	(0.171)	(0.207)	(0.289)	(0.285)	(0.097)	(0.171)	(0.207)	(0.289)
Prob(non-empl)	–1.541***	–0.148	0.513	–0.418	1.594***	–1.541***	–0.148	0.513	–0.418	1.594***
	(0.390)	(0.161)	(0.334)	(0.345)	(0.391)	(0.390)	(0.161)	(0.334)	(0.345)	(0.391)
Obs. (indv. clusters)		8147 (4606)					7232 (3007)			
Chi-squared (dg. fr.)		1085*** (116)					1065*** (108)			
Pseudo R-squared			0.187					0.216		

Notes: Authors' calculations based on ERF COVID-19 Household Monitor, rounds 0–5. AMEs shown. Governorate fixed effects controlled for. Samples weighted by individual-level weights. Heteroskedasticity and autocorrelation-robust standard errors clustered at worker level in parentheses, * $p < 0.1$, ** $p < 0.05$, *** $p < 0.01$

of establishments; self-employed or unpaid, and non-employed. These results support those in Table 5.2, but are typically weaker because of the used up degrees of freedom.[2] In any case, a number of covariates exhibit a systematic progression of coefficients across columns, providing some validation of the main results from Table 5.2. Policy stringency is associated negatively with job formality, or indeed with the different degrees of informality, and positively with remaining non-employed. Young adults have the expected negative effect on formality, and positive effect on being non-employed (except Tunisia). Coefficients on the female dummy—both standalone and in its interaction with stringency—are mixed, again failing to support the hypothesis about women's adverse fate amid harsher phases of COVID.

In Tables 5.2, 5.3 and 5.4, workers' estimated time-invariant probabilities of holding vulnerable employment statuses have unclear effects on current outcomes, but for the most part exhibit consistent signs and magnitudes of coefficients across categories of the dependent variable.

In sum, Tables 5.1, 5.2, 5.3, and 5.4 corroborate several conjectures about the dynamics of workers' employment statuses, but also fail to support other conjectures. Workers' pre-existing employment, or their estimated time-constant propensity to hold each type, has the expected effect on workers' outcomes. It shows a degree of state-dependence in workers' vulnerable status, and the difficulty for workers to shake off vulnerability. The results show that young adults experience greater risks of adverse labor market shocks and outcomes, but we do not find evidence that these effects become worse under stricter COVID conditions. The results for women are also mixed. Overall, the results highlight the disadvantaged status of young and female workers since pre-COVID times, and the importance of higher education for workers' capacity to obtain and hold decent jobs.

Risks of Experiencing Adverse Labor Market Shocks

Using the results from Tables 5.1 and 5.2, Figs. 5.4 and 5.5 show the estimated probabilities of the various labor market outcomes for young versus older workers and women versus men in the four countries, at different times during the pandemic. Specifically, each point shows the median probability in an age and sex group during a week. Figure 5.4 validates the central findings from Table 5.1, partially confirming the conjectures on the fate of younger, female and other worker groups under COVID. Among Egyptians of both sexes, young adults had a substantially higher risk of remaining inactive and a lower risk of being employed than older workers, and the gaps increased in 2021 compared to 2020. Likewise, among Jordanians of both sexes, young adults had a higher risk of remaining unemployed (or inactive, for young females), and young men had a lower risk of being employed. In Morocco, young females had a higher risk of remaining inactive even though their respective risks of being employed cannot be ranked. In Tunis, young men had a lower risk of remaining employed in the second half of 2020 and particularly in

[2] The analysis in Table 5.1 was also performed with four categories of the dependent variable: no impact—lost pay—lost hours or suspension—terminated. The results are available on request.

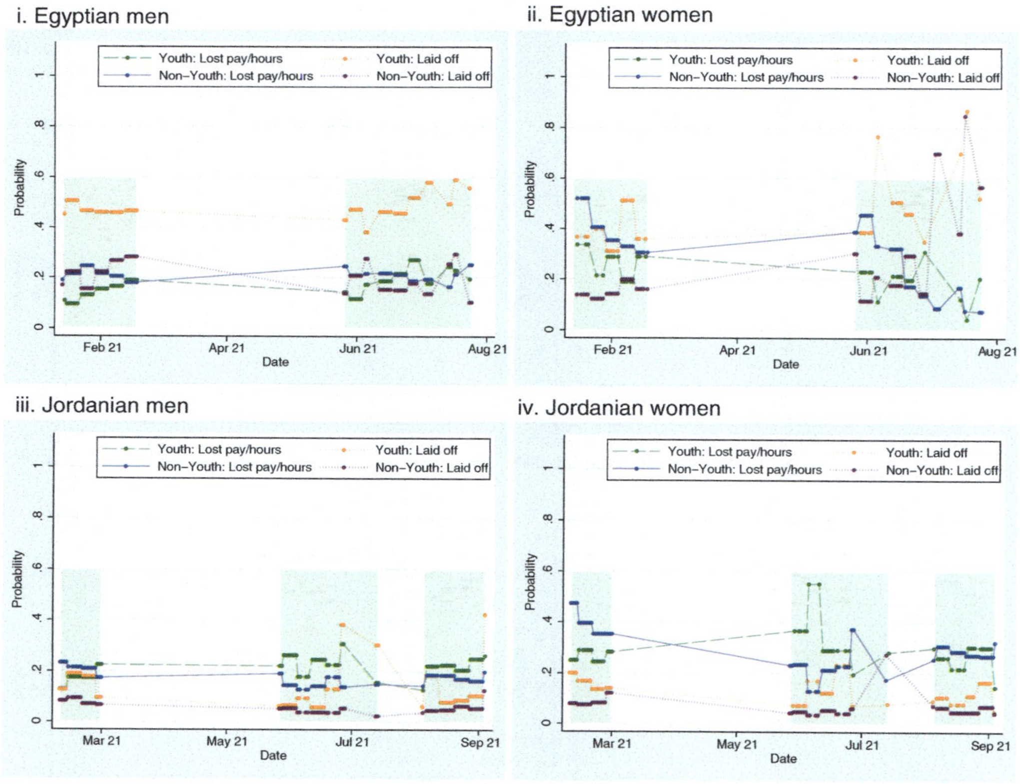

Fig. 5.4 Predicted probability of experiencing lost pay/hours and layoff by survey round, by country, by age-group and sex. Source: Authors' calculations based on ERF COVID-19 Household Monitors, rounds 1–5. Notes: Plotted probabilities during survey periods (shaded gray) are weekly medians, hence no time trend is observable within 7-day periods

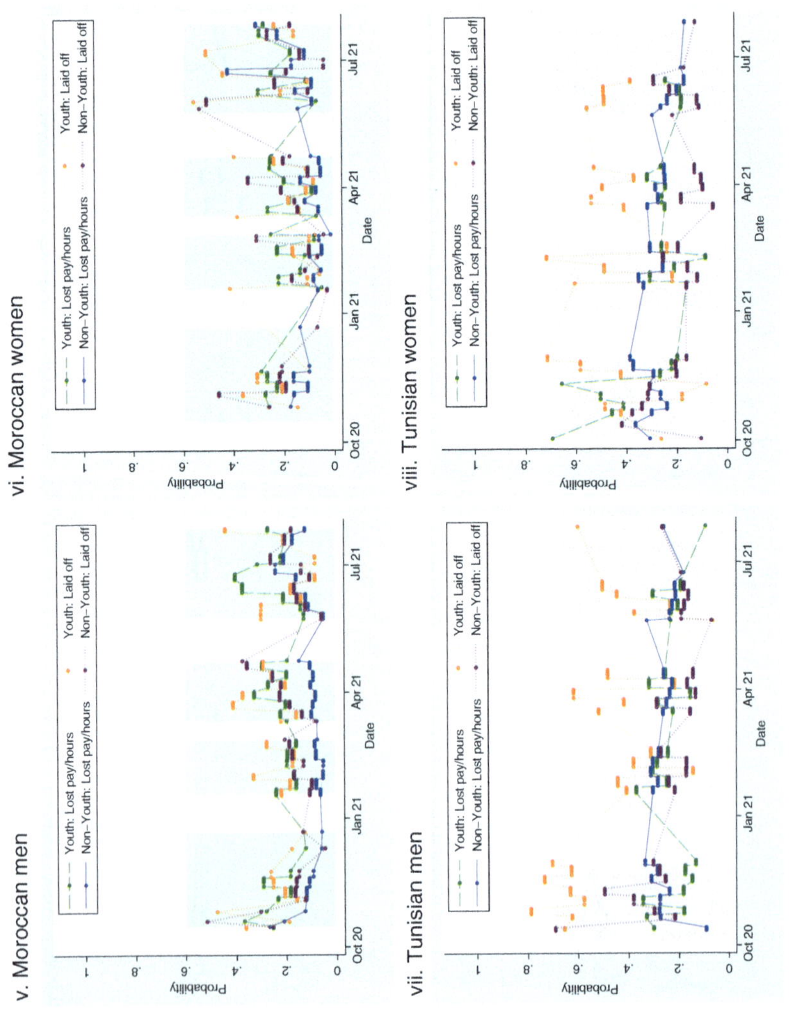

Fig. 5.4 (continued)

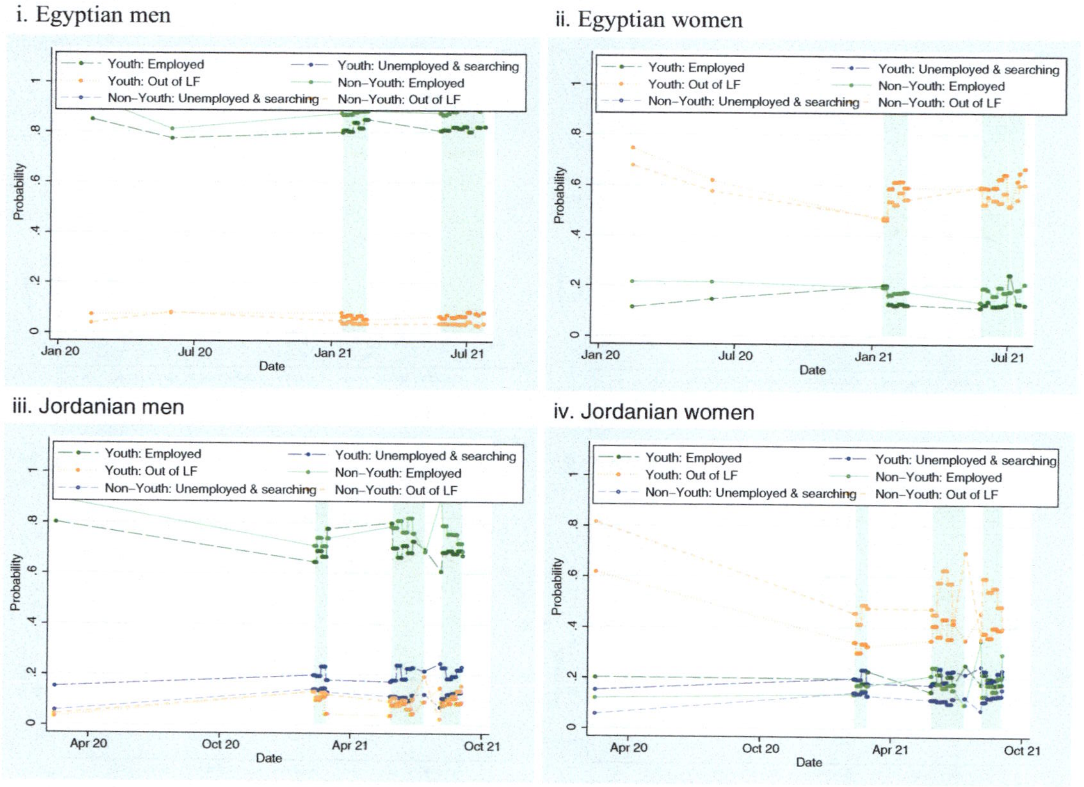

Fig. 5.5 Predicted probability of main job/activity by survey round, by country, by age-group and sex. Source: Authors' calculations based on ERF COVID-19 Household Monitors, rounds 0–5, and multinomial logit models reported in Table 5.2

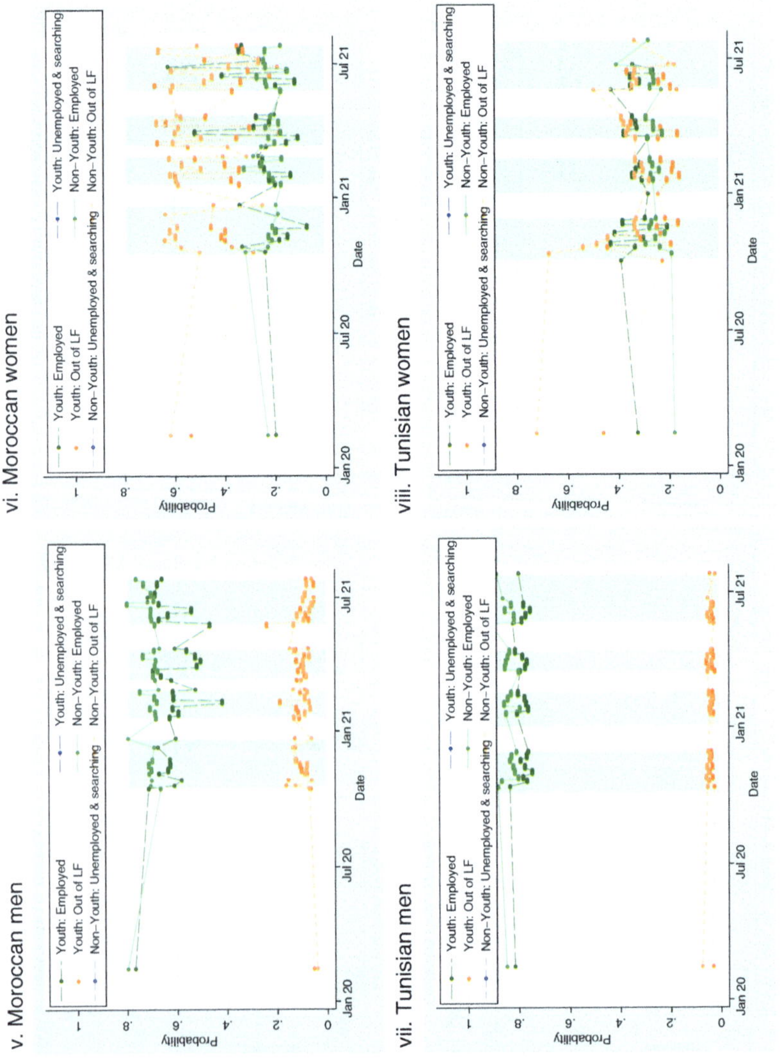

Fig. 5.5 (continued)

the first half of 2021. The outcomes of younger and older Tunisian women cannot be easily ranked.

Figure 5.5 shows the likelihoods of main employment outcomes for younger and older adults, and for women and men, across different phases of COVID. The prospect of attaining employment differs in its level between women and men. By contrast, the gap in probabilities between young and older workers is lower: among both sexes in Egypt, older workers outperform young adults in their prospect of attaining employment and in being economically active. In Jordan, older men slightly outperform younger men with regards to their employment prospects, but they also have elevated risks of remaining unemployed in search of jobs. Young Jordanian women exhibit slightly higher probabilities of being active, either employed or job searching, and lower probabilities of being inactive. In Morocco and Tunisia, older males again outperform young ones in terms of employment prospects, but among women the outcomes cannot be easily ranked between age groups.

Sensitivity Tests

The model specifications applied here have great merit, but some pitfalls must be acknowledged. Here we briefly discuss the potential issues and results of selected alternative specifications.

Most saliently, while the majority of explanatory variables in the multinomial logit regressions are validated by joint (cross-column) exclusion tests, some of the AMEs in individual columns are insignificant individually, meaning that the effects could be of either sign for particular employment outcomes. One explanation for the weak results is the heterogeneity and relatively small size of the sample. For alternative specifications, we have evaluated models disaggregated along important demographic fault lines, separately for the two sexes or age groups, or separately for workers starting in formal, informal, and inactive employment statuses (Tansel and Ozdemir 2019). Interaction of education and experience with demographic indicators was also considered. The problem with these alternative models is their lower degrees of freedom. They produced qualitatively similar but less significant results, generally corroborating the main specifications here.

Our means of controlling for panel dynamics—lagged worker status in Table 5.1, and workers' time-constant predispositions for various outcomes—could also come under criticism for being non-traditional, and could be compared against alternatives. Regressions controlling for lagged dependent variables or for individual fixed effects were estimated, but produced less consistent results (available on request) given the nature of the problem here. Namely: (1) the dependent variable does not change for a large share of workers in the limited time frame; (2) given the short time frame and a large cross section, individual-level fixed effects absorb too much of the limited variation in the dependent variable, while lagged dependent variable models exclude too many initial-period observations; and (3) multinomial logit with fixed effects is a computationally intensive, sensitive estimator.

Three, the joint use of time-invariant demographic variables, and sluggishly varying COVID stringency in regressions leads to some multicollinearity among covariates, which affects the efficiency of their coefficients. Alternative sets of covariates and sample delineations were considered, but clearly this issue of proper measurement of the slowly evolving market conditions across different phases of the pandemic calls for further analysis.

Four, the validity of multinomial logits hinges on the property of "independence of irrelevant alternatives"—the ratio of probabilities of any two outcomes should be independent of the set of available alternatives. In the case of the models reported in Tables 5.1, 5.2, 5.3, and 5.4, the Hausman specification tests fail to reject that the assumption holds, meaning that the results are not strongly systematically affected by the delineation of possible outcomes in the analysis.

5.5 Conclusion

This study investigated the impacts of the COVID pandemic and government responses to it on workers' employment outcomes in a group of developing countries characterized by high levels of labor market informality and precariousness. Focusing on young workers and women in Arab countries, we confirm that these groups were disadvantaged even before the onset of the pandemic, and that stringent policy responses to the pandemic extracted a further heavy toll on their prospects for economic participation and decent employment. Whether they were affected more adversely or more lastingly than older workers and men is, however, unclear. As of June–August 2021, men's employment prospects appeared to be recovering, among both younger and older cohorts. Women, on the other hand, continued witnessing stagnation of their employment prospects, being largely shunned by employers.

Differences were found across workers starting in different positions. In general, workers' pre-pandemic status or predisposition for specific employment types had significant effects on their later experiences and outcomes. Informal workers were seen to exit the labor market in greater numbers than formal workers. Among economically inactive workers, women faced an extreme risk of remaining inactive or unemployed, on the order of 95%, while the risk was somewhat lower, around 80%, among men. Meanwhile, formal private-sector workers—particularly from older cohorts, faced a distinctly lower risk of becoming inactive or unemployed, at 10–25%.

Experiences also differed across Arab countries. In terms of the risk of layoff, young workers of both sexes were highly disadvantaged in Egypt and Tunisia throughout the pandemic. In Jordan and Morocco, younger workers also faced somewhat elevated risks of experiencing lost pay/hours or being laid off compared to older workers. In Egypt and Jordan, women were at a greater risk than men to experience lost pay/hours, while the gaps were lower in Morocco and Tunisia. In fact, Tunisia saw fewer permanent layoffs, and less of exiting from the labor market among women.

Throughout the pandemic, younger male workers were less likely to be employed than older men in all four countries, while among women, only Egypt saw younger women being disadvantaged compared to older women. In terms of their propensity to be economically active, only Egypt—unlike other countries—saw younger workers of both sexes being less likely to be active than older workers. In Tunisia, the prospect of remaining employed was higher among older men, but so was the risk of being economically inactive, suggesting that their risk of remaining unemployed was lower than that of younger men.

In light of the differentiated trends faced by younger workers, an actionable policy-relevant question is: How should fresh graduates approach the labor market upon graduating? Should they accept the first informal employment offer in order to build their work experience, or should they hold off until decent employment opportunities present themselves? For women, the answer appears to be to accept informal employment, because historical evidence suggests that women starting in informal employment fare better down the line than those staying inactive. For male graduates this is less clear, and the recommendation may be, perversely, for them to hold off on accepting precarious work and stay "not in employment, education or training" (NEET), so as not to undermine their long-term career prospects. A brief spell of job-searching while unemployed or remaining NEET may allow them to get matched to better lifetime positions later on, perhaps because the time off serves as a signal of their latent qualities. Policymakers could help in facilitating better job matching by expanding the capacity of job centers, promoting education–industry coordination and re-skilling/upskilling of those done with formal education, and providing other information and material support to non-employed workers.

There is also a need to assist those most susceptible to career derailment, especially considering the longer-lasting COVID effects and other shocks that have arisen since the pandemic. Even before the onset of the pandemic, social protection programs and sectoral labor-market interventions provided valuable safety nets and helped to dampen informality in Arab countries, notably in Algeria, Egypt, Morocco and Tunisia (Kiaga and Leung 2020). The expansion of social protection that many Arab states undertook during the pandemic (like extending eligibility and benefits in Egypt's Takaful) is believed to have contributed to alleviating workers' hardships, and to the gradual recovery of their employment prospects. These efforts should now be maintained, regularized and further expanded for as long as the precarious labor market conditions prevail across the region.

References

AlAzzawi, S. 2023. Who can work from home in MENA? *Middle East Development Journal* 15 (1): 101–129. https://doi.org/10.1080/17938120.2023.2200729.

AlAzzawi, S., and V. Hlasny. 2022. Youth labor market vulnerabilities: Evidence from Egypt, Jordan and Tunisia. *International Journal of Manpower* 43 (7): 1670–1699.

———. 2023. Youths' employment vulnerability amidst a lingering Crisis: Evidence from the Middle East. *Hacienda Pública Española/Review of Public Economics* 247 (4): 155–186.

Assaad, R., and C.G. Krafft. 2014. *Youth transitions in Egypt: School, work, and family formation in an era of changing opportunities*. Silatech working paper no. 14-1. Doha: Silatech.

Assaad, R., R. Hendy, M. Lassassi, and S. Yassin. 2020. Explaining the MENA paradox: Rising educational attainment yet stagnant female labor force participation. *Demographic Research* 43: 817–850.

Assaad, R., C.G. Krafft, M.A. Marouani, S. Kennedy, R. Cheung, and S. Wahby. 2022. *Egypt COVID-19 country case study.* ILO/ERF report, February.

Aygun, A.H., S. Koksal, and G. Uysal. 2022. *Unpacking the effects of Covid-19 on labor market outcomes: Evidence from Turkey*. ERF working paper 1533.

Delaporte, I., and W. Peña. 2020. *Working from home under COVID-19: Who is affected? Evidence from Latin American and Caribbean countries*. CEPR COVID economics 14.

Dingel, J.I., and B. Nieman. 2020. How many jobs can be done at home? *Journal of Public Economics* 189: 104235.

Fehling, M., Z.M. Jarrah, M.E. Tiernan, S. Albezreh, M.J. VanRooyen, A. Alhokair, and B.D. Nelson. 2015. Youth in crisis in the Middle East and North Africa: A systematic literature review and focused landscape analysis. *Eastern Mediterranean Health Journal* 21 (12): 916–930.

Hale, T., A. Petherick, T. Phillips, J. Anania, B.A. de Mello, N. Angrist, R. Barnes, T. Boby, E. Cameron-Blake, A. Cavalieri, M. Di Folco, B. Edwards, L. Ellen, J. Elms, R. Furst, L.G. Ribeiro, K. Green, R. Goldszmidt, L. Hallas, N. Kamenkovich, B. Kira, S. Laping, M. Luciano, S. Majumdar, T.M. Oliveira, R. Nagesh, A. Pott, L. Ren, J. Sampaio, H. Tatlow, W. Torness, A. Wade, S. Webster, A. Wood, H. Zha, Y. Zhang, and A. Vaccaro. 2023. *Variation in government responses to COVID-19, version 15*. Blavatnik School of Government Working Paper, June. www.bsg.ox.ac.uk/covidtracker. Accessed 20 Oct 2023.

Hatayama, M., M. Viollaz, and H. Winkler. 2020. *Jobs' amenability to working from home: Evidence from skills surveys for 53 countries*. World Bank Policy Research WP 9241. Washington, DC: World Bank.

ILO (International Labour Organization). 2020a. *Global employment trends for youth 2020: Africa*. https://www.ilo.org/wcmsp5/groups/public/%2D%2D-dgreports/%2D%2D-dcomm/documents/briefingnote/wcms_737670.pdf. Accessed 20 Oct 2023.

———. 2020b. *Global employment trends for youth 2020: Arab States*. https://www.ilo.org/wcmsp5/groups/public/%2D%2D-dgreports/%2D%2D-dcomm/documents/briefingnote/wcms_737672.pdf. Accessed 20 Oct 2023.

———. 2020c. *ILO monitor: COVID-19 and the world of work. Sixth edition updated estimates and analysis*. https://www.ilo.org/wcmsp5/groups/public/@dgreports/@dcomm/documents/briefingnote/wcms_755910.pdf. Accessed 20 Oct 2023.

———. 2020d. *Preventing exclusion from the labour market: Tackling the COVID-19 youth employment crisis*. ILO Policy Brief, 27 May.

ILO and ERF (International Labour Organization and Economic Research Forum). 2021. *Rapid labour force survey on the impact of COVID-19 in Tunisia*, February, Advancing the Decent Work Agenda in North Africa (ADWA) Project. www.ilo.org/wcmsp5/groups/public/%2D%2D-africa/%2D%2D-ro-abidjan/documents/publication/wcms_791949.pdf. Accessed 20 Oct 2023.

Kiaga, A., and V. Leung. 2020. *The transition from the informal to the formal economy in Africa global employment policy.* Review background paper 4, December. International Labour Organization.

OAMDI (Open Access Micro Data Initiative). 2021. *COVID-19 MENA Monitor household survey: Egypt, Jordan, Morocco, Tunisia (CCMMHH)*. http://www.erfdataportal.com/index.php/catalog. Version 5.0 of the licensed data files; CCMMHH Nov-2020-Aug-2021. Egypt: Economic Research Forum (ERF).

Prince, H., Y. Halasa-Rappel, and A. Khan. 2018. *Economic growth, youth unemplyment, and political and social instability: A study of policies and outcomes in post-Arab Spring Egypt,*

Morocco, Jordan and Tunisia. UNRISD working paper 2018-12. Geneva: United Nations Research Institute for Social Development.

Saltiel, F. 2020. Who can work from home in developing countries. *CEPR COVID Economics* 7: 104–118.

StataCorp. 2015. *Stata statistical software: Release 14*. College Station, TX: StataCorp LP.

Tansel, A., and Z.A. Ozdemir. 2019. Transitions across labor market states including formal/informal division in Egypt. *Review of Development Economics* 23 (4): 1674–1695.

Tzannatos, Z. 2021. The youth bulge: The mismeasured, misunderstood and mistreated Arab youth. In *Routledge handbook on the Middle East economy*, ed. H. Hakimian, 302–318. London: Routledge.

UNDP. 2020. *COVID-19: Socio-economic impact*. www.undp.org/coronavirus/socio-economic-impact-covid-19. Accessed 20 Oct 2023.

UN Women, Arab States. 2021. *Assessment of the impact of COVID-19 on vulnerable women in Jordan*. https://arabstates.unwomen.org/en/digital-library/publications/2021/10/2021-assessment-of-the-impact-of-covid-19-on-vulnerable-women-in-jordan. Accessed 20 Oct 2023.

World Bank. 2020. *COVID-19 High-frequency monitoring dashboard*. www.worldbank.org/en/data/interactive/2020/11/11/covid-19-high-frequency-monitoring-dashboard. Accessed 20 Oct 2023.

Shireen AlAzzawi is a Teaching Professor, Economics Department, Santa Clara University, USA and Research Fellow at the Economic Research Forum, Egypt. Shireen's research focuses on labor and gender issues, poverty and inequality, and international trade. Her research has been published in the *Journal of African Economies, Review of Income and Wealth, International Journal of Manpower, Economic Development and Cultural Change and The Journal of International Trade and Economic Development*, among other scholarly journals. Shireen received her Ph.D. in Economics from the University of California, Davis and has Masters degrees from Stanford University and the American University in Cairo.

Vladimir Hlasny is an Associate Professor, Economics Department, Ewha Womans University, Seoul, Korea. He conducts research in labor and welfare economics, particularly in relation to Asia and the Middle East region. His research has been published in general-interest journals including the *World Bank Economic Review*, *Journal of Economic Surveys*, and *Social Science Quarterly*. He holds a doctorate in Economics from Michigan State University.

Chapter 6
The Effect of the COVID-19 Pandemic on Faculty Well-being: A Study of Academic Staff at Three Colleges in New York State

Catherine White Berheide, Megan A. Carpenter, and David A. Cotter

6.1 Job Demands, Resources, and Well-being

The public health measures that countries enacted to mitigate the spread of COVID-19, including stay-at-home orders, masking, social distancing, and school and business closures, negatively affected their citizens' well-being (Conroy et al. 2021; Passavanti et al. 2021). These negative effects on well-being fell more heavily on specific groups (Zhou and Kan 2021), including the poor (Lewin et al. 2023), women (Borrescio-Higa and Valenzuela 2021), and parents (Heers and Lipps 2022). The effects may also have varied by occupation. The pandemic's effect on faculty[1] well-being has not been adequately studied, despite the pressure they were under to adjust instructional delivery, salvage scholarly work, and increase service to address rapidly changing public health standards (Carpenter et al. 2021; Docka-Filipek and Stone 2021).

Nomaguchi and Milkie (2020, 199) defined well-being "broadly to include subjective well-being (e.g., life satisfaction, life meaning, loneliness), emotional health (e.g., anger, guilt), mental health (e.g., depression, anxiety), and physical health."

[1] In the United States, the members of the instructional staff who hold academic rank at an institution of higher education are called faculty. In some other countries, the people in these teaching positions are called academic staff. We use the terms faculty and academic staff interchangeably.

C. W. Berheide (✉)
Department of Sociology, Skidmore College, Saratoga Springs, NY, USA
e-mail: cberheid@skidmore.edu

M. A. Carpenter
Department of Psychology, St. Lawrence University, Canton, NY, USA
e-mail: mcarpenter@stlawu.edu

D. A. Cotter
Department of Sociology, Union College, Schenectady, NY, USA
e-mail: cotterd@union.edu

C. Suter et al. (eds.), *Well-being During the Pandemic*, Social Indicators Research Series 90, https://doi.org/10.1007/978-3-031-63440-6_6

This study focuses on one specific measure of each of these four dimensions of well-being. We operationalized subjective well-being as satisfaction with work-life balance, emotional health as feeling used up, mental health as depression, and physical health as sleep problems.

6.1.1 Job Demands-Resources Theory

A job demands-resources model has become common in research on workplace well-being (Demerouti and Bakker 2023; Watanabe and Falci 2016). Such models have attempted to account for the demands placed upon workers and the resources that workers had to address the demands, both of which can be psychological, organizational, temporal, or physical. In general, theoretical arguments and empirical findings have suggested that work settings that provided more resources than job demands or those where the ratio of resources to demands was balanced resulted in greater worker well-being (Bakker et al. 2023). Notably, during a crisis like COVID-19, not only must the demands and resources of the particular job and individual incumbent be considered, but organizational contexts and external demands and resources, especially family ones, also need to be taken into account (Demerouti and Bakker 2023).

When applied to academic workplaces, job demands-resources models have predicted various work outcomes, including work-life balance, exhaustion, and turnover (Naidoo-Chetty and du Plessis 2021; Watanabe and Falci 2016). The purpose of this research is to examine mechanisms leading to greater faculty well-being. Specifically, we examine the extent to which demands and resources can explain differences in work-life balance satisfaction, feeling used up, depression, and sleep problems in the first few months of the COVID-19 pandemic. For example, we expected that because women and parents experienced more demands at home, they would report less work-life balance satisfaction, feeling used up more often, more depression symptoms, and more frequent sleep problems than men and those who were not actively taking care of children at home during the shutdown in the spring and summer of 2020. We also expected that the more teaching and research resources (i.e., time, space, and concentration) a faculty member had and the fewer demands at work (e.g., emotional labor) and at home (e.g., housework responsibility) would be associated with more work-life balance satisfaction, feeling used up less often, fewer depression symptoms, and less frequent sleep problems.

6.1.2 Gendered Institutions: Higher Education and Family

The ideal worker norm that has organized managerial and professional work, such as that of a professor, has assumed that a worker can devote himself to a full-time, life-long job, unencumbered by responsibilities outside of work because someone else takes care of his personal and family's needs (Acker 1990, 2006). Gendered family and workplace arrangements usually have made it easier for men and harder for women to combine work and family. When their work and family lives have not aligned, people have experienced work-family conflict, which is a particular form of role conflict where the demands of work interfere with an individual's ability to meet the demands of family (Berheide and Anderson-Hanley 2012; Jacobs and Winslow 2004). The demands of work (e.g., number of hours worked) and the demands of home (e.g., caregiving responsibilities) have been the primary sources of work-family conflict, which can have a negative effect on employees' well-being (Odle-Dusseau et al. 2013; Walsh 2013). Odle-Dusseau et al. (2013, 27) argued that "creating an organizational culture that supports employees in both their work and family roles is important for employee well-being."

Parsons and Priola (2013) observed that higher education has been structured for workers with families supporting their careers, specifically for men with stay-at-home wives. As more women have become the primary or co-breadwinner in their families in the last few decades, these traditionally gendered workplace and family arrangements have created conflicts for workers, increasingly for men as well as women (Hill et al. 2014; Lundquist et al. 2012), including professors who have often struggled to align their work and family lives (Berheide and Anderson-Hanley 2012; Berheide et al. 2022b). Competing demands from workplace and home have created conflicts for academic staff with women faculty reporting greater work and family conflict than men (Berheide and Anderson-Hanley 2012; Berheide et al. 2022b).

6.1.3 Well-being During the COVID-19 Pandemic

6.1.3.1 Subjective Well-being During the COVID-19 Pandemic: Work-Life Balance Satisfaction

In this research, we argue that the pandemic occurred in workplaces and families with preexisting gendered divisions of labor. The pandemic exacerbated disadvantages employed parents faced (Collins et al. 2021) and reinforced the traditional gendered division of labor among US parents while upsetting it for Australian parents (Ruppanner et al. 2021). In a national survey of parents with children under the age of 18, Patrick et al. (2020) reported that the pandemic disrupted the childcare arrangements of parents with children from birth to five and six to twelve (39% and 23% respectively) more than those with teenagers (8%). School and daycare closures led to many US mothers dropping out of the labor force to take care of their children and supervise remote learning. Mothers were also four to five times more likely than fathers to reduce work hours to care for children (Collins et al. 2021). Academic women also spent more time on childcare, including facilitating their children's distance learning, than academic men (Burk et al. 2021; Carpenter et al. 2021).

While some research (e.g., Burk et al. 2021; Kotini-Shah et al. 2022; Weyandt et al. 2020) has explored the effect of the pandemic on work-life balance at research universities, academic staff at predominantly undergraduate institutions have rarely been studied, although they did constitute about a quarter of Docka-Filipek and Stone's sample (2021). This chapter seeks to remedy this gap by analyzing survey data from professors at three colleges. Compared to university faculty, academic staff at colleges in the United States have lower research expectations and higher teaching and service demands (Wolf-Wendel and Ward 2006).

6.1.3.2 Emotional Health During the COVID-19 Pandemic: Feeling Used up

The second form of well-being is emotional health, which Petcu et al. (2023, 6) defined as "the ability to generate positive thoughts and to adapt when faced with adversity and stress." According to Shen and Slater (2021), most academic staff in Northern Ireland reported poor emotional well-being during the COVID-19 pandemic with stress accounting for about one quarter of the variance in it (see also Winfield and Paris 2022). Eubank et al. (2023) concluded that faculty reported increasing levels of stress, helplessness, and negative self-efficacy across the course of the pandemic from the spring of 2020 to the spring of 2021. Kotini-Shah et al. (2022) found that this elevated stress spanned both home and work and was particularly pronounced among pre-tenure women with young children.

Kotini-Shah et al.'s (2022) study of health sciences faculty revealed high levels of work stress among 73% of respondents and high levels of home stress among 60%. Their latent class analysis identified two clusters of academic staff with high stress both at work and at home: a group most likely to be pre-tenure women faculty with young children at home and the second a group characterized by women who were tenured associate professors with children at home. A third cluster, which was more likely to consist of tenured full professors who were men without young children, exhibited moderate work stress and lower home stress. The final cluster of academic staff who exhibited low work- and home-related stress was mostly made up of men without children in visiting and lecturer positions.

Work and personal life demands have long varied by career stage for academic staff. The years immediately following receipt of the doctorate have been critical for launching one's career and for starting a family. This overlap between the prime childbearing and working years may negatively affect the well-being of faculty who want to combine a career with a family. Assistant and associate professors (who were more likely to have young children) have faced greater pressures to demonstrate high levels of productivity and skill in these domains than full professors as tenure and promotion have depended on it. Pre-pandemic, full professors, who no longer face promotion-related demands, reported less work-life conflict (Catano et al. 2010) and occupational stress (Meng and Wang 2018) than either assistant or associate professors did while assistant professors typically experienced more emotional exhaustion than other faculty (Sabagh et al. 2018). During the pandemic, full professors engaged in less emotional labor than assistant and associate professors did (Berheide et al. 2022a).

6.1.3.3 Mental Health During the COVID-19 Pandemic: Depression

According to a World Health Organization report (WHO 2022), global rates of depression increased in the first year of the pandemic as a result of social isolation, financial hardship, contracting the virus, fear of contracting the virus, grieving the deaths of friends and family, exhaustion, and loneliness. Countries with the highest COVID-19 transmission and mortality rates, such as the United States, incurred the greatest increases in psychological distress (Olff et al. 2021). The little scholarship analyzing the pandemic's effect on faculty mental health has suggested academic staff experienced worsened mental health (Docka-Filipek and Stone 2021; Ozamiz-Etxebarria et al. 2021; Weyandt et al. 2020).

Pre-pandemic, the prevalence of depression was estimated to be twice as high among women than men (Brody et al. 2018; Kuehner 2017). The gender difference in work-life conflict has been one factor that has contributed to this disparate mental health outcome (Hammarström et al. 2009). By most accounts, the pandemic has exacerbated the depression gender gap (Borrescio-Higa and Valenzuela 2021). However, it is unclear whether this gap widened among academic staff during the lockdown. While some research has found no gender differences in depression symptoms among faculty during the pandemic (Ozamiz-Etxebarria et al. 2021; Weyandt et al. 2020), other scholarship has reported gender differences, potentially as a consequence of the emotional labor expected of academic women at work and the emotion work expected of them in the home (Berheide et al. 2022a; Docka-Filipek and Stone 2021).

Research on associations between parenthood and depression symptoms has been mixed; some reports showed negative mental health consequences (Helbig et al. 2006), some claimed distinct psychological benefits (Evenson and Simon 2005), and others demonstrated no relationship (Bures et al. 2009). Pandemic era research, however, has shown parents experienced more depression symptoms during periods of social isolation as they were forced to care for and educate their children while also maintaining their paid worker roles (Xue and McMunn 2021). Among those who lost childcare because of the pandemic, 35% reported their mental health worsened (Patrick et al. 2020). Parents who adapted by working less or shifting their schedule to accommodate childcare needs were more likely to experience psychological distress (Xue and McMunn 2021). According to Russell et al. (2020), while mothers were more likely to make these compromises to their work lives, fathers tended to experience greater increases in psychological distress if they decreased their work hours because of increased childcare responsibilities. Though mothers may have done more childcare during the pandemic, fathers may have had a harder time adjusting to increased caregiving demands than mothers.

6.1.3.4 Physical Health During the COVID-19 Pandemic: Sleep Problems

Our fourth measure of well-being, sleep quality, represents one component of physical well-being. During the pandemic, rates of acute and chronic insomnia increased, as sleep quality decreased (Lin et al. 2021). Ruppanner et al. (2021) found that the pandemic negatively affected the quality of sleep for mothers, but not fathers, in the United States and for fathers, not mothers, in Australia. Among health sciences faculty at an urban research university in the United States, those who held the rank of either assistant or associate professor, were women, and had high work and home stress were especially likely to experience sleep disturbance during the pandemic (Kotini-Shah et al. 2022). The increase in sleep disturbance is particularly problematic as it is both a symptom of depression and a factor in its development (Harvey et al. 2011).

6.2 Data and Methods

6.2.1 Research Context

The three undergraduate institutions from which we drew the present study's sample are predominately white selective private liberal arts colleges in New York State. The three have similar sized student bodies (2100 to 2700 undergraduates), faculties (165 to 217), and small classes. They expect more scholarly productivity and less teaching (the equivalent of 18 semester hours per year) than most undergraduate institutions in the United States, while their shared governance systems make high service demands on faculty.

While the three colleges were very similar, there were several crucial differences. First, one of the colleges (Garnet[2]) used a trimester schedule, which meant that the transition to remote learning in March 2020 occurred at the end of the winter term for this college, but mid-semester for the other two (Scarlet and Cyan). It conducted the entire spring term online. All three colleges were fully remote from mid-March to the end of the 2019–2020 academic year. The campuses were closed to nearly all students, faculty, and staff until later in the summer of 2020.

We conducted this study between May and September 2020. Two of the three schools' institutional review boards approved this study, and the third institution's did not require additional approval. We asked the associate deans of faculty to distribute the study's recruitment email with the link to the electronic survey to their faculty. To be eligible, participants must have been employed by one of three colleges in a tenure-stream position.

Upon obtaining their consent, the survey instrument prompted respondents to complete a series of self-report measures about their position as a faculty member, the impact of the pandemic on their work and home life, familial responsibilities, mental health, and demographic data. As an incentive, we offered participants the option to enter a raffle for an iPad Pro.

---

[2] We substituted pseudonyms for the names of colleges.

Table 6.1 Participant demographics *(N* = 204*)*

	n(or *M*)	% (or *SD*)	*N*
Age, *M* (*SD*)	49.7	10.7	181
Gender, *n* (%)			194
• Cisgender women and gender non-conforming	104	53.6	
• Cisgender men	90	46.4	
Race, *n* (%)			197
• White	165	83.8	
• Black, Hispanic, Asian and other	32	16.2	
Children, *n* (%)			168
• Any children 0–12	61	36.3	
• Any children 13–18	39	23.2	
Rank, *n* (%)			204
• Assistant professor	44	21.6	
• Associate professor	75	36.8	
• Full professor	85	41.7	
Tenure-status, *n* (%)			204
• Tenure track, not yet tenured	43	21.1	
• Tenured	161	78.9	
Marital status, *n* (%)			186
• Single (never married)	17	9.1	
• Married	152	81.7	
• Widowed/separated/divorced	17	9.2	
Sexual orientation, *n* (%)			187
• Straight	166	88.8	
• Lesbian, gay, bisexual+	21	11.2	

Note. When we had fewer than five respondents in a category, we collapsed it into a broader demographic group to protect participant confidentiality, which resulted in four collapsed identity groups: cisgender women with gender non-conforming; Black, Hispanic, Asian, and other; widowed, separated, and divorced; and lesbian, gay, bisexual and other sexual orientations

As Table 6.1 shows, 204 participants responded. The average age was 50 years old (SD = 10.70). Eleven percent of the respondents identified themselves as lesbian, gay, bisexual, or another sexual orientation that is not heterosexual.

6.2.2 *Well-being Measures*

6.2.2.1 Work-Life Balance Satisfaction

To measure subjective well-being, we assessed participants' work-life balance satisfaction during the pandemic (e.g., "Since COVID-19, how satisfied are you with the balance between your professional and personal life?"). Participants rated their response on a six-point Likert scale from one (very dissatisfied) to six (very satisfied). As Table 6.2 shows, on average, participants were somewhat dissatisfied with work-life balance during the pandemic (M = 3.19, SD = 1.51).

Table 6.2 Pearson correlations, means, and standard deviations for study variables ($N = 204$)

Study variables	1	2	3	4	5	6	7	8	9	10
1 WLB satisfaction		−.44***	−.35***	−.35***	.28***	.07	.10	−.23***	.07	−.13*
2 Feeling used up			.28***	.28***	−.08	.06	.02	.20**	.09	.02
3 Depression				.36***	−.09	−.05	−.10	.06	−.06	−.01
4 Sleep problems					−.14*	.06	−.05	.04	.05	.22***
5 Cisgender man						.14*	.06	.08	−.06	−.17**
6 White							.07	.16**	−.10	−.11
7 Significant other								.20**	.08	−.14*
8 Any kids 0–12									−.06	−.01
9 Any kids 13–18										.14*
10 Other care										
11 Housework responsibility										
12 Garnet College										
13 Scarlet College										
14 Tenured										
15 Full professor										
16 On leave Spring 2020										
17 Teaching and research resources										
18 Emotional labor										
19 Scholarly productivity										
20 Worked more										
Mean	3.19	4.13	12.62	1.20	0.46	0.84	0.86	0.36	0.23	0.26
SD	1.51	0.96	8.93	1.03	0.49	0.36	0.34	0.44	0.38	0.42
Range	1–6	1–5	0–42	0–3	0–1	0–1	0–1	0–1	0–1	0–1

Study variables	11	12	13	14	15	16	17	18	19	20
1 WLB satisfaction	−.09	.18**	−.04	.14*	.36***	−.00	.60***	−.29***	.36***	−.14*
2 Feeling used up	−.04	.03	−.06	−.12*	−.20**	−.16**	−.48***	.30***	−.31***	.20**
3 Depression	.10*	−.05	.08	−.07	−.16*	.18**	−.34***	.30***	−.21***	−.05
4 Sleep problems	.01	−.08	.11	.01	−.07	.04	−.28***	.26***	−.23***	.13*
5 Cisgender man	−.14*	.10	−.07	.12*	.24***	−.04	.21***	−.24***	.07	.01
6 White	−.06	.08	−.02	.20**	.15*	.07	.03	−.19**	−.05	−.12*
7 Significant other	−.70***	.09	−.20**	−.03	.01	−.00	.06	−.16*	−.03	.00
8 Any kids 0–12	−.15*	−.06	.02	−.04	−.18**	.00	−.26***	−.03	−.12*	−.10
9 Any kids 13–18	−.11	−.06	.00	.17**	.08	−.12*	−.02	.05	−.10	.22***
10 Other care	.06	−.13*	.10	.08	−.02	.12*	−.12*	.18**	−.03	−.03
11 Housework responsibility		−.14*	.14*	−.06	−.13*	.08	−.08	.14*	.02	−.07
12 Garnet College			−.39***	.10	.16*	.07	.14*	−.17**	−.10	.03
13 Scarlet College				−.04	−.15*	.06	−.13*	.08	.04	−.13*
14 Tenured					.44***	−.02	.23***	−.16*	.10	.02
15 Full professor						−.10	.37***	−.26***	.18**	.00
16 On leave Spring 2020							−.07	.02	.01	−.44***
17 Teaching and research resources								−.32***	.44***	.03
18 Emotional labor									−.17**	.05
19 Scholarly productivity										.01
20 Worked more										
Mean	3.48	0.38	0.20	0.79	0.42	0.11	2.57	3.23	−1.26	3.97
SD	0.82	0.49	0.40	0.41	0.49	0.30	0.81	0.84	0.92	1.26
Range	1–5	0–1	0–1	0–1	0–1	0–1	1–5	1–5	−2–2	1–5

*$p < .05$, **$p < .01$, ***$p < .001$

Note: WLB: Work-Life Balance

6.2.2.2 Feeling Used up

To measure emotional health, we used one item from the General Social Survey Quality of Working Life Module. This item asked, "How often during the past month have you felt used up at the end of the day?" Response options ranged from one (never) to five (very often). The mean (4.13, *SD* = 0.96) revealed that on average respondents often felt used up.

6.2.2.3 Depression

To measure mental health, we used the seven-item depression subscale of the Depression, Anxiety, and Stress Scale (Lovibond and Lovibond 1995). We instructed participants to indicate how much each statement applied to them over the course of the *past week* (e.g., "I found it difficult to work up the initiative to do things"). Responses ranged from zero (did not apply to me at all) to three (applied to me very much or most of the time). Following standard scoring procedures for this diagnostic tool, we summed the seven items and then multiplied the sum by two, creating a range of 0 to 42 ($M = 12.62$, $SD = 8.93$). Recommended cut-off scores for depression diagnostic categories were: normal (0–9), mild (10–13), moderate (14–20), severe (21–27), and extremely severe (28+). Over half (58%) of the respondents scored high enough to meet the standard for at least mild depression (10+) and almost 10% met the criterion for extremely severe depression (28+). Internal consistency for this measure was high, $\alpha = .92$.

6.2.2.4 Sleep Problems

To measure physical health, we used one item from the Patient Health Questionnaire (PHQ-9) to assess the quality of participants' sleep (Kroenke et al. 2001). The survey asked participants "over the last *2 weeks*, how often have you been bothered by trouble falling or staying asleep, or sleeping too much?" Response options ranged from zero (not at all) to three (nearly every day). The mean ($M = 1.20$, $SD = 1.03$) indicated the respondents experienced several days of sleep problems in the last 2 weeks.

6.2.3 Demand Measures

6.2.3.1 Gender

We asked participants to indicate their gender identity from a list of options. Fewer than five faculty identified as gender non-conforming. To retain as much of the sample as possible, we chose to include the gender non-conforming faculty in the same category as cisgender women. We coded cisgender women and gender non-conforming faculty as zero and cisgender men as one, thereby creating a dummy variable for gender that contrasted all other genders to the dominant category—cisgender men. Slightly more than half (54%) identified as cisgender women or gender non-conforming.

6.2.3.2 Race

We asked participants to select all racial/ethnic identities that applied to them from a list and to type in any additional identities not on the list. Given the small number of Black, Hispanic, Asian, or other faculty and the need to protect participant confidentiality, we collapsed race/ethnic identity groups into two categories: Black, Hispanic, Asian, or other (coded as zero) and white (coded as one). Most academic staff identified as white (84%).

6.2.3.3 Parents of Children at Home

We separated children who lived in the respondent's home into two dummy variables, one for children 0 to 12 and the other for teenagers 13 to 18. The referent category were respondents who did not have minor children living at home. While just under half (48%) had no children at home at the beginning of the pandemic, 36% had children 12 or under, 23% had teenagers, and 7% had children in both age categories living with them.

6.2.3.4 Other Care

Those caring for others (not children or partners) either inside or outside the home were coded as one; those with no other caregiving responsibilities were coded as zero. Just over a quarter (26%) of the academic staff reported caring for someone other than their partner or children, such as a parent or friend.

6.2.3.5 Housework Responsibility

We measured the division of household labor by assessing five core household tasks, specifically cooking, washing dishes, grocery shopping, cleaning, and doing the laundry. To avoid a time bias, we did not ask how much time people spent on these tasks but rather who was most responsible for these tasks during the COVID-19 pandemic. Response options included: "neither of us do this task or this question is not applicable" (coded missing), "my significant other/partner always performs this task" (coded 1), "my significant other/partner usually performs this task" (coded 2), "we both share this task equally" (coded 3), "I am usually the one to perform this task" (coded 4), and "I am always the one to perform this task" (coded 5). We computed the mean score across the number of the five tasks that the respondent reported were done in their household. The 24 respondents who did not live with a significant other in the spring 2020 were coded as 5, that is as always the one to perform the task. The mean (3.48, *SD* = 0.82) denoted that the respondent was slightly more responsible for these core household tasks.

6.2.3.6 On Leave During the Onset of the Pandemic

During the shutdown, 11% (21) of the faculty respondents were on some type of leave, usually a sabbatical leave, and therefore not teaching. Those who were on leave were coded as one, and those who were teaching in spring 2020 were coded as zero.

6.2.3.7 Emotional Labor

We assessed *emotional labor demands* with a series of six questions adapted from El-Alayli et al. (2018). These six items measured whether faculty felt that they had to adjust their feelings when interacting with students (four items: e.g., "I was required to be 'artificially enthusiastic' to students") as well as whether they felt they had to help students deal with their emotions (two items: e.g., "I spent a lot of time helping students deal with stresses and difficulties"). Participants responded on a Likert-scale of 1 (strongly disagree) to 5 (strongly agree). Higher scores indicated more emotional labor. The emotional labor index had high reliability ($\alpha = .72$). On average, academic staff neither agreed nor disagreed with these six statements about emotional labor demands ($M = 3.23$, $SD = 0.84$).

6.2.3.8 Scholarly Productivity

To measure the *demands of scholarship*, we asked respondents, "To what extent have you been able to accomplish your scholarship and/or creative work during the COVID-19 pandemic?" The response options were −2 (I have been a lot less productive than before COVID-19), −1 (I have been a little less productive than before COVID-19), 0 (I have been about as productive as before COVID-19), 1 (I have been a little more productive than before COVID-19), and 2 (I have been a lot more productive than before COVID-19). A higher score indicated greater success in meeting demands for scholarly productivity. The mean (−1.26, $SD = 0.92$) denoted, however, that academic staff reported being a little less productive as scholars than before COVID-19.

6.2.3.9 Worked More

We measured changes in work schedule demands with the question: "In comparison to a typical pre-pandemic academic year, which of the following is true for the changes you made to your work schedule during the 2020–2021 academic year?" The response options ranged from one (I worked significantly less) to five (I worked significantly more) with a mean of 3.97 ($SD = 1.26$), revealing that on average faculty reported working slightly more each week following the switch to remote learning during the spring 2020 term.

6.2.4 *Resource Measures*

6.2.4.1 Lived with Significant Other

We created a dummy variable for whether the respondent was living with a significant other at least part-time during the beginning of the pandemic. Those who were living with a significant other (86%) were coded as one, those who were not were coded as zero. Almost 82% were married.

6.2.4.2 College of Employment

We created two dummy variables, one for the college on the trimester system (Garnet, 38%) and one for one of the two colleges that switched to remote instruction midway through the spring semester (Scarlet, 20%). The referent category was the third college (Cyan, 42%).

6.2.4.3 Tenured

We coded pre-tenure faculty as zero and those with tenure (79%) as one.

6.2.4.4 Full Professor

We asked participants to indicate their current rank. We coded assistant and associate professors as zero and full professors as one. Forty-two percent held the rank of full professor.

6.2.4.5 Teaching and Research Resources

To operationalize teaching and research resources, we asked six questions about whether faculty were able to dedicate "enough time" and "appropriate space" as well as whether they had "trouble concentrating" on teaching and research (e.g., "I have been able to dedicate enough time to my teaching"), reflecting material, temporal, and cognitive resources faculty felt they could deploy. The responses were a five-point Likert scale from "strongly disagree" to "strongly agree." After reverse-coding responses for the two concentration questions, we averaged the responses across the six items, with a high level of reliability ($\alpha = .77$). A higher score indicated that a faculty member reported having more time, space, and ability to concentrate for work. The mean of 2.57 ($SD = 0.81$) denoted that academic staff were slightly more likely to disagree that they had enough resources for their teaching and research.

6.2.5 Missing Data

A missing value analysis indicated 75% of cases had no missing data and another 5% only had missing data on one variable. Sixteen of the twenty variables had missing data. Little's Missing Completely at Random analysis was significant χ^2 $(63) = 97.76$, $p = .003$, indicating that the data were *not* missing completely at random. For example, all missing depression scores were from academic staff without any children 12 and under; six from cisgender men and two from cisgender women. Similarly, all seven missing values for sleep (five from cisgender men, two from cisgender women) stemmed from faculty without any children 12 and under. We replaced missing data with the grand mean.

6.2.6 Analysis Plan

We analyzed the survey data using IBM SPSS Version 28. First, we conducted descriptive and bivariate analyses (see Tables 6.1 and 6.2). Then, we ran ordinary least squares regressions to identify the significant predictors for the four measures of well-being (see Table 6.3). We performed collinearity diagnostics and found that no VIF value was greater than 2.20, indicating that there was no multicollinearity.

Table 6.3 Ordinary least squares regression predicting four measures of faculty well-being ($N = 204$)

	WLB satisfaction		Feeling used up		Depression		Sleep problems	
Variable	*b*	ß	*b*	ß	*b*	ß	*b*	ß
Cisgender man	0.50	.16**	0.02	.01	0.96	.01	−0.14	−.07
White	0.13	.03	0.30	.12	−0.94	−.04	0.33	.11
Lived with significant other	0.56	.13	−0.00	−.00	−1.21	−.05	−0.01	−.00
Children 0–12	−0.43	−.13*	0.21	.10	0.22	−.01	−0.02	−.01
Children 13–18	0.62	.16**	0.11	.04	−1.53	−.07	−0.11	−.04
Other care	−0.08	−.02	−0.03	−.01	−2.33	−.11	0.37	.15*
Housework responsibility	0.12	.07	−0.03	−.03	0.10	.01	−0.06	−.04
Garnet College	0.46	.15*	0.18	.09	−0.25	−.01	−0.05	−.02
Scarlet College	0.34	.09	−0.15	−.06	0.67	.03	0.24	.09
Tenured	−0.31	−.08	−0.06	−.03	1.05	.05	0.10	.04
Full professor	0.33	.11	−0.05	−.02	0.36	.02	0.15	.07
On leave Spring 2020	−0.26	−.05	−0.42	−.13	5.64	.19*	0.32	.10
Teaching and research resources	0.79	.42***	−0.46	−.39***	−2.61	−.24**	−0.21	−.16*
Emotional labor	−0.07	−.04	0.23	.20**	2.29	.22**	0.22	.18*
Scholarly productivity	0.28	.17**	−0.08	−.07	−0.94	−.10	−0.16	−.14
Worked more	−0.26	−.21***	0.11	.15*	0.30	.04	0.17	.20**
Constant	1.42		3.83***		10.23		−.09	
R^2	.51		.36		.21		.21	
Adj R^2	.47		.31		.14		.14	
F	12.06***		6.64***		3.02***		3.10***	

$^{*}p < .05$, $^{**}p < .01$, $^{***}p < .001$
Note: WLB: Work-Life Balance

6.3 Results

6.3.1 *Relationships Among the Four Measures of Well-being*

As Table 6.2 presents, the four measures of well-being were significantly correlated with each other. Work-life balance satisfaction was negatively correlated with feeling used up ($r = -.44$, $p < .001$), the number of depressive symptoms ($r = -.35$, $p < .001$), and the frequency of sleep problems ($r = -.35$, $p < .001$). Feeling used up, depression, and sleep problems were all positively correlated with each other.

6.3.2 *Do Demands and Resources Significantly Affect Well-being?*

As Table 6.3 shows, the only measure of well-being that gender and parental status predicted was work-life balance satisfaction. In contrast, teaching and research resources predicted all four measures of well-being, emotional labor demands predicted all of them except for work-life balance satisfaction, and working more during the pandemic than pre-pandemic predicted all of them except for depression. For three of the four well-being measures, teaching and research resources was the most powerful predictor, specifically for work-life balance satisfaction ($ß = 0.42$, $p < .001$), feeling used up ($ß = -0.39$, $p < .001$), and depression ($ß = -0.24$, $p = .005$). In contrast, for sleep problems, working more time had a stronger effect ($ß = 0.20$, $p = .008$) than resources ($ß = -0.16$, $p = .05$).

The predictors explained almost half of the variance in work-life balance satisfaction ($Adj\ R^2 = .47$, $p < .001$). In particular, parents of children 0 to 12 and faculty reporting working more hours during the pandemic than pre-pandemic reported less work-life balance satisfaction. Cisgender men, parents of teenagers, faculty working at Garnet College (the college that started a new term with the switch to remote instruction), faculty reporting more teaching and research resources, and those reporting greater scholarly productivity were more satisfied with their work-life balance.

The predictors explained a little less than a third of the variance in feeling used up ($Adj\ R^2 = .31$, $p < .001$). Academic staff who reported having more teaching and research resources felt used up less often. In contrast, those who performed more emotional labor and who worked more hours during the pandemic than pre-pandemic felt used up more often.

The predictors explained less than one-fifth of the variance in depression ($Adj\ R^2 = .14$, $p < .001$). Faculty on leave during the spring of 2020 scored almost six points higher on the 42-point depression index. For every additional point higher on the emotional labor index a faculty member scored, they were a little more than two points higher on the depression index. The more teaching and research resources faculty reported having, the lower their score on the depression index was by almost three points for each additional point on the resources index.

The predictors explained 14% of the variance in frequency of sleep problems ($Adj\ R^2 = .14$, $p < .001$). Caring for others (other than children or partner) inside or outside of the home predicted more frequent sleep problems as did performing more emotional labor and working more hours than pre-pandemic. Having more teaching and research resources and more scholarly productivity reduced the frequency of sleep problems.

6.4 Discussion

During the beginning of the pandemic in 2020, women faculty, parents of children from birth to 12, and faculty whose work hours had increased reported less work-life balance satisfaction. Almost 40% of the respondents were actively parenting children 12 and under when New York State shut down in March 2020. The presence of young children at home made it even more difficult for academic staff to get their jobs done during the shutdown. These results were consistent with those from a Swiss sample of the general population, which found that women and those with young children were especially overwhelmed by their increased responsibility for supervising their children during the pandemic (Heers and Lipps 2022). The pandemic disrupted whatever alignment academic staff had managed to achieve previously between their professional lives and their personal lives. This disruption to work-life balance fell most heavily on parents of younger children, especially women. In contrast, faculty without young children at home, particularly men, expressed higher levels of work-life balance satisfaction during the pandemic, probably because they were better able to work without interruption. In fact, about 10% reported they could get more work done during the pandemic shutdown because they spent less time on the normal interruptions of academic life—committee meetings, a student or colleague dropping by, etc. (see Carpenter et al. 2021). From the perspective of a job demands-resources model, the pandemic lowered at least some of the demands for this small subset of faculty. For most, though, a deficit of time, space, and concentration resources for their teaching and scholarship made the increased pandemic-related demands worse.

That 58% of the respondents reported enough symptoms to be categorized as experiencing at least mild depression raises important concerns about faculty mental health. Work-life balance dissatisfaction may be an important triggering factor for acute depression symptoms and as such should be considered when implementing mental health interventions for academic staff. In addition, sleep problems were significantly correlated with depression.

While the disruption to work-life balance was gendered, feeling used up, depression, and the frequency of sleep problems were not. Academic staff experiencing long-term sleep problems may be an especially important group to provide treatment to, as they may be more likely to develop chronic depression symptoms.

Gender has often been cited as a predictor of depression. Pre-pandemic estimates indicated that the prevalence of depression was twice as high among cisgender women as cisgender men (Brody et al. 2018; Kuehner 2017). There are several potential explanations for why the present study did not find a gender difference in this measure of well-being. First, it is difficult to ascertain whether college faculty ever demonstrated a gender difference in depression prevalence. It could be that college faculty are a unique population with mental health outcomes that differ from the general population. Faculty teaching in higher education have often reported struggling with work-life balance (Berheide et al. 2022b), overwork (Kinman and Wray 2014), work-related stress (Shen and Slater 2021), and burnout (Sabagh et al. 2018), all of which were associated with increased risk of depression. These work-related predictors of depression may have eclipsed any potential gender differences.

Alternatively, it may be that college faculty do typically show a gender difference in depression, but pandemic-related stressors may have closed this gap. For example, it may be the case that cisgender women faculty maintained their pre-pandemic rates of depression but cisgender men faculty experienced an increase during this time, especially cisgender men with young children, who suddenly found themselves taking on more childcare responsibilities as a result of school closures. Lending some support for this latter explanation, cisgender men with young children in our sample reported similar rates of depression to cisgender women both with and without young children. Unfortunately, we did not have large-scale empirical estimates of mental health outcomes for college faculty pre-pandemic, making it difficult to determine whether the lack of gender differences was a function of the pandemic itself or simply the typical pattern among this specific population.

Finally, although this lack of a relationship between depression and gender is inconsistent with some of the existing research on depression among academic staff during the pandemic, including Docka-Filipek and Stone's (2021) research with faculty, it is consistent with research conducted by Ozamiz-Etxebarria et al. (2021) and Weyandt et al. (2020), which also found no gender differences in depression symptoms among faculty. Given the often debilitating effects of depression, institutions of higher education should attend to the physical health, emotional health, mental health, and subjective well-being of their academic staff, indeed we would argue of their entire staff.

6.4.1 Limitations

Though the present study contributes to the growing body of literature on the consequences of the pandemic for well-being, it is not without limitations. We conducted this research with academic staff employed by three highly-ranked colleges, which differed in several meaningful ways from other types of higher education institutions in the US as well as globally with respect to resources as well as teaching, advising, and scholarly productivity demands. In addition, this study took place during the beginning of the pandemic in a part of the US that was hard hit early on.

This period covered the summer months when most academic staff normally would have been on vacation or engaged in their scholarship. Instead, many performed substantial amounts of pandemic-related service and course preparation for the fall semester. Despite these limitations, the current research is one of very few studies exploring the well-being of academic staff, and even fewer still exploring the effect of the pandemic on faculty well-being.

6.4.2 *Future Directions*

Future research must examine faculty well-being during times not defined by a global public health crisis. Institutions of higher education should track the long-term effects of pandemic-related challenges on faculty well-being, especially given the potential for negative effects on tenure and promotion cases as well as intentions to quit. These findings provide a snapshot into how the early stages of the pandemic affected the well-being of a relatively privileged group of workers. Future research needs to assess the long-term effects of the pandemic on the well-being of all workers, especially ones who did not hold secure jobs in a country of the global north that allowed them to work remotely.

6.5 Conclusion

The pandemic occurred in a gendered world, one where gendered organizations, especially workplaces and families, made it particularly easy for the challenges it created to fall most heavily on women and on parents of young children. Pre-existing gendered divisions of labor expected women to resume their traditional responsibility for the care of children even if it meant dropping out of the labor force. Employers all too often continued to expect workers to do their jobs, even remotely, without interruptions from children who were at home rather than in school or daycare. As a result, the pandemic exacerbated existing gender inequalities and worsened what little work-life alignment parents had achieved prior to the pandemic. While all three colleges gave untenured faculty the option to delay going up for tenure, that policy may not be enough to address the way differences in demands and resources affected faculty productivity. Among the select group of workers we studied, women and parents experienced greater decline in their subjective well-being, specifically their work-life balance satisfaction, during the lockdown.

These results raise the question of whether the decline in the subjective well-being of women and parents occurred simply because of their gender and the age of their children or whether it occurred because they were women and parents navigating the challenges of a pandemic within gendered organizations structured in ways that did not take into account the responsibilities of women and parents. Cisgender men and faculty without young children reported having more teaching and research resources as well as greater success in meeting scholarly productivity demands than cisgender women and parents.

These gendered organizations made it easy for one of the pandemic's biggest disruptions to fall on women and parents. As the world thinks about how to prepare for the possibility of future pandemics, it needs to consider how to restructure organizations, specifically how to degender families and workplaces, to better accommodate the needs of women and parents. Otherwise, both groups will continue to be at greater risk for declines in their well-being during any future pandemic than men and non-parents. To improve faculty well-being, colleges and universities also need to ensure they have sufficient resources to meet the demands of the job and that jobs demands, such as emotional labor, do not fall disproportionately on those faculty with the fewest resources.

Acknowledgements Start-up funds from Saint Lawrence University supported this research.

References

Acker, J. 1990. Hierarchies, jobs, bodies. *Gender & Society* 4: 139–158.

———. 2006. Inequality regimes. *Gender & Society* 20: 441–464.

Bakker, A.B., E. Demerouti, and A. Sanz-Vergel. 2023. Job demands–resources theory. *Annual Review of Organizational Psychology and Organizational Behavior* 10: 25–53.

Berheide, C.W., and C. Anderson-Hanley. 2012. Doing it all. *Advances in Gender Research* 16: 165–188.

Berheide, C.W., M.A. Carpenter, and D.A. Cotter. 2022a. Teaching college in the time of COVID-19. *Sex Roles* 86: 441–455.

Berheide, C.W., M. Watanabe, C. Falci, E. Borland, D.C. Bates, and C. Anderson-Hanley. 2022b. Gender, type of higher education institution, and faculty work-life integration in the United States. *Community, Work & Family* 25: 444–463.

Borrescio-Higa, F., and P. Valenzuela. 2021. Gender inequality and mental health during the COVID-19 pandemic. *International Journal of Public Health* 66: 1–9. https://doi.org/10.3389/ijph.2021.1604220.

Brody, D.J., L.A. Pratt, and J.P. Hughes. 2018. *Prevalence of depression among adults aged 20 and over. NCHS data brief, no 303*. Hyattsville, MD: National Center for Health Statistics. https://www.cdc.gov/nchs/products/databriefs/db303.htm. Accessed 12 Sep 2023.

Bures, R.M., T. Koropeckyj-Cox, and M. Loree. 2009. Childlessness, parenthood, and depressive symptoms among middle-aged and older adults. *Journal of Family Issues* 30: 670–687.

Burk, B.N., A.P. Mausold, and L. Oakleaf. 2021. Pandemic motherhood and the academy. *Leisure Sciences* 43: 225–231.

Carpenter, M.A., D.A. Cotter, and C.W. Berheide. 2021. I have no time for anything. *Advance Journal* 2 (3): 1–10. https://doi.org/10.5399/osu/ADVJRNL.2.3.3.

Catano, V., L. Francis, T. Haines, H. Kirpalani, H. Shannon, B. Stringer, and L. Lozanzki. 2010. Occupational stress in Canadian universities. *International Journal of Stress Management* 17: 232–258.

Collins, C., L. Ruppanner, L.C. Landivar, and W.J. Scarborough. 2021. The gendered consequences of a weak infrastructure of care. *Gender & Society* 35: 180–193.

Conroy, D.A., N.L. Hadler, E. Cho, A. Moreira, C. MacKenzie, L.M. Swanson, H.J. Burgess, J.T. Arnedt, and C.A. Goldstein. 2021. The effects of COVID-19 stay-at-home order on sleep, health, and working patterns. *Journal of Clinical Sleep Medicine* 17: 185–191.

Demerouti, E., and A.B. Bakker. 2023. Job demands-resources theory in times of crises. *Organizational Psychology Review* 13 (3): 209–236.

Docka-Filipek, D., and L.B. Stone. 2021. Twice a "housewife". *Gender, Work and Organization* 28: 2158–2179.

El-Alayli, A., A. Hansen-Brown, and M. Ceynar. 2018. Dancing backwards in high heels. *Sex Roles* 79 (3): 136–150.

Eubank, J.M., K.G. Burt, and J. Orazem. 2023. The faculty aren't alright. *Workplace: A Journal for Academic Labor* 34: 1–18. https://doi.org/10.14288/workplace.v34i.

Evenson, R.J., and R.W. Simon. 2005. Clarifying the relationship between parenthood and depression. *Journal of Health and Social Behavior* 46: 341–358.

Hammarström, A., A. Lehti, U. Danielsson, C. Bengs, and E.E. Johansson. 2009. Gender-related explanatory models of depression. *Public Health* 123: 689–693.

Harvey, A.G., G. Murray, R.A. Chandler, and A. Soehner. 2011. Sleep disturbance as transdiagnostic. *Clinical Psychology Review* 31: 225–235.

Heers, M., and O. Lipps. 2022. Overwhelmed by learning in lockdown. *Social Indicators Research* 164: 323–343.

Helbig, S., T. Lampert, M. Klose, and F. Jacobi. 2006. Is parenthood associated with mental health? *Social Psychiatry and Psychiatric Epidemiology* 41: 889–896.

Hill, P.W., M.A. Holmes, and J. McQuillan. 2014. The new STEM faculty profile. *Advances in Gender Research* 19: 3–20.

Jacobs, J.A., and S.E. Winslow. 2004. Overworked faculty. *Annals of the American Academy of Political and Social Science* 596: 104–129.

Kinman, G., and S. Wray. 2014. Work-related wellbeing in UK higher education—2014. University and College Union. https://uobrep.openrepository.com/bitstream/handle/10547/622171/HEwellbeingreport2014.pdf?sequence=3. Accessed 10 Oct 2023.

Kotini-Shah, P., B. Man, R. Pobee, L.E. Hirshfield, B.J. Risman, I.A. Buhimschi, and H.M. Weinreich. 2022. Work-life balance and productivity among academic faculty during the COVID-19 pandemic. *Journal of Women's Health* 31: 321–330.

Kroenke, K., R.L. Spitzer, and J.B.W. Williams. 2001. The PHQ-9. *Journal of General Internal Medicine* 16: 606–613.

Kuehner, C. 2017. Why is depression more common among women than among men? *The Lancet Psychiatry* 4 (2): 146–158.

Lewin, A.C., M. Shamai, and S. Novikov. 2023. Surviving in crisis mode. *Social Indicators Research* 165: 245–265.

Lin, Y.N., Z.R. Liu, S.Q. Li, C.X. Li, L. Zhang, N. Li, X.W. Sun, H.P. Li, J.P. Zhou, and Q.Y. Li. 2021. Burden of sleep disturbance during COVID-19 pandemic. *Nature and Science of Sleep* 13: 933–966.

Lovibond, P.F., and S.H. Lovibond. 1995. The structure of negative emotional states. *Behaviour Research and Therapy* 33: 335–343.

Lundquist, J.H., J. Misra, and K.A. O'Meara. 2012. Parental leave usage by fathers and mothers at an American university. *Fathering* 10: 337–363.

Meng, Q., and G. Wang. 2018. A research on sources of university faculty occupational stress. *Psychology Research and Behavior Management* 11: 597–605.

Naidoo-Chetty, M., and M. du Plessis. 2021. Systematic review of the job demands and resources of academic staff within higher education institutions. *International Journal of Higher Education* 10 (3): 268–284.

Nomaguchi, K., and M.A. Milkie. 2020. Parenthood and well-being. *Journal of Marriage and Family* 82: 198–223.

Odle-Dusseau, H.N., H.A. Herleman, T.W. Brit, D.W.D. Moore, and C.A. Castro. 2013. Family-supportive work environments and psychological strain. *Journal of Occupational Health Psychology* 18: 27–36.

Olff, M., I. Primasari, Y. Qing, B.M. Coimbra, A. Hovnanyan, E. Grace, R.E. Williamson, C.M. Hoeboer, and The GPS-CCC Consortium. 2021. Mental health responses to COVID-19 around the world. *European Journal of Psychotraumatology* 12: 1–12.

Ozamiz-Etxebarria, N., N.I. Mondragon, J. Bueno-Notivol, M. Pérez-Moreno, and J. Santabárbara. 2021. Prevalence of anxiety, depression, and stress among teachers during the COVID-19 pandemic. *Brain Science* 11 (9): 1–14. https://doi.org/10.3390/brainsci11091172.

Parsons, E., and V. Priola. 2013. Agents for change and changed agents. *Gender, Work and Organization* 20: 580–598.

Passavanti, M., A. Argentieri, D.M. Barbieri, B. Lou, K. Wijayaratna, A.S. Foroutan Mirhosseini, F. Wang, S. Naseri, I. Qamhia, M. Tangeras, M. Pelliciari, and C.-H. Ho. 2021. The psychological impact of COVID-19 and restrictive measures in the world. *Journal of Affective Disorders* 283: 26–35.

Patrick, S.W., L.E. Henkhaus, J.S. Zickafoose, K. Lovell, A. Halvorson, S. Loch, M. Letterie, and M.M. Davis. 2020. Well-being of parents and children during the COVID-19 pandemic. *Pediatrics* 146 (4): 1–8. https://doi.org/10.1542/peds.2020-016824.

Petcu, M.A., M.I. Sobolevschi-David, R.F. Crețu, S.C. Curea, A.M. Hristea, M.D. Oancea-Negescu, and D. Tutui. 2023. Telework. *International Journal of Environmental Research and Public Health* 20 (3): 1–18. https://doi.org/10.3390/ijerph20031811.

Ruppanner, L., X. Tan, W. Scarborough, L.C. Landivar, and C. Collins. 2021. Shifting inequalities? *Men and Masculinities* 24: 181–188.

Russell, B.S., M. Hutchison, R. Tambling, A.J. Tomkunas, and A.L. Horton. 2020. Initial challenges of caregiving during COVID-19. *Child Psychiatry and Human Development* 51: 671–682.

Sabagh, Z., N.C. Hall, and A. Saroyan. 2018. Antecedents, correlates and consequences of faculty burnout. *Educational Research* 60: 131–156.

Shen, P., and P. Slater. 2021. The effect of occupational stress and coping strategies on mental health and emotional well-being among university academic staff during the COVID-19 outbreak. *International Education Studies* 14 (3): 82–95.

Walsh, J. 2013. Gender, the work-life interface and wellbeing. *Gender, Work and Organization* 20: 439–453.

Watanabe, M., and C.D. Falci. 2016. A demands and resources approach to understanding faculty turnover intentions due to work–family balance. *Journal of Family Issues* 37 (3): 393–415.

Weyandt, L.L., A. Francis, E. Shepard, B.G. Gudmundsdóttir, I. Channell, A. Beatty, and G.J. DuPaul. 2020. Anxiety, depression, impulsivity, and mindfulness among higher education faculty during COVID-19. *Health Behavior and Policy Review* 7: 532–545.

WHO (World Health Organization). 2022. *COVID-19 pandemic triggers 25% increase in prevalence of anxiety and depression worldwide*. World Health Organization https://www.who.int/news/item/02-03-2022-covid-19-pandemic-triggers-25-increase-in-prevalence-of-anxiety-and-depression-worldwide.

Winfield, J.D., and J.H. Paris. 2022. A mixed method analysis of burnout and turnover intentions among higher education professionals during COVID-19. *Journal of Education Human Resources* 42 (2): 1–25. https://doi.org/10.3138/jehr-2021-0048.

Wolf-Wendel, L.E., and K. Ward. 2006. Academic life and motherhood. *Higher Education* 52 (3): 487–521.

Xue, B., and A. McMunn. 2021. Gender differences in unpaid care work and psychological distress in the UK Covid-19 lockdown. *PLoS One* 16 (3): 1–15. https://doi.org/10.1371/journal.pone.0247959.

Zhou, M., and M.-Y. Kan. 2021. The varying impacts of COVID-19 and its related measures in the UK. *PLoS One* 16 (9): 1–21. https://doi.org/10.1371/journal.pone.0257286.

Catherine White Berheide is Professor of Sociology at Skidmore College in Saratoga Springs, New York and Principal Investigator for the National Science Foundation ADVANCE PAID grant, "SUN—Skidmore Union Network: Supporting Women Faculty in STEM at Liberal Arts Colleges." A sociologist of work, she has numerous publications on women's paid work as well as women's unpaid work in the home and in the community, including three books she co-edited: *Gender Transformation in the Academy; Included in Sociology: Learning Climates That Cultivate Racial and Ethnic Diversity*; and *Women, Family, and Policy: A Global Perspective*.

Megan A. Carpenter is an Associate Professor of Psychology at Saint Lawrence University in Canton, New York. A social psychologist specializing in gender and sexuality, she studies how power dynamics influence casual sex behaviors, perceptions of sexual identities and behaviors, experiences of LGBTQ+ students on college campuses, and the impact of openly queer faculty on students' perceptions of the classroom as a "safe space."

David A. Cotter is Professor of Sociology at Union College in Schenectady, New York. A scholar of inequalities, he has published numerous articles on spatial and temporal variation in work-related gender inequalities and gender ideology as well as articles on couples' time use, rural poverty, and rural students' access to and success in STEM fields.

Chapter 7
Limited Social Contact at Work During the COVID-19 Pandemic and Shift Worker's Health and Well-being

Regina Skiba, Eileen McNeely, and Dorota Weziak-Bialowolska

7.1 Introduction

There are various types of work that require personal attendance. Shift work is conducted in enterprises where it is necessary to ensure the continuity of the production process. Work in which workers are assigned to "rotating" around-the-clock shifts (e.g. from morning to afternoon/evening to night shift; Messenger 2018) is present in many professions and occupations (Sweileh 2022). According to available data shift work in Europe is performed by about 20% of employees aged between 15 and 64 years (Eurostat 2023). In 2004 17.7%, almost 29 million employees in the EU-27, and in Poland almost 3.5 million (Eurostat 2014). Other data shows that in 2015, 21% of workers in Europe were shift workers (Eurofound 2017).

R. Skiba (✉)
Centre for Evaluation and Analysis of Public Policies, Faculty of Philosophy, Jagiellonian University, Cracow, Poland
e-mail: regina.skiba@uj.edu.pl

E. McNeely
Human Flourishing Program, Institute for Quantitative Social Science, Harvard University, Cambridge, MA, USA

D. Weziak-Bialowolska
Centre for Evaluation and Analysis of Public Policies, Faculty of Philosophy, Jagiellonian University, Cracow, Poland

Human Flourishing Program, Institute for Quantitative Social Science, Harvard University, Cambridge, MA, USA

Department of Quantitative Methods & Information Technology, Kozminski University, Warsaw, Poland

C. Suter et al. (eds.), *Well-being During the Pandemic*, Social Indicators Research Series 90, https://doi.org/10.1007/978-3-031-63440-6_7

7.1.1 Negative Effects of Shift Work

Work performed under specific conditions can have negative effects on health and various other domains of workers' lives. Many reviewed studies suggested that shift work, as work performed in rotation cycle shifts day and at night (Messenger 2018) might have serious adverse effects on physical health, well-being, and social and family life (Eurofound 2007). Night shifts cause circadian rhythm desynchronization, lack of sleep and fatigue (Leso et al. 2021). Shift work might have an impact on metabolism, and also could be a risk factor for diabetes, although the evidence is not conclusive (Szosland 2010). Working shifts outside daytime hours can have potential consequences for shift workers' mental health. Shift workers, particularly women, are at increased risk for poor mental health, especially depressive symptoms (Sweileh 2022; Torquati et al. 2019). Among shift workers, adverse health behaviors (unhealthy lifestyle habits) are also reported. Shift work can result in a low-quality diet and irregular eating patterns, increased smoking and poor sleep patterns (Nea et al. 2015). Some studies report a connection between shift or night-work and pathological consumption of alcohol consumption in different professions. The reasons for this can be self-medication of sleep problems or coping with stress and psychosocial problems typical for shift work (Richter et al. 2021). Social network, social engagement and stress are also indicated as potential mediators of disease in shift workers (Knutsson 2003). Building a social life is much more difficult when most activities are arranged according to the day-oriented rhythms of the general population. Shift work can lead to social marginalization (Kim et al. 2016). Being a shift worker or having long working hours can have negative effects on marital relationships and parental roles (Costa and Folkard 2010).

7.1.2 Limited Contact Between Workers Because of COVID-19 Pandemic

The COVID-19 disease contributed to changes in many different areas of our lives including work arrangements due to the pandemic restrictions. Recommendations and compliance with hygiene rules were implemented to prevent and manage the risk of COVID-19 infection in workplaces. It was necessary to reduce face-to-face contact between employees by changing the organization of work, for example by introducing remote work, shift work or rotational work in smaller teams and increasing use of technology, implementation of safety procedures (like physical distancing) and personal protective equipment (wearing masks and workwear; ILO 2020). According to Polish regulations, the prophylactic measures applied at the workplace should take into account the applicable legal regulations aimed at preventing, counteracting and reducing COVID-19, including restrictions and other rules of epidemic safety (Sejm Rzeczypospolitej Polskiej 2021). Thus, regardless of the generally applicable regulations, it is the employee's duty to organize work in such a way as to reduce the likelihood of an employee contracting COVID-19 as much as possible (Kancelaria Sejmu 2023). For this study, the changes in the organization of work involved modifications implemented between 2019, 2020, and 2021.

The following analyses show temporal associations between the results of employee surveys collected before the implemented changes (2019) and during the ongoing mandatory of COVID-19 restrictions (2020, 2021) and shift workers' health and well-being. The study focused on three research questions: Firstly, how does shift work impact on worker's health and well-being during COVID-19? Secondly, do work-related changes in a Polish garment factory impact on health and well-being of the workers? Thirdly, which are the health and well-being difference between rotating shift workers and only day workers?

7.2 Methods

7.2.1 Data Source

This study is based on the Worker Well-being Survey (WWBS) (Weziak-Bialowolska et al. 2020) which comprehensively assesses human flourishing at work and the state of working conditions conducted by a team of researchers from Harvard University's School of Public Health (Węziak-Białowolska et al. 2019). The concept of human flourishing encompasses five essential elements: strong social connections, both physical and mental health, happiness and life satisfaction, character and virtue, and meaning and purpose. The primary goal of this study is to measure and monitor participants' subjective well-being across workplace, medical, educational, and governmental settings using the researchers' flourishing index (Lee et al. 2021). The WWBS questionnaire focused on individual health and well-being, supportive relationships, and a set of self-reported work performance outcomes, such as self-reported work injuries, work quality, absenteeism, job satisfaction and work engagement (Weziak-Bialowolska et al. 2020).

The WWBS was tested on a sample of over 13,000 garment workers in China, Cambodia, Mexico, Sri Lanka, Poland and the United States and of over 5500 office and manufacturing employees of two Fortune 500 manufacturing companies in the U.S. For this study data from Poland was selected.

7.2.2 Participants and Sample Size

Data were collected from 660 garment industry workers from Poland in three waves: in 2019 before the COVID-19 pandemic, in 2020 and in 2021 during the spread of the coronavirus. All employees aged at least 18 years of age were eligible to participate in the survey. All participants provided their written informed consent prior to enrollment in the study. The data collection protocols (with respect to both survey and organization) were reviewed and approved by Harvard T. H. Chan School of

Public Health Institutional Review Board. More details on the sample and the study can be found in other published articles (Bialowolski et al. 2020; Lee et al. 2021; Weziak-Bialowolska et al. 2021a).

Only cases with information on shift work were included in the analysis (626), and therefore, 37 cases with no information were excluded from further analyses. The main analysis excludes only night workers (6) and office workers (27) leaving only the observations of factory floor employees (590). Table 7.1 presents the sociodemographic characteristics of the participants. Workers, who participated in the survey, had more than 10 years job tenure (76.9%), were mostly women (69.7%) and married (75.9%), with upper secondary (73.6%) or first-stage tertiary education (19.2%). Almost 60% of participants work on both day and night shifts (shift workers).

7.2.3 *Measures and Variable Specification*

7.2.3.1 Assessment of the Independent Variable

The WWBS survey questionnaire includes questions about the job type including "What is your usual work schedule/shift?" The answer categories were: "I work during the day," "I work at night," "Both". The category "Both" represents shift workers performing their duties on day and night rotations. Since there were only six participants in the group, who worked only nights, this category was excluded from the analysis.

7.2.3.2 Assessment of the Dependent Variables

The set of 26 variables chosen for this analysis corresponds to previous studies on shift workers described in the introduction part in the domain of (1) general health, (2) physical health (3) mental health, (4) well-being, (5) family life, (6) social relationships, (7) work-life balance and (8) adverse health behaviors.

Domain 1: General Health

Two questions about general health were selected: "How would you rate your general health?" (1 = poor to 5 = excellent; for the purpose of the analysis, the scale was inverted; Ware and Sherbourne 1992). "During the past 30 days, for about how many days did poor physical health or mental health keep you from doing your usual activities, such as taking care of yourself, work, or leisure?" (0–30; Moriarty et al. 2003).

Domain 2: Physical Health

The following physical health outcomes were examined by questions about self-rated physical health (0 = poor to 10 = excellent; Vanderweele 2017): number of days of poor physical health during the past 30 days (0–30 days; Moriarty et al.

Table 7.1 Characteristics of participants-garment industry workers from Poland

Characteristic	Total (N = 590) %	Day workers (N = 241) %	Shift workers (N = 349) %
What is your usual work schedule/shift?	100	40.9	59.2
Sociodemographic factors			
Gender			
Male	30.3	33.2	28.4
Female	69.7	66.8	71.6
Age			
Below 30	6.3	10.0	3.7
30–39	26.8	28.6	25.8
40–49	47.5	43.5	49.6
50–59	18.6	16.2	20.6
60+	0.8	1.7	0.3
Education			
Primary school	4.2	4.3	4.2
Lower secondary school	3.5	3.8	3.3
High school	73.9	66.7	78.9
College	8.3	9.4	7.5
University	10.1	15.8	6.1
Job tenure			
Up to 10 years	23.0	24.1	22.3
More than 10 years	77.0	75.9	77.7
Marital status			
Married	75.8	73.9	77.1
Widowed	3.0	1.8	3.8
Divorced	7.1	7.8	6.6
Separated	0.7	0.9	0.6
Single, never married	8.4	10.1	7.2
Non-married partner	5.0	5.5	4.7
Having children under the age of 18 years old			
0	38.2	38.9	37.8
1	33.0	32.4	33.4
2	25.6	24.1	26.6
3+	3.2	4.6	2.2
Taking care of an elderly			
0	60.5	58.4	61.9
1	27.4	29.4	26.1
2	9.6	8.9	10.1
3+	2.5	3.3	1.9

Source: Worker Well-being Survey (WWBS), Poland (Weziak-Bialowolska et al. 2020)

2003), number of days of impairing pain during the past 30 days (0–30; Moriarty et al. 2003), number of days with poor physical health or mental health, henceforth referred to as disability days (0–30). The measurement of scales listed above was included in the flourishing index (Vanderweele 2017) adapted from the set of healthy days questions of the Health-Related Quality of Life instrument (Moriarty et al. 2003). Questions about feeling at work pain and tiredness (1 = never to 4 = all the time) were included in the domain of physical health (Van Katwyk et al. 2000).

Domain 3: Mental Health
Two categories are included: mental health ("How would you rate the health of your mind (mental health)?" 0 = poor to 10 = excellent; flourishing index, Vanderweele 2017), and number of days of poor mental health ("Now thinking about your mental health, which includes stress, depression, and problems with emotions, for how many days during the past 30 days was your mental health not good?" 0–30; Moriarty et al. 2003).

Domain 4: Well-being
This domain focuses on the assessment of life satisfaction ("Overall, how satisfied (content) are you with your life these days?" 0 = not at all satisfied to 10 = extremely satisfied; Vanderweele 2017; Weziak-Bialowolska et al. 2021b), and the frequency of experiencing emotions such as sadness, depression, stress, and tiredness ("How often did you feel the following at work yesterday (or the last day you worked) on a scale of 1=never to 4=all the time?" Watson and Clark 1988; for the purpose of the analysis, the scale was inverted). All indices are included in the flourishing index (Vanderweele 2017).

Domain 5: Family Life
Family life domain was measured using a single question: "Please tell us how much you agree with the following: Demands of my job interfere with my home life" (on a scale of 1 = strongly disagree to 4 = strongly agree; Netemeyer et al. 1996; flourishing index, Vanderweele 2017).

Domain 6: Social Relationships
Participant's reported about their relationships outside the workplace, such as general overall satisfaction with relationships (on a scale of 0 = strongly disagree to 10 = strongly agree; Vanderweele 2017), the satisfaction with friend relations (on a scale of 0 = strongly disagree to 10 = strongly agree; Vanderweele 2017), availability of neighbor's help ("Do you have neighbors who can help you when you need them?" 0 = no, 1 = yes, 2 = not sure; the last category has been excluded from analyses; Keyes 1998) and also how often they feel lonely (on a scale of 1 = never, to 4 = all the time; Goodman et al. 2016; Vanderweele 2017).

Domain 7: Work Life
For the work-related domain, the following questions from the flourishing index (Vanderweele 2017) were selected: having friends at work ("Some of my coworkers are personal friends"), availability of coworkers' support ("I can depend on my coworkers for help"), feeling part of a team ("I feel part of a team at work").

Responses were provided using a 4-point Likert scale (from 1 = strongly disagree to 4 = strongly agree). For the final question, supervisor help ("My supervisor is helpful") the Likert scale ranged from 1 = never to 4 = all the time. These measurements are an adapted version of the Positive and Negative Affect Scale (PANAS; Watson and Clark 1988) referring to the work domain from the Job-Related Affective Well-Being Scale (Van Katwyk et al. 2000).

Domain 8: Adverse Health Behaviors

As shift work is associated with higher risk of non-healthy behaviors such as heavy drinking, smoking and poor sleep patterns (Nea et al. 2015), the three following questions from the survey were included in the analysis: "In general, how many days per week do you drink alcoholic beverages, such as wine, beer or liquor?" (0–7; Vanderweele 2017), "Do you currently smoke tobacco or cigarettes?" (0 = no, 1 = yes; Vanderweele 2017), and "During the past 30 days, how many days did you not get enough rest or sleep?" (0–30; Moriarty et al. 2003; Vanderweele 2017). Table 7.2 presents the distribution by frequency of all outcomes' characteristics in the baseline wave (2019).

Table 7.2 Distribution of outcome characteristics at baseline wave (2019) of participants-garment industry workers from Poland

	Total (N = 590)		Day workers (N = 241)		Shift workers (N = 349)	
Outcomes	%	Mean (SD)	%	Mean (SD)	%	Mean (SD)
General health						
General health rate (1–5)		2.87 (0.89)		2.86 (0.88)		2.87 (0.88)
Disability days (0–30)		3.51 (5.36)		3.10 (5.01)		3.80 (5.58)
Physical health						
Physical health rate (0–10)		6.61 (1.87)		6.59 (1.78)		6.63 (1.93)
Days of poor physical health (0–30)		5.66 (7.018)		5.49 (7.16)		5.78 (6.91)
Feeling pain at work (1–4)		2.38 (0.84)		2.35 (0.83)		2.40 (0.84)
Fatigue (1–4)		2.65 (0.71)		2.62 (0.71)		2.67 (0.71)
Mental health						
Mental health rate (0–10)		7.18 (2.16)		7.25 (2.15)		7.13 (2.17)
Days of poor mental health (0–30)		5.73 (7.32)		5.54 (7.01)		5.85 (7.53)

(continued)

Table 7.2 (continued)

Outcomes	Total (N = 590) %	Total (N = 590) Mean (SD)	Day workers (N = 241) %	Day workers (N = 241) Mean (SD)	Shift workers (N = 349) %	Shift workers (N = 349) Mean (SD)
Well-being:						
Life satisfaction (1–10)		7.08 (1.86)		7.13 (1.94)		7.05 (1.81)
Sad (1–4)		2.09 (0.67)		2.13 (0.64)		2.21 (0.68)
Depressed (1–4)		2.05 (0.70)		2.05 (0.71)		2.13 (0.74)
Stressed (1–4)		2.37 (0.80)		2.48 (0.78)		2.50 (0.80)
Tired (1–4)		2.73 (0.73)		2.63 (0.69)		2.80 (0.72)
Family life:						
Work-family conflict (1–4)		2.01 (0.65)		2.01 (0.38)		2.00 (0.59)
***Social relationships*:**						
Neighbor help						
Yes	75.69		73.06		82.07	
No	13.81		13.70		17.93	
Loneliness (1–4)		1.69 (0.72)		1.75 (0.76)		1.66 (0.70)
Friendship satisfaction (1–10)		7.17 (2.09)		7.45 (2.09)		7.50 (2.02)
Relationship satisfaction (1–10)		7.49 (2.02)		7.16 (2.08)		7.17 (2.11)
Work life						
Friends at work (1–4)		2.78 (0.80)		2.78 (0.81)		2.77 (0.80)
Coworkers support (1–4)		2.91 (0.55)		2.93 (0.55)		2.90 (0.55)
Feel as a part of a team (1–4)		2.99 (0.67)		3.00 (0.68)		2.98 (0.66)
Supervisor help (1–4)		3.06 (0.69)		3.08 (0.67)		3.05 (0.70)
Behavioral lifestyle:						
Drinking alcohol		0.83 (1.30)		0.90 (1.40)		0.77 (1.22)
Smoking						
Yes	24.22		23.74		24.54	
No	75.78		76.26		75.46	
Days of no sleep days (0–30)		9.26 (7.99)		9.39 (8.18)		9.15 (7.88)

Notes: SD = standard deviation
Source: Worker Well-being Survey (WWBS), Poland (Weziak-Bialowolska et al. 2020)

7.2.4 *Covariates*

Covariates included the following sociodemographic characteristics: participant age, gender, and highest educational attainment (response categories presented in Table 7.1). All models were controlled for prior sociodemographic variables and baseline values of all outcome variables simultaneously (to limit the risk of reverse causation and residual confounding).

7.2.5 *Statistical Analysis*

Data from three-time points (2019, 2020 and 2021) were used. All 26 outcomes were included in the analysis from each of the three waves of the survey. Covariates and information about type of shift were mainly taken from 2019 but the missing values (for age, gender and type of shift) were completed by available values, marked by the respondent from another database's wave. To account for missing other covariate variables, outcomes and exposure variables the multiple imputations were applied using chained equations (with ten sets of imputed data) (White et al. 2011).

In order to represent a multivariate data table, summary indices, principal component analysis (PCA) with orthogonal varimax rotation were used. PCA allows for synthesis of multiple variables (indicators) with a single result (new variables as linear combinations of multivariate set) specific to each studied dimension (Sagan 2003). Prospective associations between shift work and each of the eight domains were examined using generalized estimating equations. In order to create indexes with the direction of a consistent value, some variables were recoded from the original scales.

Three sets of analyses were conducted to measure prospective associations between work-related changes implemented in the Polish garment factory during the COVID-19 pandemic and shift worker's health and well-being. First, we measured the association between shift work in 2019 and subsequent outcomes in 2020. Second, the associations between shiftwork in 2020 and outcomes in 2021 were examined. Finally, the 2-year lag was considered and associations between shift work in 2019 and outcomes in 2021 were also analyzed. All models were controlled for participant demographics: age, gender, educational attainment. Each model was also adjusted for the prior values of the 26 outcome variables, all simultaneously in each regression model, and for the prior value of the exposure variable. Statistical analyses were performed using Stata-SE—Standard Edition 17.

7.3 Results

In this study, the associations between eight domains of life and shiftwork were examined. The data presented in Table 7.3 show a time comparison of the results of the linear regression models examining the associations between shift work and

Table 7.3 Associations between shift work and eight domains of life

Statistics	2019–2020 β CI p-value	2020–2021 β CI p-value	2019–2021 β CI p-value
General health[a]	0.02 (−0.322–0.403) 0.826	0.20 (0.0481–0.846) 0.028***	0.07 (−0.176–0.474) 0.367
Physical health[a]	0.22 (0.122–0.776) 0.008***	0.06 (−0.293–0.552) 0.543	0.10 (−0.0746–0.489) 0.148
Mental health[a]	0.057 (−0.176–0.399) 0.444	0.18 (0.0294–0.712) 0.034***	0.12 (−0.0576–0.507) 0.118
Well-being[b]	3.67 (−1.240–1.630) 0.091	−0.09 (−0.514–0.136) 0.251	−0.08 (−0.520–0.189) 0.355
Family life[a]	0.17 (−0.00338–0.405) 0.0539	0.08 (−0.108–0.278) 0.382	0.07 (−0.105–0.271) 0.385
Social relationships[b]	−0.10 (−0.611–0.213) 0.339	−0.23 (−0.875–0.003) 0.048***	−0.11 (−0.578–0.171) 0.283
Work life[b]	−0.07 (−0.444–0.143) 0.313	−0.01 (−0.403–0.343) 0.873	−0.05 (−0.409–0.218) 0.548
Adverse health behaviors[b]	−0.01 (−0.392–0.329) 0.863	−0.21 (−0.833–0.009) 0.055	−0.09 (−0.544–0.167) 0.296

Notes:β the standardized effect size, CI = 95% confidence interval, 0 = day shift, 1 = shift work, ***$p < 0.05$

[a]The higher score show poorer assessment

[b]The higher score show positive assessment

Sample size: 2019: N = 590, 2020: N = 156, 2021: N = 195.

Source: Worker Well-being Survey (WWBS), Poland (Weziak-Bialowolska et al. 2020)

general health, physical health, mental health, wellbeing, family life, social relationships, work life and adverse health behaviors.

The findings indicate that between 2020 and 2021 shift workers rated poorer their general health (β=0.20, 95% CI = 0.0481/0.846, p = 0.028), mental health (β=0.18, 95% CI = 0.0294/0.712, p = 0.034), and social relationships (β = −0.23, 95% CI = −0.875/−0.003, p = 0.048). Comparing data collected in 2019 and 2020, shift workers rated worse their physical health (β=0.22, 95% CI = 0.122/0.776, p = 0.008). In a 2-year perspective between 2019 and 2021 no statistically significant association could be observed.

Longitudinal study at three time points can show us the difference between and during COVID-19 time. Based on a comparison of results on the same workers in the different time over time we can assume that the COVID-19 pandemic time (2020, 2021) has a negative impact on shift workers' general health and mental health. This study conducted at three distinct time points can provide insights into the variations before, during, and after the COVID-19 pandemic. By comparing the results of the same group of workers across these different time periods, we can infer that the COVID-19 pandemic, particularly in the years 2020 and 2021, has adversely affected the overall health and mental well-being of shift workers. Moreover, workers evaluated their social relationships as worsening during that time. Results differ between shift workers and only day workers. When comparing self-reported health measures of those working only day shifts and those working rotating shifts, COVID-19 appears to have a negative impact on shift worker's health.

7.4 Discussion and Conclusion

Shift work as a job performed in unfavorable conditions due to disruption of day and night rhythms could be associated with negative consequences. The results of previous research indicate that shift work has a negative impact on workers' physical health, mental health, well-being, family life, social relationships (Eurofound 2007), work-life balance (Costa and Folkard 2010) and health behaviors (Nea et al. 2015). In this particular data analysis, the statistically significant differences between day workers and shift workers are prospectively noticeable only in some of the aforementioned aspects. This may be due to the fact that shift workers adapt to shift working conditions (Postnova et al. 2013) and the negative influence may depend on workers' tolerance to shift work (Costa 2003; Nachreiner 1998). COVID-19 may change habits and may have influenced the changes shown in results presented here. The results of the analysis show that for shift workers, the pandemic and the changes implemented due to the pandemic led to more difficulties in the domains of general health, mental health, and social relationships. When explaining the changing results over time, differences can be seen when COVID-related restrictions were applied. Before the pandemic between 2019 and 2020, rotating shift workers rated their physical health as being poorer compared to day shift workers. The shift workers in the surveyed factory are mainly manual workers. Physical work can be associated with experiencing physical health problems. Working conditions for blue-collar workers were improved at the factory after the first wave of the WWBS. The factory introduced physical activities for workers during work time, and associations between shift work and worse physical health in the following year were not noticeable. Between 2020 and 2021 the results for shift workers in the domains of self-assessed general health, mental health and social relationship satisfaction were noticeably worse than those of other workers. The associations between shift work and mental health during 2019 and 2020 were not noticeable in 2021. In 2020, all factory workers faced the introduction of new restrictions consistent with the guidelines at the national level that, in particular, limited the possibility of contact (GIP 2020). Other COVID-19 studies reported that physical distancing could have increased mental health problems (Fischer et al. 2020; Li Duan 2020; Hamouche 2021) and that social disconnection can cause feelings of loneliness, which worsens mental health (Bowins 2021). Shift workers at the factory, as shown in this study experienced limited social relationships. In the survey, in open-ended questions, some workers provided their subjective impressions that production workers felt "isolated" from office workers: "Contact between office and production workers is limited," "Office workers isolate themselves from production workers" (Source: open-ended questions in WWBS, translated citation). Thus, the COVID-19 situation may not only have been reflected in a poorer assessment of general health and social relationships but may have had further consequences on self-esteem and mental health. For shift workers, sleep desynchronization may not be the only source of negative effects. The restrictions that were put in place to restrict social contact, however, due to the nature of their work, shift workers have experienced similar constraints before the pandemic.

These results are consistent with the findings of other studies. Thus, the living, working, and COVID-19 e-survey (Eurofound-ETF 2022) findings show that 75% of respondents from the EU neighboring countries (aged between 18 and 44) were at risk of depression (Eurofound-ETF 2022). Problematically low levels of well-being were reported with pessimism, limited resilience, fatigue, and health risks, all likely exacerbated by the COVID-19 pandemic (Eurofound-ETF 2022). The epidemiological situation has caused different stressors, including changes implemented at workplaces described in the Introduction section of this chapter, that could trigger negative effects.

Shift workers are a special group of employees, working under unfavorable conditions due to the rotating time of work type and their social life can be limited because of that. Among shift workers there is a known the phenomenon called the social jetlag (Wittmann et al. 2006). According to the results of the study on shift work and social life, poor social networks and less social engagement are indicated as potential mediators of disease in shift workers (Knutsson 2003). Social isolation and lockdowns implemented to alleviate the epidemiological situation reduced contacts in general and resulted in a reduced possibility of socializing during free time. Furthermore, changes implemented in the factory reduced social contact at work.

Work relationships are worth considering when organizing the work of shift workers. Connections at work can be especially important for shift workers who, outside of the work environment, may not have the opportunity to establish friendly relationships.

Happiness and well-being are important to people both in general and in the workplace, and have implications for mental and physical health (Fisher 2014). Moreover, how people are treated at work affects their health, well-being, performance (McNeely 2020) and productivity (Węziak-Białowolska et al. 2019). Factors like support and the assistance of supervisors, and availability of favorable social areas (common areas like the cafeteria for the social activity of workers) must be taken into account when organizing workplace facilities in order to raise the conditions that provide opportunities for work-related socialization. It is very important as other research indicates that social networks and positive relationships in general favorably affect health and well-being (Umberson and Karas Montez 2010).

7.5 Future Studies

More studies are needed to examine the impact of work conditions including restrictions on direct contact of employees (e.g., extend the working time, reduction of shift groups, number of members of teams, the extension of working hours from 8 to 12 h shifts). More longitudinal studies are needed to examine the implications of short-term social disconnection, especially if some negative outcomes could be reversible. Additionally, not every shift worker is affected by the negative effects of shift work. Although the present outcomes do not show the causality of implemented specific restrictions, the background presented here suggests a direction for further research. Future studies on shift workers may include more questions about leisure activities, and diet, and deepen information on close relationships and relations at work. By observing the behaviors of shift workers that prevent the negative effects of shift work despite unfavorable conditions, we can create recommendations that will help with negative results in unfavorable circumstances for all types of workers.

Acknowledgements This research was supported by the Levi Strauss Foundation under the grant No. 44057265 "The Impact of new work designs on worker well-being—Plock, Poland Factory Workers" and the Norwegian Financial Mechanism 2014–2021 (UMO-2020/37/K/HS6/02772).

References

Bialowolski, P., E. McNeely, T.J. Vanderweele, and D. Weziak-Bialowolska. 2020. Ill health and distraction at work: Costs and drivers for productivity loss. *PLoS One* 15 (3): 1–15. https://doi.org/10.1371/journal.pone.0230562.

Bowins, B. 2021. Social connectedness. In *States and processes for mental health*, 41–48. Academic Press. https://doi.org/10.1016/B978-0-323-85049-0.00004-0.

Costa, G. 2003. Shift work and occupational medicine: An overview. *Occupational Medicine* 53 (2): 83–88. https://doi.org/10.1093/occmed/kqg045.

Costa, G., and S. Folkard. 2010. Shift work and extended hours of work. In *Hunter's diseases of occupation*, ed. P.J. Baxter, P.H. Adams, T.-C. Caw, A. Cockcroft, and J.M. Harrington, 10th ed., 1233–1245. London: CRC Press. https://doi.org/10.1201/b13467.

Eurofound. 2007. Shift work, *European industrial relations dictionary*. Dublin: Eurofound. https://www.eurofound.europa.eu/observatories/eurwork/industrial-relations-dictionary/shift-work. Accessed 10 Feb 2024.

———. 2017. *Living and working in Europe*. Luxembourg: Publications Office of the European Union. ISBN 978-92-897-1721-2. https://doi.org/10.2806/603802.

Eurofound-ETF. 2022. *Living, working and covid-19 in the European Union and 10 EU neighbouring countries*. Luxembourg: Publications Office of the European Union. ISBN 978-92-897-2301-5. https://doi.org/10.2806/442725.

Eurostat. 2014. *Regional yearbook*. Luxembourg: Publications Office of the European Union. ISBN 978-92-79-38906-1. https://doi.org/10.2785/54659.

———. 2023. The European Union Labour Force Survey-Metadata Structure (ESMS). https://ec.europa.eu/eurostat/databrowser/view/LFSA_EWPSHI/default/map?lang=en. Accessed 10 Feb 2024.

Fischer, I., S. Avrashi, T. Oz, R. Fadul, K. Gutman, and D. Rubenstein. 2020. The behavioural challenge of the COVID-19 pandemic: Indirect measurements and personalized attitude changing treatments (IMPACT). *Royal Society Open Science* 7: 201131. https://doi.org/10.1098/rsos.201131.

Fisher, C.D. 2014. Conceptualizing and measuring wellbeing at work. In *Wellbeing: A complete reference guide, work and wellbeing*, ed. P.Y. Chen and C.L. Cooper, 9–34. New York: John Wiley & Sons. https://doi.org/10.1002/9781118539415.wbwell018.

GIP. 2020. Bezpieczenstwo i ochrona zdrowia osob pracujacych w czasie epidemii COVID-19 Ogolne wytyczne i lista kontrolna. Warszawa: Centralny Instytut Ochrony Pracy – Państwowy Instytut Badawczy (Główny Inspektor Pracy). https://m.ciop.pl/CIOPPortalWAR/file/89970/2020051833329&Koronawirus-zalecenia-ogolne-2020-05-18.pdf. Accessed 10 Feb 2024.

Goodman, A., J. Wrigley, K. Silversides, and N. Venus-Balgobin. 2016. *Measuring your impact on loneliness in later life, campaign to end loneliness report, 40*. London: Campaign to End Loneliness. https://www.campaigntoendloneliness.org/wp-content/uploads/Loneliness-Measurement-Guidance1.pdf. Accessed 10 Feb 2024.

Hamouche, S. 2021. Human resource management and the COVID-19 crisis: Implications, challenges, opportunities, and future organizational directions. *Journal of Management & Organization* 29 (5): 799–814. https://doi.org/10.1017/jmo.2021.15.

ILO. 2020. Standards and COVID-19, Labour standards, 2.1 (May 2020), 38. International Labour Organization. https://www.ilo.org/wcmsp5/groups/public/%2D%2D-ed_norm/%2D%2D-normes/documents/genericdocument/wcms_739937.pdf. Accessed 10 Feb 2024.

Kancelaria Sejmu. 2023. Art. 207 § 2 oraz art. 304 Kodeksu pracy, 1–103. https://isap.sejm.gov.pl/isap.nsf/download.xsp/WDU20230001465/T/D20231465L.pdf. Accessed 10 Feb 2024.

Keyes, Corey Lee M. 1998. Social well-being. *Social Psychology Quarterly* 61 (2): 121–140. https://doi.org/10.2307/2787065.

Kim, W., T. Hyun Kim, T. Hoon Lee, J. Woo Choi, and E. Cheol Park. 2016. The impact of shift and night work on health related quality of life of working women: Findings from the Korea health panel. *Health and Quality of Life Outcomes* 14 (1): 1–6. https://doi.org/10.1186/s12955-016-0564-x.

Knutsson, A. 2003. Health disorders of shift workers occupational. *Occupational Medicine* 53 (2): 103–108. https://doi.org/10.1093/occmed/kqg048.

Lee, M.T., P. Bialowolski, D. Weziak-Bialowolska, D. Kay, Ph.J. Lerner, E. McNeely, and T.J. Vanderweele. 2021. Self-assessed importance of domains of flourishing: Demographics and correlations with. *The Journal of Positive Psychology* 16 (1): 137–144. https://doi.org/10.1080/17439760.2020.1716050.

Leso, V., L. Fontana, A. Caturano, and I. Vetrani. 2021. Impact of shift work and long working hours on worker cognitive functions: Current evidence and future research needs. *International Journal of Environmental Research and Public Health* 18 (12): 6540. https://doi.org/10.3390/ijerph18126540. PMID: 34204504; PMCID: PMC8296479.

Li Duan, G.Z. 2020. Psychological interventions for people affected by the COVID-19 epidemic. *The Lancet Psychiatry* 7: 300–302. https://doi.org/10.1016/S2215-0366(20)30073-0.

McNeely, E. 2020. Well-being and equity as a business imperative summary of the Harvard sustainability and health initiative (SHINE) Research on Worker Well-being Report, Harvard T.H. Chan School of Public Health. https://www.levistrauss.com/wp-content/uploads/2021/05/Harvard-SHINE_WWB-Impact-Study-Summary-Report_12-October-2020.pdf. Accessed 10 Feb 2024.

Messenger, J. 2018. Working time and the future of work, *ILO future of work research paper series* 6. ISBN 978-92-2-132218-4 (print); 978-92-2-132219-1 (web pdf).

Moriarty, D.G., M.M. Zack, and R. Kobau. 2003. The centers for disease control and prevention's healthy days measures—Population tracking of perceived physical and mental health over time. *Health and Quality of Life Outcomes* 1: 37. https://doi.org/10.1186/1477-7525-1-37. PMID: 14498988; PMCID: PMC201011.

Nachreiner, F. 1998. Individual and social determinants of shiftwork tolerance. *Scandinavian Journal of Work, Environment & Health* 24: 35–42. https://doi.org/10.2486/indhealth.SW-5. Ind Health. 2019 Apr 1;57(2):201–212. Epub 2019 Jan 31. PMID: 30700671; PMCID: PMC6449641.

Nea, F.M., J. Kearney, M.B.E. Livingstone, L.K. Pourshahidi, and C.A. Corish. 2015. Dietary and lifestyle habits and the associated health risks in shift workers. *Nutrition Research Reviews* 28 (2): 143–166. https://doi.org/10.1017/S095442241500013X.

Netemeyer, R.G., J.S. Boles, and R. McMurrian. 1996. Development and validation of work-family conflict and family-work conflict scales. *Journal of Applied Psychology* 81 (4): 400–410. https://doi.org/10.1037/0021-9010.81.4.400.

Postnova, S., P.A. Robinson, and D.D. Postnov. 2013. Adaptation to shift work: Physiologically based modeling of the effects of lighting and shifts start time. *PLoS One* 8 (1): e53379. https://doi.org/10.1371/journal.pone.0053379.

Richter, K., A. Rodenbeck, and G. Weess. 2021. Shiftwork and alcohol consumption: A systematic review of the literature. *European Addiction Research* 27 (1): 9–15. https://doi.org/10.1159/000507573.

Sagan, A. 2003. Skale i indeksy jako narzedzia pomiaru w badaniach marketingowych. *Zeszyty Naukowe / Akademia Ekonomiczna w Krakowie* 640: 21–36. YADDA ID: bwmeta1.element.ekon-element-000044907806.

Sejm Rzeczypospolitej Polskiej. 2021. Rozporządzenie Rady Ministrów z dnia 6 maja 2021 r. w sprawie ustanowienia określonych ograniczeń, nakazów i zakazów w związku z wystąpieniem stanu epidemii, Dz.U.2021.861, *Dziennik ustaw 1360*, 47:1–10. https://isap.sejm.gov.pl/isap.nsf/download.xsp/WDU20210000861/O/D20210861.pdf. Accessed 10 Feb 2024.

Sweileh, W.M. 2022. Analysis and mapping of global research publications on shift work (2012–2021). *Journal of Occupational Medicine and Toxicology* 17 (22): 1–14. https://doi.org/10.1186/s12995-022-00364-0.

Szosland, D. 2010. Shift work and metabolic syndrome, diabetes mellitus and ischaemic heart disease. *International Journal of Occupational Medicine and Environmental Health* 23 (3): 287–291. https://doi.org/10.2478/v10001-010-0032-5.

Torquati, Luciana, Gregore I. Mielke, Wendy J. Brown, Nicola W. Burton, and Tracy L. Kolbe-alexander. 2019. Shift work and poor mental health: A meta-analysis of longitudinal studies. *American Journal of Public Health* 109 (11): 13–20. https://doi.org/10.2105/AJPH.2019.305278.

Umberson, D., and J. Karas Montez. 2010. Social relationships and health: A flashpoint for health policy. *Journal of Health and Social Behavior* 51: S54–S66. https://doi.org/10.1177/0022146510383501.Social.

Van Katwyk, P.T., S. Fox, P.E. Spector, and E.K. Kelloway. 2000. Using the job-related affective well-being scale (JAWS) to investigate affective responses to work stressors. *Journal of Occupational Health Psychology* 5 (2): 219–230. https://doi.org/10.1037/1076-8998.5.2.219.

Vanderweele, T.J. 2017. On the promotion of human flourishing. *Proceedings of the National Academy of Sciences of the United States of America* 114 (31): 8148–8156. https://doi.org/10.1073/pnas.1702996114.

Ware, J.E., and C.D. Sherbourne. 1992. The MOS 36-item short-form health survey (SF-36): I. Conceptual framework and item selection. *Medical Care* 30 (6): 473–483.

Watson, D., and L.A. Clark. 1988. Development and validation of brief measures of positive and negative affect: The PANAS scales. *Journal of Personality and Social Psychology* 54 (6): 1063–1070. https://doi.org/10.1037/0022-3514.54.6.1063. PMID: 3397865.

Węziak-Białowolska, D., P. Białowolski, and E. McNeely. 2019. Workers well-being. Evidence from the apparel industry in Mexico. *Intelligent Buildings International* 11 (3–4): 158–177. https://doi.org/10.1080/17508975.2019.1618785.

Weziak-Bialowolska, D., P. Bialowolski, P.L. Sacco, T.J. Vanderweele, and E. McNeely. 2020. Well-being in life and Well-being at work: Which comes first? Evidence from a longitudinal study. *Frontiers in Public Health* 8: 1–12. https://doi.org/10.3389/fpubh.2020.00103.

Weziak-Bialowolska, D., P. Bialowolski, T.J. Vanderweele, and E. McNeely. 2021a. Character strengths involving an orientation to promote good can help your health and well-being. Evidence from two longitudinal studies. *American Journal of Health Promotion* 35 (3): 388–398. https://doi.org/10.1177/0890117120964083.

Weziak-Bialowolska, D., P. Bialowolski, M.T. Lee, Y. Chen, T.J. Vanderweele, and E. McNeely. 2021b. Psychometric properties of flourishing scales from a comprehensive well-being assessment. *Frontiers in Psychology* 12: 1–15. https://doi.org/10.3389/fpsyg.2021.652209.

White, I.R., P. Royston, and A.M. Wood. 2011. Multiple imputation using chained equations: Issues and guidance for practice. *Statistics in Medicine* 30: 377–399. https://doi.org/10.1002/sim.4067.

Wittmann, M., J. Dinich, M. Merrow, and T. Roenneberg. 2006. Social jetlag: Misalignment of biological and social time. *Chronobiology International* 23 (1–2): 497–509. https://doi.org/10.1080/07420520500545979.

Regina Skiba is a PhD student enrolled at the Doctoral School of Social Sciences at Jagiellonian University, Poland. She holds a master's degree in Sociology with a specialization in Social Research and Data Analysis. Her research is centered on exploring the connections between social factors and health. Specifically, she examines the social factors that can either mitigate negative impacts on health and well-being or positively influence them. Within this framework she investigates adaptive behaviors among shift workers.

Regina Skiba is currently participating in the "Positive Health Program," a research initiative funded by the National Science Center. Further information about the project can be found at: https://positivehealth.project.uj.edu.pl/.

Eileen McNeely is Executive Director at Harvard SHINE (Sustainability and Health Initiative for NetPositive Enterprise), Human Flourishing Program, Institute for Quantitative Social Science, Harvard University. She is a researcher and consultant in the fields of worker well-being and health, corporate social responsibility and sustainability. Her research is dedicated to the exploration of well-being, with a particular emphasis on unveiling the impacts of business on individuals, the planet, and the surrounding environment. She is committed to the pursuit of sustainability and flourishing for all through her work.

Dorota Weziak-Bialowolska is an Associate Professor of Sociology at Kozminski University Warsaw, Poland. With a research focus on methodology, including impact assessment, evaluation, psychometrics, composite scales, and indicators, her recent work centers on positive health and human flourishing. Previously, she served as a research scientist at the Harvard T.H. Chan School of Public Health (2017–2021) and worked at the European Commission Joint Research Centre in Italy (2011–2017). Currently, she contributes to the Global Flourishing Study, a collaboration between scholars at the Human Flourishing Program at Harvard, Baylor's Institute for Studies of Religion, Gallup, and the Center for Open Science.

Part III
Sociability, Civic Participation and Solidarity During the Pandemic

Chapter 8
The Pandemic Effects on Sociability and Well-being of Low-Income Adolescents in Mexico

Gonzalo A. Saraví

8.1 Introduction

The first responses to control the COVID-19 pandemic were social. In most parts of the world, governments implemented very similar measures of confinement, social distancing, and the suspension of many educational, commercial, and recreational activities, both in public and private spaces. Their consequences radically reconfigured social life, transforming the dynamics and rhythm of our daily activities, as well as the most basic patterns of sociability that had previously structured our life in society. What have been the effects of these alterations in social life on people's socio-emotional well-being?

This chapter specifically explores this relationship between sociability and socio-emotional well-being in adolescents from low-income sectors. In particular, the analysis focuses on the repercussions of confinement and the pandemic in general, on the relationships, interactions, and social ties of adolescents from lower social class background, and how this disruption of sociability patterns affected their socio-emotional well-being.

Adolescents' experiences, conditions and perceptions of the pandemic and confinement have remained relatively invisible (Branquinho et al. 2020). On the one hand, they are not among the main risk groups (unlike the adult and elderly population), and on the other hand, they enjoy a certain independence and autonomy that frees their families from their care (unlike young children). On many occasions and different countries, they have also been stigmatized by the media and public opinion (and even by some politicians) for their alleged irresponsibility and reluctance to

G. A. Saraví (✉)
Center for Research and Graduate Studies in Social Anthropology (Ciesas), Mexico City, Mexico
e-mail: gsaravi@ciesas.edu.mx

C. Suter et al. (eds.), *Well-being During the Pandemic*, Social Indicators Research Series 90, https://doi.org/10.1007/978-3-031-63440-6_8

comply with the lockdown measures, blaming them for being active super-spreaders of the virus (Bengtsson et al. 2021a, 2021b; Mora Salas and Urbina 2021). This stigmatization has also contributed to silence the suffering of young people during the pandemic.

However, at the same time, this segment of the population has been particularly affected by measures of confinement and social distancing. The closure of schools, a central institution at this stage of life, radically disrupted the daily life and social life of adolescents, particularly in countries such as Mexico, where this measure lasted almost 2 years. The suspension of recreational activities in public and private spaces as well as the confinement at home with the rest of the family, had also severe implications in young people' well-being. Interaction with peers and gaining independence from adults are key dimensions for the development and psycho-social well-being of adolescents (Crosnoe and Johnson 2011).

Moreover, the effects of the pandemic have not been homogeneous throughout society as a whole: "the crisis has hit people who were already struggling the hardest" (OECD 2021a, 23). Its impact, both in terms of mortality (OECD 2021a) and socio-emotional well-being (Rose 2020), differed across multiple categories of inequality. Low-income sectors, for instance, have had to face confinement in contexts of social precariousness and economic limitations that further accentuate many of its consequences. The equipment and size of the home, the quality of electronic devices and internet access, the employment conditions, the characteristics of the neighborhood, or the disposition of financial savings have had unequal effects on the experience of confinement and its consequences.

Not only were the effects of the pandemic on adolescents and youth initially underestimated, it also silenced their voices. In an article entitled *Hey, we also have something to say,* Branquinho et al. (2020) highlight the importance of studies that capture young people's concerns, needs and experiences of the lockdown as an important contribution to the design of social policies for the well-being of young people. This chapter is based on the analysis of some of the results obtained from a participatory-research on Adolescence and the COVID-19 Pandemic. Following the guidelines of the Youth Participatory Action Research (YPAR) young people were invited to be involved as co-researchers and thus, to co-create a research process driven by their lived experiences of the pandemic (Cook and Krueger-Henney 2017; Smith et al. 2021). Unlike other qualitative studies, we did not limit ourselves to consulting and listening to young people's experiences through surveys and/or interviews, but rather we proposed to a group of students from a secondary school located on the outskirts of the metropolitan area of Mexico City to be active collaborators in all stages of the research: (a) defining the research questions; (b) designing and implementing tools of data collection; (c) and analyzing findings. They also collectively generated different audio-visual products of their own authorship and in their own languages to communicate and share their main findings with the public (Saraví et al. 2014).

8.2 Adolescent Confinement and Well-being

From a comprehensive review of the literature on youth well-being, Helen Cahill (2015) concludes that there is a certain consensus in attributing a determining weight to the social, emotional, and relational aspects of well-being, thus defining a field of interest and analysis focused on the psycho-social elements of well-being. The COVID-19 pandemic has been a historical and global event whose consequences are not limited to the medical and economic dimensions. Recent studies have begun to focus on the consequences of the pandemic itself, and on the measures of confinement and social distancing, on these psycho-social dimensions of well-being (in many cases under the concept of mental health). Most of these studies report a negative effect, with a generalized increase in psycho-emotional distress throughout the population but particularly among adolescents and young people. The World Health Organization (WHO) estimated that the COVID-19 pandemic has led to a 27.6% increase in cases of major depressive disorder and a 25.6% increase in cases of anxiety disorders (AD) worldwide during the first year of this global crisis (WHO 2022). According to this international study, females were more affected than males, and younger people, especially those aged 20–24 years, were more affected than older adults; additionally, it also mentions that many low- and middle-income countries were majorly affected.

Focusing on youth, the Organization for Economic Cooperation and Development (OECD 2021b), for example, reports available data from Belgium, France and the United States showing that the percentage of young people experiencing symptoms of anxiety and depression during the pandemic was more than double the percentage recorded before the onset of the COVID-19 crisis. These data not only suggest a very substantial increase in these conditions among young people due to the pandemic, but also show that this is a segment of the population that is particularly sensitive to the emotional distress caused by the lockdown: the level of prevalence of symptoms of "anxiety" and "depression" in young people in these same countries was found to be between 30% and 80% higher than in the general population (OECD 2021b). According to Marchini et al. (2021), data for Italy show that in this country there does not seem to be a higher prevalence of "fear" and "anxiety" among young people, but feelings of "loneliness" and "boredom" are evident.

Some studies on the subject seem to suggest that the factors associated with the pandemic that affect the well-being of adolescents and young people are mainly related to its social dimensions (Marchini et al. 2021; Panarese and Azzarita 2021). While in the adult population factors such as fear of contagion or death, economic difficulties or loss of employment are causes of discomfort, among adolescents the main causes are associated with disruptions in social life and daily routines. This coincides with Cahill's (2015) observations regarding the determining weight of social and relational factors in adolescent well-being.

In this regard, Panarese and Azzarita (2021) point out that it is very likely that school closures and physical distancing measures have had a very significant impact on young people, especially adolescents, due directly to the absence of face-to-face interactions with peers, and indirectly to increased family stress. Branquinho et al. (2020) citing a study in The Lancet also emphasize the possible negative effects of restricting face-to-face peer interactions on the emotional well-being of adolescents.

Other studies have drawn attention to the potential effect of the changes brought about by confinement on daily habits and routines. The temporality and rhythm of daily life were radically disrupted for adolescents, including the structure of leisure time (Bengtsson et al. 2021a, 2021b). Many of their daily activities lost temporal order and spatial differentiation (Aymerich-Franch 2020; OECD 2021b; Panarese and Azzarita 2021).

In Latin America, studies on these aspects are still very scarce, and most of them are surveys (self-applied by internet) conducted by international organizations or governmental agencies. The United Nations Children's Fund (UNICEF 2022), for example, conducted a survey in 2020 with young people aged 13–29 years, and preliminary results show that the pandemic had a significant impact on the mental health of Latin American adolescents and young people. According to this regional survey, 27% of participants reported feelings of anxiety and 15% depression; almost half (46%) reported having less motivation to perform activities they usually enjoyed and 36% said they felt less motivated to perform their daily activities.

The Population Council together with the Government of Mexico (the Ministry of Welfare and the Ministry of Health) conducted a much more extensive survey in Mexico between November 2020 and February 2021, online and self-administered, with young people (15–24 years old) (Larrea-Schiavon et al. 2021). This survey is more comprehensive and methodologically rigorous than the one conducted by UNICEF. The results show that 40% presented moderate to severe symptoms of depression and 31% presented moderate to severe symptoms of anxiety. These percentages are more or less the same between young people (20 to 24 years old) and adolescents (15 to 19 years old), and between different socioeconomic strata, but show very significant differences between genders. Females presented symptoms of depression and anxiety in a much higher proportion than males (45% vs. 33% and 36% vs. 25%, respectively); in the non-binary or other gender-identified population, the percentages with symptoms of both conditions were significantly higher (70% depression and 56% anxiety).

Beyond these and other surveys, and some journalistic reports that provide a descriptive overview of the situation, there are still very few studies in the region that analyze the relationship between confinement and these and other conditions of socio-emotional distress. It is important to consider that school closures in Latin American countries have been among the most extensive in the world. In Mexico, for example, the suspension of face-to-face classes began on March 19, 2020, and it was not until September–October 2021 that a gradual return to classrooms began (a few days a week) and only at some levels (at the end of 2021 the university was still without face-to-face classes). On the other hand, the deep socio-economic gaps prevailing in the region (among the most unequal in the world) make the conditions and possibilities of confinement, education and work during the pandemic differ substantially among different sectors of the population (Oxfam 2021; Rose 2020). Undoubtedly, these aspects may have had an impact on the socio-emotional discomfort experienced by adolescents and young people.

8.3 Methods

The empirical information on which the analysis presented in this article is based comes mainly from a Youth Participatory Action Research whose fieldwork was conducted between the months of October 2020 and August 2021, that is, in the middle of the period of confinement and suspension of classes due to the COVID-19 pandemic. In collaboration with a high school teacher from a school located in the municipality of Ciudad Nezahualcóyotl,[1] we invited students from four different classrooms (of approximately 50 students each) to participate in a research project on the experience of the pandemic in adolescence; in other words, this chapter analyzes a rich corpus of empirical materials produced by "adolescents researching adolescents."

After several introductory sessions, a total of 61 adolescents were voluntarily involved in this project; they were organized into 13 different work-teams. All of them were between 17 and 19 years old at the time, 25 boys (41%) and 36 girls (59%), and were in their last year of high school. To conduct their research, each team applied different techniques with their own classmates, or other friends and acquaintances between the ages of 15 and 19. These techniques included, among others, short surveys, recorded interviews, individual letters, personal diaries, or field notes about their own experiences of the pandemic, and photographs. Finally, each team produced a product in different languages expressing the results of their research; these products included videos, drama, podcasts, literature, photographic samples, and music, most of which were later edited into audiovisual format by the research team.[2]

Throughout this process the students were advised and trained in some basic skills regarding how to define a research problem, how to elaborate interview guides, survey questionnaires, and other information gathering techniques, and how to elaborate and edit their products. At the conclusion of each of these three stages, the teams shared with the project coordinators the results obtained, i.e.: (a) the

[1] Nezahualcóyotl is one of the most populated municipalities in Mexico, with a little more than 1.1 million inhabitants. Its urbanization dates back to the 1960s and was a product of the popular processes of informal urbanization typical of Latin America cities, associated with flows of internal migration (from the countryside and from Mexico City itself after the 1985 earthquake). It is currently a consolidated municipality but maintains its popular character.

[2] These products can be viewed at: https://youtube.com/playlist?list=PLYifbJ7Q5WQea17mj911_xtuYGvzPc8-5.

definition and justification of their research problem; (b) the material obtained through the techniques applied; and (c) the adolescent-authored products. This methodological strategy made it possible to develop a qualitative research "on the pandemic during the pandemic," which is absolutely exceptional in the context of the studies that are emerging and which are, due to the very limitations of the context, mostly of a quantitative type through surveys (many of them by telephone or virtual).

This chapter is based on the analysis of all that empirical material, mainly the interviews, letters, diaries or field notes and some of the audio-visual products generated. Except for the latter, all of them (if not written) were transcribed and subsequently coded. This diversity of methods resulted in a very broad and rich set of qualitative materials that were analyzed from a sociological perspective treating "texts as a window into human experience" (Ryan and Bernard 2000, 769).

Finally, it should be noted that all the names of the adolescents mentioned in this article are fictitious in order to preserve their anonymity. The research was carried out with the authorization of the school, the collaboration as project co-coordinator of Mario Obispo Quezada, a teacher at the school, and the voluntary willingness of the adolescents themselves to participate and/or withdraw when they wished to do so. Since all the research was carried out during the confinement, there was no face-to-face interaction between the coordinators and the students at any time. In mid 2022, once the confinement was over, we held a face-to-face meeting with the young co-researchers at the school. During this meeting, in addition to getting to know each other and sharing a lunch, we recorded a television program about the research project and its findings, which was later broadcast by a national channel. This was a source of social recognition and pride for the participating adolescents whose voices and experiences are seldom heard.

8.4 Changes in Adolescent Sociability During the Pandemic

Three main areas of adolescent sociability have been substantially affected by the pandemic and confinement: (a) peer relationships; (b) coexistence with family or household members; and (c) use of public space. In each of these spheres of social interaction, the adolescents identified significant changes, mostly (although not all) considered negative.

The suspension of face-to-face classes and their replacement by virtual modalities of education is the issue that adolescents associate with the pandemic with most insistence and concern. The closure of schools in their traditional format is discussed in their empirical materials from multiple angles: the limitations in the teaching-learning process, the technological restrictions and inequalities it revealed, the disorganization of schools and administrators to adapt to the new situation, the limited skills of teachers to adapt to virtuality, and the excessive homework required of them, among many others. But among all these aspects, a particularly relevant one highlighted by adolescents is precisely the cancellation of a key space for interaction between peers.

> During the pandemic we have realized that relationships between friends have been affected due to the distance, because generally our social interaction was based on going to school and enjoying free time together. Now, we no longer see each other every day, with some luck every two months and in video calls that are not necessarily to see each other and talk about us, but were video calls for team work, which is quite stressful because we do not have the time we had to enjoy the company …, not even company at a distance (Team 6, several adolescents, justification of the research problem).

During this stage of the life course, school represents a fundamental space for encounters between peers and the construction of relationships of friendship, courtship, companionship, or casual interaction with an equivalent other. The school, even for the popular sectors, constitutes part of the institutionalization of adolescence. In the previous quote, two interesting aspects emerge: one of them is the reference to free time "at" school and the other is the questioning of video calls or communication through social networks in general.

The mention of free time at school is a first piece of information that allows us to question a widespread common sense that contrasts school with free time. What the quote makes clear is that there is free time "in" school. And what is meant by this is not only the break periods between class-hours, but also the multiple and micro interstices located within strictly academic practices and which are also part of the school experience. Luis refers to them even more explicitly:

> The virtual classes were a total disaster, and it is ugly because we missed the company of our friends, the relaxation we had, the jokes we made, the chatting among other things, little by little we were separating and people began to fall into depression, anxiety, because of the confinement … (Team 6, Luis, letter).

Chatting, jokes and relaxation are an essential part of adolescent sociability, and this is one of the aspects that the closing of schools has radically and abruptly cancelled. Virtuality seems unable to replace or replicate this aspect of sociability. Video calls on different platforms were initially exalted as the great solution and were overused throughout the pandemic. However, although they made it possible to replace—partially—classes in their academic dimension, they have been unable to do the same with their social dimension: "they are not necessarily to see each other and talk about us" said the members of Team 6. Face-to-face schooling opens interstices for sociability that the efficiency of virtuality suppresses.

> Technology has kept us in touch with our friends and classmates, however, obviously, it is not the same; now they send you a sticker saying: "virtual hug" and at the beginning it felt nice … how, from a distance, affection can still be shown, but, as expected, with time that would not be enough … I have not seen my friends, I have not seen my boyfriend, they are important people in my life and I feel very ugly in my chest because this stage [adolescence] will end before the pandemic. We will all go our separate ways (Team 6, Ana Laura, letter).

Virtuality also suppresses another essential aspect of adolescent sociability: corporeality. Corporeality, both in terms of physical presence in front of the other and physical contact with the other, is suppressed or at least strongly limited and disrupted. If this aspect, directly linked to affectivity, is central to the human condition, it is decisive in adolescence due to its importance for adolescent psycho-social development: in the construction of identity, affective bonds, subjectivation, body recognition, etcetera.

> During these months, almost a year that the pandemic has lasted, it has been a Russian roulette of emotions for me, since the fact of being alone in my house every day is very frustrating, because I tend to be a person who loves to live with people, since I am too sociable and although there are social networks and I can talk through them with my friends, it is not the same as being with them physically (Team 10, Fernando, letter).

> What happens to me the most is that I get bored, it is not the same to talk to a person face to face as it is to talk to a person through the screen of your cell phone or computer (Team 11, Alejandra, field notes).

Once again, the difference generated by physical presence is noted. Not only is it not the same as virtual communication, but the absence of these spaces of sociability in which face-to-face interaction and corporeality come into play, has repercussions on feelings and moods such as boredom, loneliness and sometimes depression. At the same time, an aspect that also appears associated with confinement is the feeling of helplessness that adolescents often express as frustration. These feelings of discomfort and distress may explain the frequent transgressions of lockdown measures by youngsters, which were used by the public opinion in their stigmatization.

The other side of school closure and its replacement by distance learning has been an intensification of coexistence at home, mostly with other family members such as parents and siblings. As pointed out by the adolescents themselves, confinement has meant a substantial change in terms of daily routines and family dynamics: the schedules and activities outside the home of all members of the household were altered, and in general terms were limited, which in turn implied new experiences (and negotiations) of coexistence. The imposed co-presence of the family for most of the day meant for many adolescents an unexpected situation with diverse repercussions.

In low-income sectors, working hours outside the home tend to be long. Distances and transfers in large urban conglomerates such as Mexico City also tend to take several hours, forcing people to leave very early in the morning and return very late in the evening. In other words, in the pre-pandemic daily life, family gatherings during the week were scarce for many households; but the lockdown changed this and imposed an intense coexistence. For some, as in the cases of Johanna and Ruby, this meant a rediscovery of family ties, and even a strengthening and improvement of the relationship and dialogue with parents, siblings or other members of the household.

> Personally, I think I learned to live more with the people I live with, because before I was more antisocial, I didn't talk to anyone, neither with my parents nor with my siblings, with anyone; so I think that to a certain extent I have learned to dialogue more with them, to work more on trust, and to communicate more (Team 5, Johanna, interview).

> Well, yes, a little bit. With my grandmother I didn't really talk much, and with this pandemic we've been able to communicate more with her .... With my mom it has always been like that, we have always been in 100% communication, she is my best friend as well .... And my siblings a little bit ... the truth is that being united like that is not something we do, and sometimes there were fights and things like that (Team 5, Ruby, interview).

But Ruby's last quote subtly hints that such an intense coexistence can also have its negative nuances, especially for those who were not used to it. In another of the interviews conducted by Team 5, Naomi notes "I think what has affected me the most [from confinement] has been intolerance"; and then adds in the same vein as Ruby did:

> Well, I think it's because of being with the same people all year long and not being able to go out or see other people ... it's like so much living together overwhelmed me. Being cooped up for so long, there are times when living so much together overwhelms you ... because there are fights and many things ... (Team 5, Naomi, interview).

The intensification of coexistence can trigger boredom and stress, but also conflicts. In this regard, we must take into account two other elements that contribute to gives certain specificity to our target population; I am referring to the social condition and the age condition. On the one hand, the precariousness of the housing conditions of the popular sectors translates, among other characteristics, not only into situations of (more or less) overcrowding, but also into limitations in the availability of open, independent, and comfortable spaces.

These features of low-income housing accentuate encounters and interactions, constrain autonomy and privacy, increase reciprocal interference, and multiply the possibilities of conflict. Results of the survey conducted by the Population Council Mexico (2021) show that for 43.5% of young people aged 15 to 24 years it was "very stressful" to stay at home during the pandemic.[3] However, beyond this high percentage in average, the differences according to the socio-economic level of households are especially relevant: while in households in the wealthiest quintile 38% of young people said they felt "very stressed," in households located in the lowest income quintile the percentage of "very stressed" young people was 52%. These results may be associated with the contrasting housing conditions of both groups (Population Council Mexico 2021).

The same Population Council survey shows that the high level of stress attributed to confinement is slightly higher among adolescents. Just as peer relationships become preeminent in adolescence, relationships with the family, especially with parents, also tend to be strained. The very process of subjectivation, that is, of positioning oneself in the world and recognizing oneself as an autonomous subject, implies a certain distancing from the close family, and the search for interaction with peers, but also with other adults. Home confinement with the nuclear family censored these possibilities.

> We are going through a variety of mixed emotions: happy to sleep, stressed from homework and online classes, homework at home, yelling or fighting from our family members that make us frustrated, getting sad about not going out and seeing our friends, and even missing our school. (Team 11, several teens, justification of the research problem).

> With my family I have had a rapprochement, but at the same time a distancing. Although I have been able to connect a little more with my family, but I do consider that the fact of

[3] For 18.1% it was "stressful," for 26.6% "a little stressful" and only 11.7% said it was "not stressful at all."

> being daily seeing your family, living with them, there comes a time that like everything there is a limit, then as you have to be close there also comes a time when you have to think about yourself, that you will not always be comfortable with your own family, sometimes you need a moment where being alone is a good time; I do not know .... I don't know ... a rest more than anything, because it is very nice to have the support of your family, to have them living with you and everything, but there comes a time when the routine of it is also a little bit tiring. So it's never a bad thing to withdraw a little bit from that family nucleus, even if it's just for a day, and give yourself time (Team 4, Paul, interview).

Paul's quote is eloquent regarding this need of adolescents for a relative distancing from the family, but also the demand for a space and time of intimacy and privacy. Without implying a rejection of the family, excessive cohabitation in small spaces can end up being perceived as harassment. Obviously, the negative connotations of this situation are accentuated in authoritarian families, conflictive environments, or homes where adolescents' needs and interests are devalued or not recognized. It is also worth noting the numerous references made by adolescents to the loss of close family members, the stressful care of sick relatives in small spaces, economic hardships and job losses in their families; all these factors also add tension to intrafamily relations.

A third dimension linked to changes in sociability that emerges from adolescents' experiences is the limited used of public space. While this aspect is directly related to the closure of schools that was one of the most important daily activities outside the home, it also refers to the alterations of what we could call "urban sociability": the use of public space and casual interaction with known and unknown people.

Many male adolescents involved in this research highlighted the closure of gyms, public spaces and other sports activities. Miguel notes: "I have felt desperate, since the pandemic has cancelled the games and the sport center, and that is where I spent part of my time outside of school" (Team 11, field notes). In many of the audiovisual products generated by the adolescents as part of this research project there are countless references to public spaces: empty streets, parks with closed areas and benches, street markets (*tianguis*) with few people, sports areas at night, public transportation, etc. showing the importance that lower-class youth attach to life in the city. These adolescents miss the possibility of privacy and the chance to get out of adult surveillance. Young people from lower social classes often find these opportunities in juvenile public spaces given the precariousness and small size of their residential spaces. Identity, aesthetics, languages, bodily affectivity are very often experienced in public spaces of youth sociability.

The cancellation of activities in public spaces led to a radical reconfiguration of their daily routines. But it is also linked to a feeling of being trapped in their homes, which is a cause of tedium, boredom and anxiety.

> Sometimes I feel sad because I miss my classmates, I have also felt closed in because I feel that my days have become routine, every day I repeat the same thing (Team 11, Miguel, field notes).

> I have felt closed in, I feel like I wasted time of my life, I felt sad on many occasions and I think the most important one is that I felt sad most of the time (Team 11, Alejandra, field notes).

Miguel and Alejandra associate this disruption of daily routines, but above all the monotony and lack of sociability derived from confinement, with a feeling of sadness. It is also important to dwell on what Alejandra expresses in the last quote; the idea that the pandemic meant "taking time away" from their lives. It seems to be about the suspension of a social-historical time that combines with the continuity of a chronological and biological time. The adolescents feel that adolescence itself escapes them without having lived it.

8.5 Sociability and Well-being in Adolescence

The pandemic and confinement meant a drastic change in the daily routines and habits of the general population (Aymerich-Franch 2020). Our fieldwork, and all sources of empirical information generated throughout this work, show that, in the specific case of adolescents, one of the most important areas affected by this rupture in daily life has been sociability. In particular, three spheres of sociability have been affected: peer sociability, family sociability, and urban sociability.

Each of these three spheres is particularly important in the socio-emotional development and well-being of adolescents. Adolescence is a life stage in which the relationship with peers and other adults outside the family of origin is fundamental in the process of subjectivation and identity construction. Distancing from parents in the search for emotional autonomy for decision making and the formation of one's own positioning in the social world is also essential at this stage of life (Crosnoe and Johnson 2011). Both dimensions, the distancing or search for autonomy from the nuclear family, on the one hand, and integration into peer groups and interaction with them and other adults, on the other, complement each other in this process of psycho-social development. Both, however, have been closed or at least substantially altered due to the confinement measures.

The closure of schools in their face-to-face modality has been a critical aspect in this alteration of sociability among peers and in the mental health of adolescents and young people (OECD 2021a). The suspension of traditional schooling made us see clearly that school is not only relevant in its academic-cognitive function, but also for the development and psycho-social well-being of children and adolescents in their process of identity construction and subjectivation.

Face-to-face interaction and the corporeality of co-presence and physical contact are also essential to this peer sociability in the school as well as in youth public spaces. Identities and self-recognition, the construction of affective bonds, youth aesthetics, tastes and preferences independent of the nuclear family, and many other aspects of adolescent development are dependent on this peer sociability. The closure of sociability and interaction is associated with feelings of loneliness and isolation, which in turn are precursors, for young people, of other mental health problems (Orgilés et al. 2020). But our research suggests that the cancellation of face-to-face and subsequent peer sociability is also associated with sadness and depression. Adolescents themselves perceive that the pandemic and confinement imply the loss of school as a space for youthful life and, therefore, of essential aspects of adolescent development. In other words, sadness derives from the feeling of a lost adolescence as a result of an advancing chronological time and a social time that has been suspended.

Virtuality, beyond its contributions to school continuity in its academic dimension, has not been capable of replacing this social dimension. The pandemic teaches us that social networks can be a new space for relationships, links and social interactions that complement or add new forms of sociability (Bengtsson et al. 2021a, 2021b), but (at least in our case study) they do not replace face-to-face sociability among peers. While some studies (Orben et al. 2020) suggest that young people may have been more resilient to confinement than adults thanks to their status as digital natives, others, in line with our own findings, point out that this mitigation has been partial; Panarese and Azzarita (2021), for example, state that in reality, the intense online activity of young people can be interpreted rather as a response to an exceptional situation. In our case, we focused on young people from a lower-class background with severe economic restrictions, a condition that could make it more difficult for them to socialize in this digital "third space" (Bengtsson et al. 2021a, 2021b).

Some young people identified, on the other hand, relationships with household members as a resilience factor in the face of confinement. The exchange of experiences and feelings, companionship, or expressions of affection with siblings, grandparents, or parents, and even with pets, has been highlighted by many adolescents. But the intensification of cohabitation has also meant an alteration, not always positive, of family sociability. The constant surveillance (intentional or not) of the parents and the lack of spaces and moments of intimacy were the cause of emotional discomfort among the adolescents. Indeed, confinement may have generated the strengthening of certain family ties, but also, and apparently mostly, conflicts and other tensions in family sociability. In other words, the family can be a support but also represent a stressful environment for adolescents (Panarese and Azzarita 2021). The results presented in the previous section showed that, indeed, family conflicts, fights and tensions in which adolescents, due to confinement, were involved or involuntary witnessed, are a cause for concern and stress. Excessive cohabitation and lack of intimacy also make the home a suffocating, at times overwhelming, space. These situations can be greatly exacerbated in family spaces where conflictual or violent relationships prevail, and particularly for women, minorities, or other youth identities that are often rejected within their own families.

Interesting in this regard are the results of a survey conducted by Panarese and Azzarita (2021) in Italy, which show that young people under 25 years of age were more likely than the rest of the population to report that personal privacy decreased and that tensions within the home and reciprocal interference and annoyance increased, all as a consequence of the pandemic and confinement. These results are consistent with our findings, and support the importance of spaces of privacy and autonomy from the nuclear family at this stage of life.

The socio-emotional discomforts derived from the intensification of family sociability have a direct relationship with the socio-economic conditions of habitability. In popular sectors, as in our case of analysis, housing conditions tend to be characterized by overcrowding, precariousness, and the absence of independent and open spaces. All these factors accentuate the possibilities of conflict and limit privacy, leading in turn to greater stress.

The lockdown and the restrictions on many activities triggered a substantial limitation of urban sociability. For adolescents from low-income sectors, urban public space continues to play a significant role in their daily experiences, both voluntarily (sports or leisure activities) and involuntarily (work, transportation, leisure). The confinement, derived from all these limitations, not only meant a radical alteration of daily routines, but also were a cause of feelings of frustration, anxiety and helplessness.

Some studies suggest that young females are more likely than males to express feelings of anxiety and depression (Branquinho et al. 2020; WHO 2022); complementarily, the results of our research seem to suggest that frustration and despair would be especially present among males. In any case, gender differences in the way that alterations in peer, family and urban sociability affect the socio-emotional well-being of adolescents is a topic that requires further study, and on which our research does not provide sufficient information.

8.6 Conclusion

The COVID-19 pandemic and, especially, the lockdown had a significant effect, initially little recognized, on the socio-emotional well-being of individuals. Our findings contribute to provide an interpretation of this association between pandemic and well-being for a specific life stage such as adolescence. Confinement measures radically altered adolescent sociability practices (family, urban and peer) with repercussions on their socio-emotional well-being. The results presented in the previous sections seem to support this mediating character of sociability. Face-to-face sociability is so central in this stage of life that its cancellation is perceived by adolescents as a suppression or cancellation of adolescence itself. In different products generated in this research, adolescents stated that "this stage is going to end before the pandemic," "I feel that I lost time of my life" or "life feels stagnant," expressions that summarize the feeling of an unlived youth experience. Many socio-emotional discomforts experienced by these adolescents during the pandemic, such as anxiety, depression, or sadness, may be associated with this inconsistency between a stopped biographical time and a chronological time that kept moving forward. This raises the need for further research on the possible implications of the pandemic for the processes of transition to adulthood.

References

Aymerich-Franch, L. 2020. COVID-19 lockdown: Impact on psychological Well-being and relationship to habit and routine modifications. *PsyArXiv Preprints*. https://doi.org/10.31234/osf.io/9vm7r. Accessed 12 May 2022.

Bengtsson, T., S. Blackman, H. King, and J. Østergaard. 2021a. Distancing, disease and distress: The young and COVID-19: Exploring young people's experience of inequalities and their resourcefulness during the pandemic. *Young* 29 (4S): S5–S10.

Bengtsson, T., L.H. Bom, and L. Fynbo. 2021b. Playing apart together. Young people's online gaming during the COVID-19 lockdown. *Young* 29 (4S): S65–S80.

Branquinho, C., C. Kelly, L.C. Arevalo, A. Santos, and M. Gaspar de Matos. 2020. "Hey, we also have something to say": A qualitative study of Portuguese adolescents' and young people's experiences under COVID-19. *Journal of Community Psychology* 48: 2740–2752.

Cahill, H. 2015. Approaches to understanding youth well-being. In *Handbook of children and youth studies*, ed. J. Wyn and H. Cahill, 95–113. London: Springer.

Cook, A., and P. Krueger-Henney. 2017. Group work that examines systems of power with young people: Youth participatory action research. *The Journal for Specialists in Group Work* 42 (2): 176–193.

Crosnoe, R., and M.K. Johnson. 2011. Research on adolescence in the twenty first century. *Annual Review of Sociology* 37: 439–460.

Larrea-Schiavon, S., L. López-Lalinde, I. Vieitez Martínez, R. Regules, J.P. Gutiérrez, R. Nevárez, C. Mac Gregor, P. López, N. Haberland, and T. Ngô. 2021. *Findings from the violence outcomes in COVID-19 era study (VoCes-19): Baseline results*. Mexico: Population Council.

Marchini, S., E. Zaurino, J. Bouziotis, N. Brondino, V. Delvenne, and M. Delhaye. 2021. Study of resilience and loneliness in youth (18–25 years old) during the COVID-19 pandemic lockdown measures. *Journal of Community Psychology* 49: 468–480.

Mora Salas, M., and G. Urbina. 2021. Las juventudes populares mexicanas frente a la COVID-19: Estigmas, apremios y prácticas de prevención. *Última Década* 56: 104–148.

OECD (Organization for Economic Cooperation and Development). 2021a. COVID-19 and well-being. Life in the pandemic. https://doi.org/10.1787/1e1ecb53-en. Accessed 15 Sep 2022.

———. 2021b. Supporting young people mental's health through the COVID-19 crisis. https://www.oecd.org/coronavirus/policy-responses/supporting-young-people-s-mental-health-through-the-covid-19-crisis-84e143e5/#contactinfo-d7e2442. Accessed 15 Sep 2022.

Orben, A., L. Tomova, and S. Blakemore. 2020. The effects of social deprivation on adolescent development and mental health. *Lancet Child Adolescent Health* 4: 634–640.

Orgilés, M., A. Morales, E. Delvecchio, C. Mazzeschi, and J.P. Espada. 2020. Immediate psychological effects of the COVID-19 quarantine in youth from Italy and Spain. *Frontiers in Psychology* 11: 579038. https://doi.org/10.3389/fpsyg.2020.579038. Accessed 20 June 2022.

Oxfam. 2021. *The inequality virus. Bringing together a world torn apart by coronavirus through a fair, just and sustainable economy*. Oxford, UK: Oxfam GB.

Panarese, P., and V. Azzarita. 2021. The impact of the COVID-19 pandemic on lifestyle: How young people have adapted their leisure and routine during lockdown in Italy. *Young* 29 (4S): S35–S64.

Population Council Mexico. 2021. *VoCes-19*. https://vocescontralaviolencia.org/data-viz-y-publicaciones/. Accessed 01 Feb 2023.

Rose, N. 2020. Social suffering. *RSA Journal* 166 (2): 30–33.

Ryan, G.W., and H.R. Bernard. 2000. Data management and analysis methods. In *Handbook of qualitative research*, ed. N. Denzin and Y. Lincoln, 2nd ed., 769–802. London: Sage.

Saraví, G.A., P. Abrantes, and M. Bertely. 2014. Rights and indigenous adolescence in Mexico. New subjects, new dilemmas. *The International Journal of Children's Rights* 22 (2): 313–338.

Smith, R., M. Danford, S.C. Darnell, M.J. Lima Larrazábal, and M. Abdellatif. 2021. "Like, what even is a podcast?" Approaching sport-for-development youth participatory action research through digital methodologies. *Qualitative Research in Sport, Exercise and Health* 13 (1): 128–145.

UNICEF (The United Nations Children's Fund). 2022. The impact of COVID-19 on the mental health of adolescents and youth. https://www.unicef.org/lac/en/impact-covid-19-mental-health-adolescents-and-youth. Accessed 07 Jan 2023.

WHO (World Health Organization). 2022. Mental health and COVID-19: Early evidence of the pandemic's impact: Scientific brief. https://www.who.int/publications/i/item/WHO-2019-nCoV-Sci_Brief-Mental_health-2022.1. Accessed 07 Jan 2023.

Gonzalo A. Saraví is a researcher at the Center for Research and Graduate Studies in Social Anthropology (CIESAS) in Mexico and member of the National System of Researchers with the highest category. He holds a B.A. in Social Anthropology from the University of Buenos Aires, Argentina and Ph.D. in Sociology from the University of Texas at Austin, USA. Saraví has been a visiting researcher at the Latin American Center (LAC) from the University of Oxford, U.K. and at the IDAES from the National University of San Martin, Argentina. His main areas of interest include youth studies, class inequality, sociology of education, and urban studies in Latin America.

Chapter 9
The Latent Classes of the Volunteer Satisfaction Index and Donation During the Pandemic in Singapore

Joonmo Son, Pildoo Sung, and Benjamin Tay

9.1 Introduction

Volunteering and donation are two distinct prosocial behaviors that may often be interconnected (Lee and Chang 2007; Yeomans and Al-Ubaydli 2018). However, locating studies that tested a plausible association between volunteering and donation is hard. Moreover, the literature has not identified the relationship between the evaluation of volunteer satisfaction and donative behaviors. That is, it is plausible that not all volunteers but those satisfied with volunteer activities organized by voluntary associations may be more likely to donate to various causes. This question loomed larger during the COVID-19 pandemic because numerous voluntary associations experienced a lack of volunteer workforce and donations due to the pandemic's social and economic impacts (Nowakowska 2023). Specifically, many governments enforced social gathering restrictions to prevent the virus's human-to-human transmission. These restrictive orders also reduced volunteer activities that naturally involve face-to-face social interactions (Dederichs 2023). The pandemic also brought serious barriers to the economic activities of employed or self-employed individuals and numerous firms. Therefore, voluntary associations and social welfare agencies in many countries have observed a drastic reduction in donations (Brañas-Garza et al. 2022).

The chapter's research question is whether a high degree of volunteer satisfaction was related to donative behaviors during the pandemic. The study examined the

J. Son (✉)
National University of Singapore, Singapore, Singapore
e-mail: socioson@nus.edu.sg

P. Sung
Hong Kong Baptist University, Kowloon Tong, Hong Kong

B. Tay
National Volunteer & Philanthropy Centre, Singapore, Singapore

C. Suter et al. (eds.), *Well-being During the Pandemic*, Social Indicators Research Series 90, https://doi.org/10.1007/978-3-031-63440-6_9

research question using Galindo-Kuhn and Guzley's (2001) Volunteer Satisfaction Index (VSI). The VSI comprises 26 items under four subdomains, capturing various aspects of volunteer satisfaction. Further, the chapter employed a person-centered approach using the Latent Class Analysis. This person-centered approach assumes that people vary in how they combine multiple items of volunteer satisfaction. The problem then becomes whether people can be sorted into various classes based on the pattern of their composition of volunteer satisfaction indices.

In categorizing volunteer satisfaction indices, the study employed an analytical plan that considers that a particular item of volunteer satisfaction is only one of several or many with which a volunteer agrees that they were satisfied or dissatisfied. The chances are that these multiple items are interconnected through the subdomains of volunteer satisfaction. People compose various "repertoires" from prosocial activities, presumably based on their satisfaction with them (Oser 2017, 2022). As a result, different groups of volunteers may exhibit involvement in disparate classes of volunteer satisfaction items and subdomains.

In turn, volunteers are more likely to contribute money to charities when they are more satisfied with the activities organized by voluntary associations (Piersma et al. 2017; Smith 1994). This study identifies and analyzes the association between several latent classes composed of the volunteer satisfaction index and a set of donative behaviors.

How is the association between the latent classes of volunteer satisfaction and donative behaviors established? It is plausible that satisfied volunteers may become proponents of the cause, more likely to decide to be donors and donate more money than unsatisfied volunteers or nonvolunteers. Further, the satisfied volunteers may try to share their positive experiences with others in their networks, emanating a spillover effect on a larger pool of potential donors.

In particular, volunteers' perception of their participation efficacy in bringing necessary changes to the intended recipients of their services may be associated with the chance of making donations. When they believe that their time investment through voluntary organizations paid off by making a significant difference, they may determine that monetary donation would be another way to strengthen the cause (Basil et al. 2008; Carroll and Kachersky 2019). Further, if volunteers are satisfied with their social relationships with other volunteers in an organization, they may take the additional role of a donor due to the mutual recognition among covolunteers (Brooks 2005).

Theoretically, Galindo-Kuhn and Guzley (2001) wanted to establish the relationship between volunteer satisfaction and volunteer retention measured by the intent to remain in volunteer workforce. The present study proposes that positive evaluation of volunteer activities spills over to being associated with a separate type of prosocial act of donation, explaining how volunteers become donors or vice versa. Thus, the study contributes to the literature by providing a plausible pathway between volunteering and donation, the two distinct prosocial acts.

In order to examine the association between the latent classes of volunteer satisfaction and donative behaviors, the study used a nationally representative dataset from the Individual Giving Study (IGS) in Singapore that was administered during the pandemic.

9.2 Methods

This study aims to see if different classes of Volunteer Satisfaction Index exist in a random sample of the Singaporean population and if the latent classes are associated with donative behaviors. To check the presence of the latent classes, a person-centered analysis is undertaken on the assumption that people vary in the ways that they combine one dimension of volunteer satisfaction with another. The issue then becomes whether current or former volunteers can be sorted into various classes based on the pattern of their agreement with various items concerning volunteer satisfaction.

The latent class analysis (LCA) sorts people into subgroups or classes based on their attributes, in this case, their agreement or disagreement with various items on volunteer satisfaction (Hofmans et al. 2020; Oser 2022). The method acknowledges that a volunteer population comprises individual members who configure their volunteer satisfaction holistically rather than one at a time (Ahlquist and Breunig 2012; Wang and Wang 2019). Current or former volunteers in one class may be agreeable to a broad range of volunteer satisfaction subdimensions, while those in another confine themselves to one or only a few subdimensions. LCA provides reliable criteria for determining the optimal number of latent classes by objective goodness of fit indices (Nylund et al. 2007; Sinha et al. 2021).

Once the number of latent classes has been identified, they are used as independent variables to check their associations with various measures regarding their donative behaviors, controlling for possible confounding factors. The study used a logit regression for a dichotomous outcome variable and OLS for ordinal or continuous outcome variables (Long and Freese 2014).

9.3 Data

The present research used the Individual Giving Study survey in 2021, a nationally representative data set from Singapore. The IGS is a biannual cross-sectional survey project of the National Volunteer & Philanthropy Center initiated in 2000 (NVPC Knowledge & Insights Team 2021). The survey period was between April and September 2021, amid the COVID-19 pandemic. Due to the serious development of the pandemic with an increased number of cases, the survey could not continue for about a month between May and June.

The survey respondents were citizens, permanent residents, foreign workers with work passes and their spouses, or international students with relevant passes. Citizens and permanent residents account for 91% of the sample; 81% of the survey respondents were citizens, while 10% were permanent residents. The respondents had to be at least 15 years old to be eligible to participate in the survey.

Despite the difficulties stemming from the pandemic, the IGS 2021 had 2004 respondents with a response rate of 66.8%, similar to those of previous IGS data.

This study employed a sample of 1093 respondents who were current or former volunteers, excluding those who belonged to self-interest groups or involved in informal gatherings. This is because the major objective of the study was concerning the relationship between volunteers' satisfaction in formal organizations and their donations for various causes.

9.4 Measures

The study used three sets of measures in the analysis. First, five variables that measured varied aspects of donative behaviors were used as outcome measures in multivariable regression analyses. Second, 26 items measuring various subdimensions of volunteer satisfaction were employed in the latent class analysis. Third, control variables that may affect donative behaviors were included in multivariable regressions, along with the latent classes of volunteer satisfaction.

9.4.1 Outcome Variables

Donation behavior has several aspects to consider, from whether a person is a donor to the total amount of donations one makes in a certain period.

Donor status was a dichotomous variable where 1 = donated for any cause in the past few years, 0 = did not.

Donation recency was an ordinal variable: "0. Never," "1. More than 2 years ago," "2. 1–2 years ago," "3. In the past 12 months," "4. In the past 6 months," "5. In the past 3 months," "6. Past 4 weeks," or "7. Past week."

Donation frequency was an ordinal variable: "0. Never," "1. Less than once a year," "2. Annually," "3. Biannually," "4. Quarterly," "5. Monthly," or "6. Weekly."

Number of organizations donated to counted the number of voluntary organizations a person donated to in the past 12 months. It ranges between 0 and 7 or more.

Total amount of donations was a continuous variable indicating the amount of money given to various causes in the past 12 months.

9.4.2 Volunteer Satisfaction Index

The study used the Volunteer Satisfaction Index (VSI) to measure whether volunteers in Singapore were satisfied with the organizations they engaged with for various causes (Galindo-Kuhn and Guzley 2001). The specific 26 items are presented in Appendix. The VSI is a multidimensional scale that measures volunteer's degree of satisfaction in four areas. First, the organizational support dimension is composed of 12 items that ask whether a volunteer is satisfied with various supports provided by the organization, including the relationship with paid staff and the acknowledgment of volunteer work by the organization. Second, the participation efficacy dimension comprises seven items that probe how much progress and changes were made by a volunteer's engagement. Third, the empowerment dimension has three items that concern the degrees of decision-making power, information access to organizational matters, and utilization of one's knowledge and skills in volunteer work. Fourth, the group integration dimension comprises four items regarding the quality and quantity of relationships among volunteers in the organization. The Cronbach alpha coefficients of the four dimensions were 0.95, 0.94, 0.84, and 0.95, respectively, indicating that each dimension of the VSI was reliable. These VSI items were used in creating latent classes reported in the next section.

9.4.3 Control Variables

It is necessary to account for other likely confounders of donative behaviors, such as demographic and socioeconomic characteristics and religiousness, to isolate the relationship between volunteer satisfaction latent classes and donation (Campbell and Yonish 2003; Musick and Wilson 2008; De Abreu et al. 2015).

Age was a continuous variable ranging from 15 to 85.

Gender was a dichotomous variable where 1 = Female, 0 = Male.

Ethnicity was measured by a set of dichotomous variables that reflect the multi-ethnic composition of the Singaporean population: Chinese (1 = Chinese, 0 = other), Malay (1 = Malay, 0 = other), Indian (1 = Indian, 0 = other), or Other (1 = Other, 0 = Chinese, Malay, or Indian). Chinese is the reference category in the multivariable analyses.

Marital status was a dichotomous variable where 1 = Married, 0 = Non-married.

Education was an ordinal variable of educational level: "1. No formal education," "2. PSLE," "3. Secondary N- or O-level certificate," "4. College/ITE/Pre-University/A-level certificate," "5. Polytechnic diploma or equivalent," or "6. University degree or higher."

Due to the high portion of missing values in income variables, it has been a practice in Singapore to use housing type instead as a socioeconomic status variable (e.g., Tan et al. 2022).

Housing type was an ordinal variable of various housing types: "1. HDB (Housing Development Board) 1–2-room flat," "2. HDB 3-room flat," "3. HDB 4-room flat," "4. HDB 5-room flat/Executive flat," "5. Condominium/Private flat," "6. Landed property."

Work status had three dichotomous variables as follows: Full-time work (1 = Full-time work [i.e., 35 h or more working hours per week], 0 = other), Part-time work (1 = part-time work [i.e., less than 35 working hours per week], 0 = other), or Unemployed (1 = Unemployed, 0 = other). Unemployed was a reference category in multivariable analyses.

Religious affiliation comprised a series of dichotomous variables: Buddhist (1 = Buddhist, 0 = other), Christian (1 = Christian, 0 = other), Muslim (1 = Muslim, 0 = other), Hindu (1 = Hindu, 0 = other), Other religion (1 = other religion, 0 = Buddhist, Christian, Muslim, or Hindu), or No religion (1 = no religion; 0 = any religion). No religion was a reference category in multivariable analyses.

9.4.4 Sample Description

A majority of the study sample (60%) engaged in donative behaviors in the past few years (Table 9.1). However, these respondents were current or former volunteers. Thus, the percentage of donors reduces to 41.5% among no volunteers. The respondents in the study sample donated in the past 6 months on average in terms of donation recency. Their average frequency of donation was biannually. The average number of organizations they donated to was about 1. The total amount of donations the study sample made in the past year was S$516. The amount fell to S$216 among no volunteers. The sample description of the VSI latent classes is done in the next section.

As for the control covariates, the respondents in the study sample were 46 years old on average. Fifty-seven percent of them were women, and 69% were Chinese. Fifty-six percent were married. The average educational level was a polytechnic diploma or equivalent, while the average housing type was an HDB four-room flat. About 67% of the respondents worked full-time. Buddhism and Christianity were the largest religious affiliations in the study sample.

Table 9.1 Variables in the analyses

Measure	N	Mean/Percent (S.D.)	Range
Outcome variables			
Donor status	1093	60%	0–1
Donation recency	1093	4.08 (2.28)	0–7
Donation frequency	1093	3.22 (1.74)	0–6
Number of organizations donated to	1093	1.13 (1.10)	0–7+
Total amount of donations in the past year	1093	516.22 (1561.87)	0–24,000
Latent classes of volunteer satisfaction index[a]			
Highest overall satisfaction	1093	14%	0–1
High participation efficacy & group integration	1093	13%	0–1
High organizational support	1093	10%	0–1
Medium participation efficacy	1093	19%	0–1
Lowest overall satisfaction (reference)	1093	44%	0–1
Controls			
Age	1093	45.96 (14.66)	15–85
Female	1093	57%	0–1
Chinese (reference)	1093	69%	0–1

Table 9.1 (continued)

Measure	N	Mean/Percent (S.D.)	Range
Malay	1093	13%	0–1
Indian	1093	14%	0–1
Other ethnicity	1093	4%	0–1
Married	1093	56%	0–1
Education	1091	4.96 (1.33)	1–6
Housing type	1093	3.33 (1.26)	1–6
Full-time work	1091	67%	0–1
Part-time work	1091	6%	0–1
Unemployed (reference)	1091	27%	0–1
Buddhist	1093	26%	0–1
Christian	1093	24%	0–1
Muslim	1093	16%	0–1
Hindu	1093	10%	0–1
Other religion	1093	5%	0–1
No religion (reference)	1093	19%	0–1

Note: Mean and standard deviation are reported for non-dichotomous variables, while percent is reported for dichotomous variables

[a] Refer to Appendix for the subdomains and specific indicators of the VSI

9.5 Results

9.5.1 Latent Classes of Volunteer Satisfaction Index

The study applied a Latent Class Analysis to the 26 items of the Volunteer Satisfaction Index. Each item had seven response categories from 1 = very dissatisfied to 7 = very satisfied. The Latent Class Analysis dichotomized them into 0 = not satisfied (combining original response categories 1 to 5) and 1 = satisfied (combining original response categories 6 and 7).

Determining the number of latent classes is crucial in a person-centered approach to volunteer satisfaction. Three types of model fit statistics of the LCA appear in Table 9.2. First, information criteria indicators such as the Akaike Information Criterion (AIC), Bayesian Information Criterion (BIC), and sample-size-adjusted BIC (ssaBIC) were employed. The lower the values in these criteria, the better the model fit. Second, both the Vuong-Lo-Mendell-Rubin (VLMR) likelihood ratio test and the Lo-Mendell-Rubin (LMR) adjusted likelihood ratio test evaluate if an LCA model with a certain number of classes (*k* classes) is better than a model with one fewer classes (*k*-1 classes) (Cheng et al. 2022). Specifically, significant *p*-values denote that *k* classes should be chosen over *k*-1 classes. Third, entropy indicates classification accuracy, although it should not be used in deciding the optimal number of latent classes (Lubke and Muthén 2007; Morin et al. 2011). It ranges between 0 and 1, with a higher value meaning a more accurate assignment of individuals into latent classes.

Table 9.2 Latent class analysis model fit statistics of the volunteer satisfaction index

	AIC	BIC	ssaBIC	VLMR test	LMR test	Entropy
1-class	33,395.18	33,525.09	33,442.51	–	–	–
2-class	21,803.07	22,067.90	21,899.56	−16,671.59***	11,584.78***	0.96
3-class	19,521.43	19,921.16	19,667.07	−10,848.54***	2323.35***	0.96
4-class	18,918.83	19,453.48	19,113.62	−9680.72***	653.14***	0.94
5-class	18,627.04	19,296.59	18,870.98	−9352.42*	343.97*	0.92
6-class	18,467.10	19,271.57	18,760.20	−9179.52	212.81	0.92

Note: AIC: Akaike Information Criterion, BIC: Bayesian Information Criterion, ssaBIC: Sample-size-adjusted BIC. VLMR test: Vuong-Lo-Mendell-Rubin likelihood ratio test. LMR test: Lo-Mendell-Rubin adjusted likelihood ratio test
* $p < .05$; *** $p < .001$ (two-tailed)

According to the model fit tests, the six-class model recorded the smallest AIC, BIC, and ssa BIC values. However, the gaps between the five- and six-class models were narrow (e.g., only a 25-point difference in the BIC values compared to a 157-point gap between the four- and five-class models). Moreover, the VLMR and LMR likelihood ratio tests showed that the five-class model fits the data better than the six-class model. Additionally, the non-significance of the VLMR and LMR log-likelihood values in the six-class model indicates that the five-class model is optimal. The entropy value of the five-class model is 0.92, indicating excellent classification accuracy. Therefore, the study employs the five-class model as the best-fitted LCA model.

Specifically, the LCA identified five subgroups of the current and former volunteers, as shown in Fig. 9.1 and Table 9.1. They are as follows: (1) highest overall volunteer satisfaction (14%), (2) high Participation Efficacy and Group Integration (13%), (3) high Organizational Support (10%), (4) medium Participation Efficacy (19%), and (5) lowest overall satisfaction (44%). The study used these latent classes as the main independent variables that may be associated with donative behavioral outcomes.

9.5.2 *Regression of Donative Behaviors by the VSI Latent Classes*

The five latent classes comprised a set of the main independent variables, putting the lowest overall satisfaction in the hidden reference category. The five behavioral practices concerning donation were the outcome measures in the multivariable regression analyses. Due to the dichotomous nature of the donor status variable, the study applied a logit regression to it, whereas it used the OLS model for the other four outcome measures in Table 9.3.

Most of all, the multivariable regression results confirmed that the latent classes of volunteer satisfaction were associated with donative behaviors except donation frequency. What mattered most were the two latent classes—the highest overall

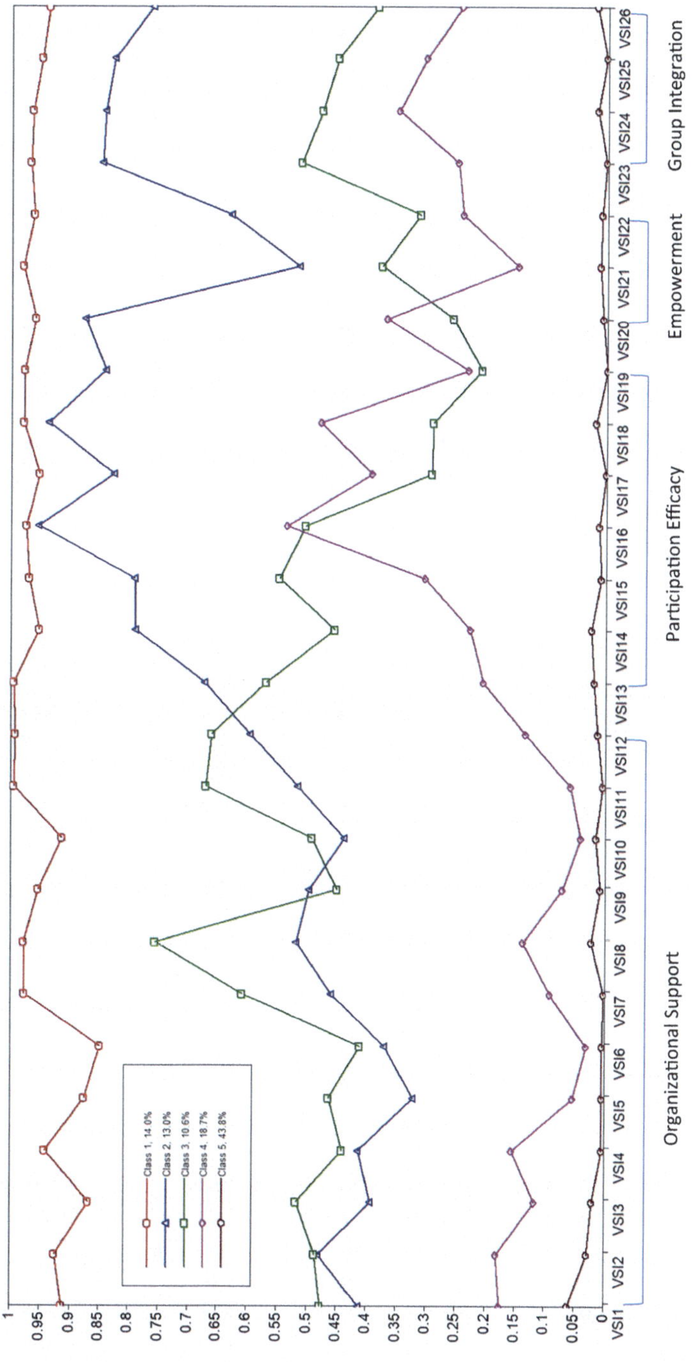

Fig. 9.1 Five latent classes of volunteers based on the voluntary satisfaction index and its subdomains

Table 9.3 Multivariable regression of donative behaviors by the VSI latent classes

	Model 1 (Logit regression)	Model 2 (OLS)	Model 3 (OLS)	Model 4 (OLS)	Model 5 (OLS)
	Donor status	Donation recency	Donation frequency	Number of organizations donated to	Total amount of donations
Latent classes of VSI					
Highest overall satisfaction	0.49^{*}	0.56^{**}	0.20	0.34^{***}	345.32^{*}
	(0.21)	(0.20)	(0.15)	(0.10)	(144.24)
High participation efficacy & group integration	0.62^{**}	0.54^{**}	0.26	0.16	214.22
	(0.22)	(0.21)	(0.16)	(0.10)	(147.92)
High organizational support	0.18	0.22	−0.08	0.06	129.07
	(0.24)	(0.23)	(0.17)	(0.11)	(162.64)
Medium participation efficacy	0.11	0.26	0.03	0.07	46.65
	(0.18)	(0.18)	(0.14)	(0.09)	(127.47)
(reference category: Lowest overall satisfaction)					
Controls					
Age	0.01^{*}	0.02^{***}	0.02^{***}	0.01^{***}	16.51^{***}
	(0.01)	(0.01)	(0.00)	(0.00)	(3.71)
Female	−0.02	0.13	−0.02	0.01	25.41
	(0.14)	(0.13)	(0.10)	(0.06)	(94.69)
Malay	0.24	0.25	0.37	−0.10	-686.41^{*}
	(0.48)	(0.44)	(0.34)	(0.22)	(318.66)
Indian	0.20	−0.08	0.09	0.06	−376.26
	(0.42)	(0.39)	(0.30)	(0.19)	(280.34)
Other	0.68	0.28	0.19	0.26	−93.90
	(0.40)	(0.33)	(0.26)	(0.16)	(240.23)
Married	0.29^{*}	0.34^{*}	0.17	0.08	−52.29
	(0.15)	(0.15)	(0.11)	(0.07)	(104.92)
Education	0.34^{***}	0.37^{***}	0.24^{***}	0.18^{***}	127.15^{**}
	(0.06)	(0.06)	(0.05)	(0.03)	(42.45)
Housing type	0.16^{**}	0.15^{**}	0.12^{**}	0.11^{***}	125.23^{**}
	(0.06)	(0.05)	(0.04)	(0.03)	(39.42)
Full-time work	0.38^{*}	0.56^{***}	0.43^{***}	0.27^{***}	171.79
	(0.17)	(0.16)	(0.13)	(0.08)	(118.06)
Part-time work	−0.02	−0.00	−0.05	−0.09	6.26
	(0.29)	(0.29)	(0.22)	(0.14)	(207.77)
Buddhist	0.32	0.33	0.26	0.08	−55.96
	(0.19)	(0.20)	(0.15)	(0.10)	(140.28)
Christian	0.93^{***}	0.98^{***}	0.85^{***}	0.17	538.83^{***}

Table 9.3 (continued)

	Model 1 (Logit regression)	Model 2 (OLS)	Model 3 (OLS)	Model 4 (OLS)	Model 5 (OLS)
	Donor status	Donation recency	Donation frequency	Number of organizations donated to	Total amount of donations
	(0.21)	(0.20)	(0.15)	(0.10)	(144.50)
Hindu	0.58	0.81	0.55	0.13	413.13
	(0.49)	(0.46)	(0.35)	(0.22)	(329.09)
Muslim	1.35**	1.65***	1.02**	0.55*	799.17*
	(0.49)	(0.45)	(0.34)	(0.22)	(320.49)
Other religion	1.19***	1.05**	0.48	0.19	−8.10
	(0.34)	(0.33)	(0.25)	(0.16)	(237.28)
Intercept	−3.59***	−0.64	−0.23	−0.98***	−1537.67***
	(0.48)	(0.44)	(0.34)	(0.22)	(315.70)
N	1089	1089	1089	1089	1089
R^2	0.10[a]	0.16	0.16	0.12	0.08

Note: Standard errors in parentheses
[a] Pseudo R^2 from a logit regression model
* $p < 0.05$, ** $p < 0.01$, *** $p < 0.001$

satisfaction and the high Participation Efficacy and Group Integration satisfaction. The other two latent classes (the high Organizational Support satisfaction and the medium Participation Efficacy) were related to none of the donative behaviors.

Specifically, Model 1 shows that after accounting for other confounders, those who belonged to the high Participation Efficacy and Group Integration or the highest overall satisfaction latent class were more likely to be donors than others in the latent class of the lowest overall satisfaction. Likewise, Model 2 indicates that respondents in the high overall satisfaction or the high Participation Efficacy and Group Integration latent class tended to donate more recently than others in the lowest overall satisfaction latent class. However, none of the VSI latent classes was related to the donation frequency.

Then Model 4 reports that those respondents in the highest overall satisfaction latent class tended to donate to more organizations than others in the lowest satisfaction latent class. Further, Model 5 shows that those who belonged to the highest overall satisfaction latent class donated about S$345 more than others in the lowest overall satisfaction latent class. Though statistically insignificant, the respondents in the other three latent classes also donated more (i.e., from S$47 to S$214) than those in the lowest overall satisfaction latent class.

Apart from the main independent variables of the VSI latent classes, certain individual characteristics were remarkably related to the donative behavioral outcomes. First, socioeconomic status measured by education, housing types, and full-time work status were consistently associated with the five donative behaviors except for the nonsignificant relationship between full-time work status and the total amount of donations. In particular, those with a higher educational level or more expensive and spacious housing were more likely to be donors and tended to have donated more recently and frequently to a greater number of organizations in larger amounts than others with a lower level of education or less expensive or smaller housing. Being older was also consistently associated with the five outcome measures of donation. Those who were married were more likely to be donors and have donated recently than the non-married. Concerning religiosity, being a Muslim was consistently associated with all five donative behaviors, while being a Christian was also related to most donative behaviors except for the number of organizations they donated to. There was no significant association between ethnicity and donative behaviors.

9.6 Discussion

The IGS 2021 gathered the data during the COVID-19 pandemic in Singapore. It was when the state directives limited face-to-face activities, including work and formal education, to prevent the further spread of the virus (Wong et al. 2023). Instead, non-contagious online media were recommended as alternative communication tools. Therefore, volunteerism had to suffer because most volunteering activities involve intimate face-to-face interactions between volunteers and the recipients of their services (Gray et al. 2024; Luksyte et al. 2021). Due largely to this barrier, Singapore also saw a 7% drop in volunteer rates between 2018 and 2021, while the nation experienced a 19% decrease in donations during the same period (NVPC Knowledge & Insights Team 2021). Therefore, it is crucial to analyze what kind of volunteers are more likely to turn to donative behaviors when interpersonal activities involving physical contact are discouraged due to public health crises such as a pandemic.

The present study showed that the volunteers who experienced a higher overall satisfaction with the organizations tended to donate more money to multiple organizations than those who were generally dissatisfied. Among the four subdimensions of volunteer satisfaction, the participation efficacy and group integration satisfaction were more important than the other two (the organizational support and empowerment satisfaction) in turning volunteers into donors. First, those who realized that what they contributed through participating in volunteer activities made a significant difference among the recipients of their services were more likely to be donors. This particular type of efficacy is also called response efficacy because it concerns "the ability of the advocated behavior to solve the focal problem or issue" (Basil et al. 2008, 7). In other words, the practical changes their activities brought mattered more than their sense of empowerment in the relationship with voluntary organizations. Second, the mutual bonding among volunteers (i.e., group integration) mattered more than how the organizations treated them and whether they were satisfied by the organizational support. The mutual bonding may indicate bridging social capital embedded in the volunteers' networks that helps increase their chances of donating when someone in the networks asks them to (Musick and Wilson 2008; Son and Lin 2008; Wang and Graddy 2008).

These roles of volunteer satisfaction should be further clarified in two regards. First, the associations between the latent classes of volunteer satisfaction and donative behaviors were observed despite the strong relationship among socioeconomic status, religiosity, and donation in Singapore. Whether one occupies a volunteer role should be considered separately from one's socioeconomic status and religious affiliation in considering the likelihood of one's donative behaviors. More specifically, it is critical to know if one evaluates positively on various dimensions of volunteer satisfaction. In short, volunteers who report higher satisfaction with their prosocial activities conducted through voluntary associations are also more likely to donate. Second, in the opposite sense, some volunteers whose experiences with voluntary associations are evaluated to be poor are no more likely to donate than nonvolunteers. Thus, the lack of volunteer satisfaction may turn volunteers into nonvolunteers and nondonors. There is no reason to expect those dissatisfied with an organization's activities to donate to the organization or others similar to it. Therefore, volunteer satisfaction is a double-edged sword that does not allow a simplistic understanding of the relationship between volunteering and donation.

9.7 Limitations

The study suffers from several limitations. First, the cross-sectional data do not guarantee a causal relationship between volunteer satisfaction and donation. The approach taken in the study was to check the association between the latent classes of volunteer satisfaction and a set of donative behaviors. Nonetheless, it is plausible that some donors can also become volunteers. Alternatively, it is also possible that some respondents were volunteering donors. For example, they may be active members of a religious congregation who volunteer for some religious causes. At the same time, they may donate regularly or periodically to religious establishments through dana (Buddhism), tithe (Christianity), zakat (Islam), or prasada (Hinduism). However, the study's finding that dissatisfied volunteers may reduce or stop donating applies to the case of religious volunteers, too. In addition, the study controlled for religious affiliations when checking the association between the VSI latent classes and donation.

Second, because the study focused on the relationship between volunteer satisfaction and donation, it could not consider nonvolunteers and their donative behaviors. Although nonvolunteers recorded a lower percentage of donors and smaller means in the other four donative behaviors of the study, some of the nonvolunteers were donors. Still, the study is limited in what it can say about the nonvolunteers.

Third, considering that the study sample included only current and former volunteers, the results may suffer from the sample selection bias. The problem can intensify if volunteers and donors share the same prosocial traits. Arguably, it is not that certain latent classes of volunteer satisfaction are related to donative behaviors but that both the VSI latent classes and donative behaviors are affected by the same prosocial traits. However, the correlation coefficient between volunteer status and donor status was 0.21, a modest level. Therefore, it is hard to maintain that the study results were spurious.

9.8 Conclusion

The present study showed that the organic association between volunteer satisfaction and donation existed during the COVID-19 pandemic in Singapore. Not all volunteers donate, nor do all donors volunteer. The study's latent class analysis investigation indicated that a minority of volunteers with the highest overall satisfaction (14%) or the high participation efficacy and group integration satisfaction (13%) were more likely to donate. In contrast, those volunteers who expressed a high degree of organizational support satisfaction (10%) or a medium level of participation efficacy satisfaction (19%) were no more or less likely to donate than those who showed the least overall satisfaction (44%). Therefore, volunteer satisfaction concerning the perceived efficacy of volunteer activities and the social bonding with covolunteers may particularly translate into donative behaviors.

In summary, the chapter demonstrated that volunteer satisfaction may encourage a minority of volunteers to donate generously to more charitable causes despite global-scale catastrophes such as the COVID-19 pandemic. Future studies are warranted to examine the association between volunteer satisfaction and donation in other countries.

Appendix: Volunteer Satisfaction Index, its Subdomains, and Indicators

Organizational support
1. The ability of getting help when I need it.
2. The realism of the picture I was given of what my volunteer experience would be like.
3. My relationship with paid staff.
4. The support network that is in place for me when I have volunteer-related problems.
5. The way in which the agency provides me with performance feedback.
6. The flow of communication coming to me from paid staff and board members.
7. The support I receive from people in the organization.
8. The amount of information I receive about what the organization is doing.
9. How often the organization acknowledges the work I do.
10. The amount of permission I need to get to do the things I need to do on this job.
11. The degree of cohesiveness I experience within the organization.
12. The degree to which the organization communicates its goals and objectives to volunteers.
Participation efficacy
13. The progress that I have seen in the clientele served by my organization.

14. The difference my volunteer work is making.
15. My ability to do this job as well as anyone else.
16. The opportunities I have to learn new things.
17. The fit of the volunteer work to my skills.
18. How worthwhile my contribution is.
19. The amount of effort I put in as equaling the amount of change I influence.
Empowerment
20. The chance I have to utilize my knowledge and skills in my volunteer work.
21. The access I have to information concerning the organization.
22. The freedom I have in deciding how to carry out my volunteer assignment.
Group integration
23. My relationship with other volunteers in the organization.
24. The friendships I have made while volunteering here.
25. The amount of interaction I have with other volunteers in the organization.
26. The amount of time spent with other volunteers.

Note: The response categories were from 1 = very dissatisfied to 7 = very satisfied

References

Ahlquist, J.S., and C. Breunig. 2012. Model-based clustering and typologies in the social sciences. *Political Analysis* 20: 92–112. https://doi.org/10.1093/pan/mpr039.

Basil, D.Z., N.M. Ridgway, and M.D. Basil. 2008. Guilt and giving: A process model of empathy and efficacy. *Psychology & Marketing* 25: 1–23. https://doi.org/10.1002/mar.20200.

Brañas-Garza, P., D. Jorrat, A. Alfonso, A.M. Espín, T. García Muñoz, and J. Kovářík. 2022. Exposure to the COVID-19 pandemic environment and generosity. *Royal Society Open Science* 9: 210919. https://doi.org/10.1098/rsos.210919.

Brooks, A.C. 2005. Does social capital make you generous? *Social Science Quarterly* 86: 1–15. https://doi.org/10.1111/j.0038-4941.2005.00287.x.

Campbell, D.E., and S.J. Yonish. 2003. Religion and volunteering in America. In *Religion as social capital: Producing the common good*, ed. C. Smidt, 87–106. Waco, TX: Baylor University Press.

Carroll, R., and L. Kachersky. 2019. Service fundraising and the role of perceived donation efficacy in individual charitable giving. *Journal of Business Research* 99: 254–263. https://doi.org/10.1016/j.jbusres.2019.02.051.

Cheng, G.H.-L., P. Sung, A. Chan, S. Ma, and R. Malhotra. 2022. Transitions between social network profiles and their relation with all-cause mortality among older adults. *Social Science & Medicine* 292: 114617. https://doi.org/10.1016/j.socscimed.2021.114617.

De Abreu, M.E., R.M.S. Laureano, R.V. Da Silva, and P. Dionísio. 2015. Volunteerism, compassion and religiosity as drivers of donations practices. *International Journal of Nonprofit and Voluntary Sector Marketing* 20: 256–276. https://doi.org/10.1002/nvsm.1526.

Dederichs, K. 2023. Volunteering in the United Kingdom during the COVID-19 pandemic: Who started and who quit? *Nonprofit and Voluntary Sector Quarterly* 52: 1458–1474. https://doi.org/10.1177/08997640221122814.

Galindo-Kuhn, R., and R.M. Guzley. 2001. The volunteer satisfaction index. *Journal of Social Service Research* 28: 45–68. https://doi.org/10.1300/J079v28n01_03.

Gray, D., J. Randell, R. Manning, and M. Cleveland. 2024. Helping in times of crisis: Examining the social identity and wellbeing impacts of volunteering during COVID-19. *Journal of Community & Applied Social Psychology* 34: e2699. https://doi.org/10.1002/casp.2699.

Hofmans, J., B. Wille, and B. Schreurs. 2020. Person-centered methods in vocational research. *Journal of Vocational Behavior* 118: 103398. https://doi.org/10.1016/j.jvb.2020.103398.

Lee, Y.-K., and C.-T. Chang. 2007. Who gives what to charity? Characteristics affecting donation behavior. *Social Behavior and Personality* 35: 1173–1180. https://doi.org/10.2224/sbp.2007.35.9.1173.

Long, J.S., and J. Freese. 2014. *Regression models for categorical dependent variables using Stata*. 3rd ed. College Station, TX: Stata Press Publication, StataCorp LP.

Lubke, G., and B.O. Muthén. 2007. Performance of factor mixture models as a function of model size, covariate effects, and class-specific parameters. *Structural Equation Modeling* 14: 26–47. https://doi.org/10.1080/10705510709336735.

Luksyte, A., P.D. Dunlop, D. Holtrop, M. Gagné, D. Kragt, and H.M. Farid. 2021. The challenges of volunteering during the COVID-19 pandemic. *Industrial and Organizational Psychology* 14: 286–289. https://doi.org/10.1017/iop.2021.62.

Morin, A.J.S., C. Maïano, B. Nagengast, H.W. Marsh, J. Morizot, and M. Janosz. 2011. General growth mixture analysis of adolescents' developmental trajectories of anxiety: The impact of untested invariance assumptions on substantive interpretations. *Structural Equation Modeling* 18: 613–648. https://doi.org/10.1080/10705511.2011.607714.

Musick, M.A., and J. Wilson. 2008. *Volunteers: A social profile*. Bloomington, IN: Indiana University Press.

Nowakowska, I. 2023. Age, frequency of volunteering, and present-hedonistic time perspective predict donating items to people in need, but not money to combat COVID-19 during lockdown. *Current Psychology* 42: 17329–17339. https://doi.org/10.1007/s12144-021-01993-0.

NVPC Knowledge & Insights Team. 2021. *NVPC individual giving study 2021*. Singapore: National Volunteer & Philanthropy Center. https://cityofgood.sg/resources/nvpc-individual-giving-study-2021/. Accessed 19 Nov 2021.

Nylund, K.L., T. Asparouhov, and B.O. Muthén. 2007. Deciding on the number of classes in latent class analysis and growth mixture modeling: A Monte Carlo simulation study. *Structural Equation Modeling* 14: 535–569. https://doi.org/10.1080/10705510701575396.

Oser, J. 2017. Assessing how participators combine acts in their "political tool kits": A person-centered measurement approach for analyzing citizen participation. *Social Indicators Research* 133: 235–258. https://doi.org/10.1007/s11205-016-1364-8.

———. 2022. Protest as one political act in individuals' participation repertoires: Latent class analysis and political participant types. *American Behavioral Scientist* 66: 510–532. https://doi.org/10.1177/00027642211021633.

Piersma, T.W., R. Bekkers, E.F. Klinkenberg, W.L.A.M. de Kort, and E.-M. Merz. 2017. Individual, contextual and network characteristics of blood donors and non-donors: A systematic review of recent literature. *Blood Transfusion* 15 (5): 382. https://doi.org/10.2450/2017.0064-17.

Sinha, P., C.S. Calfee, and K.L. Delucchi. 2021. Practitioner's guide to latent class analysis: Methodological considerations and common pitfalls. *Critical Care Medicine* 49: e63–e79. https://doi.org/10.1097/CCM.0000000000004710.

Smith, D.H. 1994. Determinants of voluntary association participation and volunteering: A literature review. *Nonprofit and Voluntary Sector Quarterly* 23: 243–263. https://doi.org/10.1177/089976409402300305.

Son, J., and N. Lin. 2008. Social capital and civic action: A network-based approach. *Social Science Research* 37: 330–349. https://doi.org/10.1016/j.ssresearch.2006.12.004.

Tan, S.B., B.L. Dickens, A. Sevtsuk, S. Zheng, K. Zeng, Y.S. Lee, F. Yap, S.-Y. Chan, J.K.Y. Chan, K.H. Tan, Y.-S. Chong, J.G. Eriksson, M.F.-F. Chong, and M.C. Arcaya. 2022. Exploring how socioeconomic status affects neighbourhood environments' effects on obesity risks: A longitudinal study in Singapore. *Landscape and Urban Planning* 226: 104450. https://doi.org/10.1016/j.landurbplan.2022.104450.

Wang, L., and E. Graddy. 2008. Social capital, volunteering, and charitable giving. *VOLUNTAS: International Journal of Voluntary and Nonprofit Organizations* 19: 23–42. https://doi.org/10.1007/s11266-008-9055-y.

Wang, J., and X. Wang. 2019. *Structural equation modeling: Applications using Mplus*. Hoboken, NJ: John Wiley & Sons.

Wong, A., C. Zoller, A. Fouda, and F. Paolucci. 2023. Are we past the COVID-19 pandemic? Insights from Singapore. *Health Policy and Technology* 13 (1): 100779. https://doi.org/10.1016/j.hlpt.2023.100779.

Yeomans, M., and O. Al-Ubaydli. 2018. How does fundraising affect volunteering? Evidence from a natural field experiment. *Journal of Economic Psychology* 64: 57–72. https://doi.org/10.1016/j.joep.2017.11.004.

Joonmo Son is an Associate Professor of Sociology in the Department of Sociology and Anthropology at the National University of Singapore. He studies social capital, social networks, volunteerism, health and aging, and religion. His works appeared in journals such as *Journal of Health and Social Behavior*, *Aging & Mental Health*, *Social Networks*, *Social Indicators Research*, *Social Science Research*, *Journal for the Scientific Study of Religion*, and *Sociological Forum*. He recently published a book titled *Social Capital* in the Polity's Key Concepts Series. He was elected president of the International Sociological Association Research Committee 55 (Social Indicators) from 2023 to 2027.

Pildoo Sung is an Assistant Professor of Sociology at Hong Kong Baptist University. He studies the impact of social relationships on health and well-being, mainly among older adults and their informal caregivers. His research has been published in journals such as *The Journals of Gerontology*, *Journal of Aging and Social policy*, *Gerontology*, and *Journal of Aging and Health*.

Benjamin Tay currently works for the National Volunteer & Philanthropy Centre, Strategy & Policy. He has a keen interest in conducting research for emerging, unmet, and underserved needs in the social and community sector and has been involved in national studies to better understand the giving behaviours and motivations of individuals and corporates. His prior research includes understanding the respite needs of caregivers, the quality of life of vulnerable populations in Singapore, and attitude studies towards persons with disabilities and persons recovering from mental health conditions.

Chapter 10
COVID-19 and Community-Based Volunteerism: How the Rohingya Volunteers Acted for Community Engagement to Fight against the Pandemic in Rohingya Refugee Camps of Bangladesh

Md. Fakhrul Alam

10.1 Background

The global outbreak of COVID-19 (SARS-CoV-2) in 2020 disrupted the world and negatively impacted the life and livelihood of people. Especially, the first wave of COVID-19 seriously affected the public health system and society at large (Miao et al. 2021). The marginalized and disadvantaged communities, such as the refugees living under vulnerable conditions, were adversely affected. Globally, 89.3 million people were forcibly displaced, of which 27.1 million were refugees, and low- and middle-income countries hosted around 83% of these global refugees (UNHCR 2022). Since developing countries struggled to manage COVID-19 and serve their citizens, the refugees were found more vulnerable to the pandemic. The refugees experienced the worst impacts of the pandemic in their daily lives, access to work, safety, and financial means because of their harsh living conditions (World Health Organization 2020a).

Bangladesh hosts around 1 million Rohingya refugees from neighboring Myanmar (Jubayer et al. 2020). It is a densely populated and poverty-stricken country, which was seriously affected by COVID-19 (Gautam et al. 2022). The country's healthcare system was found incompetent to battle the pandemic (Al-Zaman 2020). The shortage of protective equipment and testing kits, limited testing facilities, and resource constraints exacerbated the health crisis during the first wave of COVID-19 (Al-Zaman 2020). Despite the challenges, the government in collaboration with international organizations responded promptly to protect the Rohingya refugees. The Rohingyas are a Muslim ethnic group from the Rakhine state of Myanmar. Around 740,000 Rohingyas fled to Bangladesh in 2017 to protect their lives from

Md. F. Alam (✉)
Department of Social Work, Shahjalal University of Science and Technology,
Sylhet, Bangladesh
e-mail: fakhrul-scw@sust.edu

C. Suter et al. (eds.), *Well-being During the Pandemic*, Social Indicators
Research Series 90, https://doi.org/10.1007/978-3-031-63440-6_10

brutal military crackdowns and violence, sexual abuse, and persecution in Rakhine (Ergül 2020a; Sahana et al. 2019). They took shelter in 34 congested refugee camps in Cox's Bazar (Jubayer et al. 2020). The Rohingyas and local host communities live side by side with little restriction on movement from the camp to the host community, though the refugees are not allowed officially to move outside the camps (Khan et al. 2020). Therefore, it was difficult to control the community-level transmission of COVID-19.

It was anticipated that COVID-19 could spread quickly in the refugee camps because of the high population density (40,000 refugees live per km^2), non-availability of space for physical distance and self-isolation, Rohingya's poor knowledge about COVID-19, unhygienic living conditions, and inadequate access to water, sanitation, and health care facilities (Islam and Yeasir Yunus 2020; Khan et al. 2020). It was also challenging to engage the Rohingya community in COVID-19-related programs and services because of the information gap, limited access to telecommunication, infected people's fear of being stigmatized and killed, rumors, ignorance, and misconception (Islam and Yeasir Yunus 2020; Khan et al. 2020). Moreover, health workers' increased risk of infection, limited financial aid, inadequate COVID-19 testing and treatment facilities, and shortage of medical equipment and hospital beds made the situation worse (Islam and Yeasir Yunus 2020). Against this backdrop, the UN organizations and humanitarian agencies in collaboration with the Government of Bangladesh took rapid actions, such as providing training, increasing hospital capacities, establishing isolation and quarantine facilities, and promoting lab testing facilities (Islam and Yeasir Yunus 2020; Khan et al. 2020). The Rohingya volunteers were educated about COVID-19 to make all-out efforts for increasing community-level awareness and civic engagement.

Global studies on disaster management highlight the importance of community engagement for raising community awareness, strengthening community response and resilience, and executing emergency actions (Johnston et al. 2012; Ryan et al. 2020; Satizábal et al. 2022). In recent years, there has been increased emphasis on community engagement as an effective strategy to manage the COVID pandemic and protect people's well-being (Adebisi et al. 2021; Khan et al. 2022; Larmar et al. 2021; Miao et al. 2021; Mondal 2021). Since multiple stakeholders act jointly and collaboratively for community engagement (Satizábal et al. 2022), it is necessary to investigate the roles of young volunteers recruited from a culturally sensitive, disadvantaged, and marginalized community, and how they contribute to raise civic responsibilities, strengthen community solidarity, and encourage and motivate people for civic engagement during a period of heightened risks and uncertainty. Data from some recent studies (Ekzayez et al. 2020; Ha et al. 2021; Miao et al. 2021) also suggest that collaborative actions of local volunteers, communities, and other stakeholders were useful for pandemic management. Despite the importance of community engagement in participatory emergency management (Satizábal et al. 2022), there remains a paucity of evidence on community engagement activities at refugee camps led by refugee volunteers in the pandemic situation. To date, no previous studies have investigated how the refugees or young refugee volunteers were engaged in risk communication and community engagement (RCCE) activities, how they collaborated with different stakeholders to overcome the barriers and challenges of people's participation in pandemic management, and how they worked to raise civic responsibilities to slow the rate of infection in refugee camps where congested living arrangements, resource crisis, illiteracy, religious misinterpretation, public health behavior, and rumor could increase community-level infection rapidly (Islam and Yeasir Yunus 2020; Khan et al. 2020).

Considering the research gap, the current study aims to highlight the actions undertaken by humanitarian organizations to curb the spread of COVID-19 with the active involvement of young Rohingya volunteers and refugee leaders, how the volunteers were made capable of fighting against the risks and challenges of civic engagement in the absence of humanitarian workers, and how they helped the refugees during the first wave of COVID pandemic. More specifically, it seeks to discover and explain the actions performed by Rohingya volunteers and other refugees in facilitating COVID-19-related awareness programs and health services, and the outcome of those actions.

10.2 Community Engagement for Pandemic Management: A Review of Recent Evidence

Much of the literature on community engagement comes from studies related to disaster management. Various studies argue that community engagement is crucial for disaster planning, mitigation, preparedness, response, recovery, and strengthening people's compliance with top-down policies (Ryan et al. 2020; Satizábal et al. 2022). It is a process where the government, civil society groups, businesses, and stakeholders act collaboratively, share capacity, and develop a trustworthy relationship through which the demands, needs, expectations, concerns, and values of the community are integrated into policies, decisions, service delivery, and evaluation (Satizábal et al. 2022). It builds a resilient and healthy community, changes human behavior, promotes social support, empowers the community, strengthens social networks, enhances mutual respect, and raises people's awareness about the purpose and means of community-level actions (den Broeder et al. 2021). Since community engagement helps understand the experience, problems, needs, and resources of the local community, it could be effective for health promotion and community resilience during a crisis in disadvantaged communities (den Broeder et al. 2021; Mehta et al. 2022). A community faces multiple risks and receives contrasting messages from formal and informal sources during a pandemic which creates dilemmas in decision-making. Therefore, effective community engagement, collaboration of stakeholders, and interactive risk communication can develop the strength of community-based organizations, build community trust, leverage community participation, and encourage and incentivize volunteers in pandemic planning, response, and risk reduction (Cheng et al. 2020; Khan et al. 2022).

To date, several studies on disaster management have highlighted the importance of community engagement and collaborative actions of different stakeholders. A recent study by Ryan et al. (2020) concluded that community engagement was found useful in disaster preparedness activities and in improving knowledge. In fact, multiple actors of community engagement were involved in planning, community access, trust building, risk and behavioral change communication, surveillance, tracing, and administrative actions in the past outbreaks of Ebola, SARS, Zika, and H1N1 (Gilmore et al. 2020). Evidence also shows that interventions through community engagement had a range of positive outcomes in health behavior, health consequences, and health behavior self-efficacy across diverse conditions in OECD countries (O'Mara-Eves et al. 2015).

Comparatively, very few empirical studies examined the role of community-based volunteers in civic engagement during the COVID-19 pandemic. Utilizing community conference calls, the Department of Spiritual Care and Chaplaincy in the John Hopkins Bayview Medical Center encouraged participation from congregation and faith-based organizations. This medical-religious community engagement helped explore the ways to solve the challenges of quarantine, isolation, health disparities, and mental health, and the resources needed for helping the community (Galiatsatos et al. 2020). Similarly, the University of Arkansas for Medical Sciences strengthened community engagement to build trust between partners of community stakeholders and the health centers. The partners collaboratively developed COVID-19 response strategies of health education, contact tracing, COVID-19 testing, quarantine, and case management for the Latinx and Pacific Islander communities, and thus, community-based participatory research and programmatic networks were found effective in addressing COVID-19 problems (McElfish et al. 2021). Analyzing the Australian context, Maher and Murphet (2020) argue that continuous effective community engagement, cyclical and repetitive communication, information preparedness and sharing, and trust building for behavioral changes could be the primary ways of arresting the spread of COVID-19. Reviewing multifarious community actions in the UK and The Netherlands, den Broeder et al. (2021) claim that citizens, communities, and community-based organizations can build community resilience and empower the community through community engagement, which will help promote health and manage COVID-19. Similarly, Mughal et al. (2022) also report that community engagement activities executed by different cultural groups, charities, community-based organizations, and mutual aid groups provided support for the social, physical, and mental well-being of individuals in response to COVID-19 in the UK. Taking cultural and structural contexts into consideration, RCCE (Risk communication and community engagement) with participatory approaches were found effective in disseminating COVID-19-related scientific information to the affected migrant workers' communities, encouraging bottom-up RCCE efforts, mobilizing peer-led supports, creating an enabling environment, and ensuring feedback from the affected communities in Singapore (Tam et al. 2022).

Analyzing the situation of COVID-19 in China, Hu and Qiu (2020) suggest developing a risk communication system, stakeholder coordination, and community engagement to confront uncertainty, refute rumors, strengthen cooperation, take local actions, provide health education, and act jointly. Miao et al. (2021) found that the collaborative approach was applied to strengthen networks of public organizations, civil society groups, and community volunteers in Zhejiang Province of China, where the volunteers played dynamic roles in protecting people from COVID-19 and filled gaps in public health and other services. In Vietnam, local communities, especially the migrant workers executed activities related to early detection, isolation, quarantine, and COVID-19 treatment in collaboration with multi-sectoral committees and organizations. The active engagement of migrant communities mobilized resources, strengthened capacity, facilitated better communication, and built trust in state interventions (Ha et al. 2021). The community-based campaign called "Volunteers against Corona" in Syria encouraged and involved thousands of local volunteers in community awareness programs, disinfection campaigns, referrals, communication, information sharing, and local resource mobilization for pandemic management (Ekzayez et al. 2020). In Tanzania, a medical college worked collaboratively with the municipality response team for community engagement in COVID-19 programs. Mass public health campaigns providing updated information, tackling rumors and misinformation, and ensuring community compliance with interventions, and stakeholder coordination were found effective in pandemic management (Mboya et al. 2020). RCCE techniques used through training, capacity development, risk communication, coordination, information sharing, and public communication were found helpful in controlling COVID-19 transmission in some African countries (Adebisi et al. 2021).

In summary, existing global literature shows that community engagement is essential for managing a pandemic like COVID-19, and volunteers can play a significant role in disaster risk mitigation. But little is known about how the global humanitarian agencies engaged community-based volunteers from the refugee camps for RCCE activities, and how they played dynamic roles in mitigating disaster risks, developing community trust and resilience, strengthening a sense of civic responsibilities of the refugees to follow health safety rules and participate in health programs designed to protect the refugees.

10.3 Methodology

10.3.1 Nature of the Study

By using qualitative design (Creswell 2013) this exploratory study discloses and elucidates the contexts of Rohingya volunteers' involvement in community engagement during the first wave of COVID-19 in Rohingya refugee camps. A qualitative design was found effective in exploring service providers' views, experiences, and knowledge about COVID-19 and its impacts, and the management and delivery of emergency services (Neely-Barnes et al. 2021). This study explored and explained the real-life experiences of Rohingya refugees, Rohingya volunteers, and humanitarian workers regarding their involvement in community engagement during COVID-19.

10.3.2 Study Participants

All humanitarian agencies execute field-based programs and services at refugee camps of Cox's Bazar, Bangladesh with the help of local Rohingya volunteers. The volunteers are not recruited as employees, but they get some remuneration for volunteering in humanitarian activities (Ergül 2020a). This study recruited Rohingya refugees, Rohingya volunteers, and humanitarian workers as study participants. Official permission to visit refugee camps and interview the refugees was granted by the office of the Refugee Relief and Repatriation Commissioner (RRRC). Two Rohingya volunteers were recruited to act as gatekeepers and help the field investigators select potential refugee respondents. Since purposive sampling is widely used in qualitative research for matching the sample with the research objectives and developing rigor and trustworthiness of the data (Campbell et al. 2020), the refugee respondents were selected purposively. Likewise, after identifying major humanitarian agencies in Cox's Bazar, Bangladesh, the agency personnel (humanitarian workers) with direct experience in serving the refugees during the pandemic were selected purposively. Table 10.1 shows different categories of respondents and the size of the samples. Although the study focused on the actions of humanitarian agencies, it recruited one government employee who mainly worked coordinating different agencies at the refugee camps and had work experience during the pandemic situation.

10.3.3 Data Collection

In-depth interviews help explore participants' experiences and views about the COVID-19 pandemic (Hirani and Wagner 2022). This study used in-depth interviews using semi-structured interview guidelines, one guideline for humanitarian workers and another for Rohingya refugees. Three NGO workers serving Rohingya

Table 10.1 Research participants and sample size

Respondents	Number
Rohingya refugees	21
Rohingya teachers	03
Rohingyas working for NGOs or UN organizations	04
Rohingya community leaders (*Majhi* and *Imam*)	04
Community-based Rohingya volunteers	17
Sub-total	**49**
Field-level officers from national NGOs	04
Field-level officers from international NGOs	27
Field-level officers from UN organizations	10
Field-level government employee (administration)	01
Sub-total	**42**
Total	**91**

refugees were recruited as field investigators with training in ethical issues and in-depth interviews. They conducted face-to-face interviews with the help of Rohingya volunteers and recorded interviews after obtaining prior permission. On average, each interview lasted for 30 to 40 min. The interviews were transcribed and translated into the Bengali language by one Research Assistant experienced in the Rohingya language. Similarly, the field investigators purposively selected the humanitarian workers for interviews in Cox's Bazar. They recorded the interviews and transcribed them verbatim. All interview transcripts were checked by the Research Assistants and the researcher. Considering the COVID-19 situation, the fieldwork was completed between October 2020 to January 2021.

10.3.4 Data Analysis and Interpretation

The study adopted thematic analysis techniques of qualitative data analysis (Braun and Clarke 2006). All transcripts were prepared in Bengali language and then translated into English. The Research Assistants and the researcher went through the transcripts and read and reread them to develop the initial ideas about the data. Then the interesting features of the data were identified for coding and relevant data were collated according to the codes (for example, misconceptions, misbeliefs, rumors, training, awareness sessions, public trust, and knowledge of COVID-19, etc.). After further checking and reviewing, the researcher finalized the codes and collated them with the potential themes, and gathered data pertinent to each potential theme. The generated themes were reviewed according to their workability to the codes and extracted data. The researcher then defined and named themes through investigating the essence of each theme, and then supported the themes coherently and consistently with accompanying quotes from the respondents. The themes reflect the views and experiences of research participants and provide a logical and meaningful explanation of the data.

10.3.5 Ethical Considerations

A researcher needs to overcome several ethical challenges while researching refugees in a crisis (Mackenzie et al. 2007). This study followed the ethical principles prescribed under the guidelines of the Australian Government (National Statement on Ethical Conduct in Human Research, 2007 updated 2018)[1] and the WMA Declaration of Helsinki.[2] It was peer-reviewed and funded by a public university in

[1] https://www.nhmrc.gov.au/about-us/publications/national-statement-ethical-conduct-human-research-2007-updated-2018#block-views-block-file-attachments-content-block-1.

[2] https://www.wma.net/policies-post/wma-declaration-of-helsinki-ethical-principles-for-medical-research-involving-human-subjects/.

Bangladesh. It also received ethical clearance from the same university. Interviews were conducted following COVID-19 rules, and no interviewees were asked any personal questions to reduce personal harm. Participation was voluntary and interviews were conducted to align with the respondent's convenience. Written or oral informed consent was taken after respondents were supplied with the Information Sheet. Attempts were also made to ensure anonymity and confidentiality. Moreover, all refugee participants were given TK200 (US$2.5) or materials of the same value to compensate for their time (Mackenzie et al. 2007). The respondents also benefitted through participation as the interview questions helped develop awareness of COVID-19-related risks and health services.

10.4 Findings

Following the study's purposes, the findings unveil and explain the risks and challenges of community engagement, vulnerabilities of the refugees to COVID-19, actions of agencies and stakeholders to leverage community participation, voluntary activities of Rohingya volunteers and refugees, and the outcome of community engagement. The findings summarized in Fig. 10.1 show how the UN and humanitarian agencies and the government of Bangladesh acted to address the risks and challenges of COVID-19 in Rohingya camps, the community engagement activities of the Rohingya volunteers, and the outcome of agency-community collaboration. Then the findings are presented under each theme.

10.4.1 Challenge of Risk Communication and Community Engagement

The highly congested living environment, lack of physical space, and inadequate access to water, sanitation, and health facilities at refugee camps made the Rohingya refugees vulnerable to the risks of COVID-19. Lockdown and movement restrictions made it difficult to organize regular awareness sessions at the camps.

> Once the army did not allow us to enter the block. We took an awareness session after their exit. While I advised people to maintain distance, they replied that there was no space to maintain physical distance. A person caught with a fever does not find any space for physical isolation inside a house. (Respondent 84, Female Rohingya volunteer, Save the Children)

The Rohingya refugees did not have any idea about COVID-19 during its onset in 2020. The limited access to telecommunication made it difficult to receive scientific information about COVID-19, the way it spread, and the protection and treatment measures. Many Rohingyas failed to realize the actual danger of COVID-19 by doubting its existence. Moreover, religious misconceptions and misbeliefs hindered awareness activities.

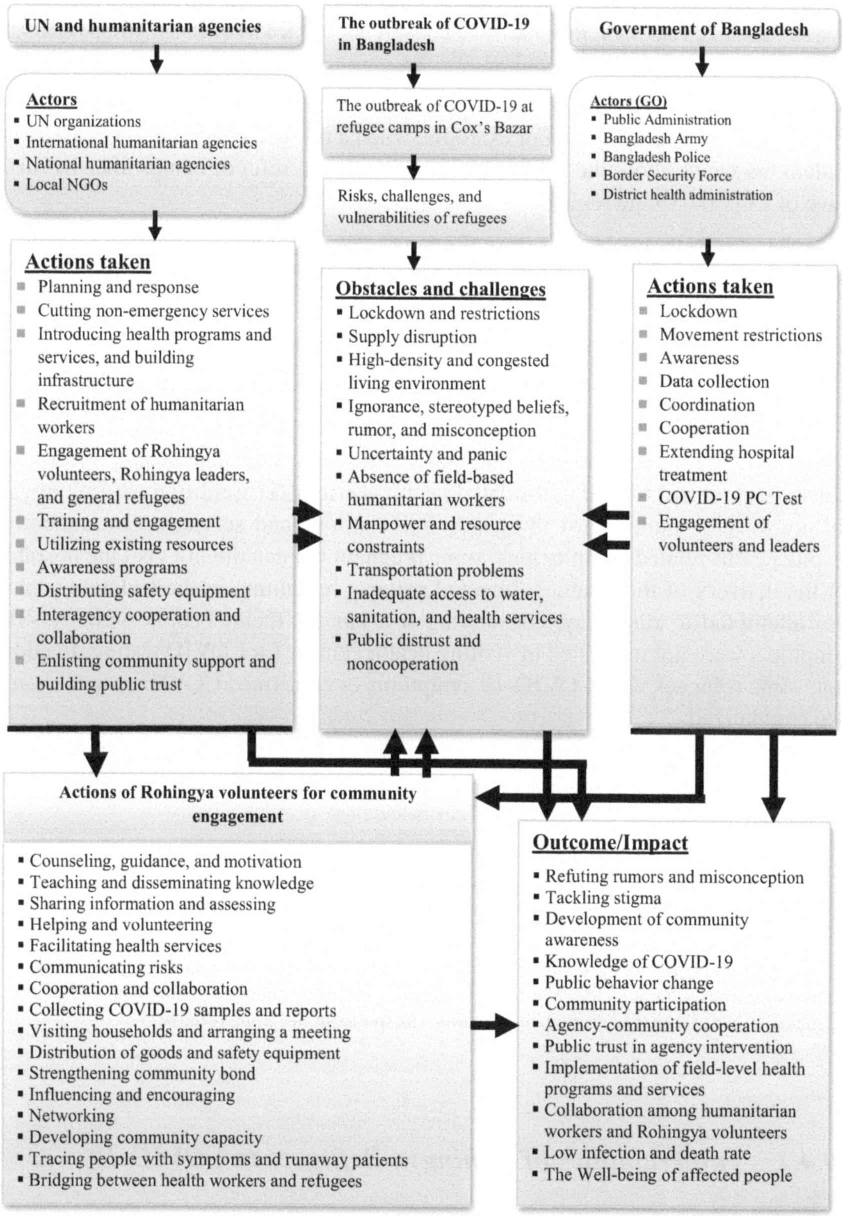

Fig. 10.1 Community engagement through Rohingya volunteers in COVID-19 pandemic management at Rohingya refugee camps in Bangladesh

> People said, "What is corona? Corona has not come for Rohingya. The poor are not infected with corona". Others said, "Religious Rohingyas are not infected with corona." (Respondent 88, Male refugee and Guard, Save the Children)

In fact, religious prejudice and stereotyped ideas were identified as the strong barriers to COVID-19 campaigns. For example, when a refugee of 65 years was asked to explain his views about the lower number of deaths at refugee camps after the first wave of COVID-19, he replied:

> Nobody died in the camps for Corona. If someone says so, we will not believe it. Corona has appeared for those who tortured us. We are oppressed. Allah is saving us. Did you find anyone died for Corona? (Respondent 70, Male refugee)

When he was informed about two or three deaths in the camps, he answered:

> Those people did not die of corona. It was publicized as Corona's death. (Respondent 70, Male refugee)

Community ignorance, rumors, and panic situations impeded agency efforts to deliver general and COVID-19-related health services. Therefore, most Rohingyas did not develop public trust in agency interventions and services. Consequently, despite health-related complexities, some pregnant women did not visit the hospital for the delivery of their babies. Infected patients remaining in the isolation center also attempted to run away, considering it a jail for them. People with COVID symptoms were not interested in visiting health centers for COVID testing. In addition, some refugees with COVID-19 symptoms or confirmed COVID patients were also stigmatized.

> We did not go to the hospital. They (agencies) would confine us there (health centers) treating us as corona patients. We heard from people that patients were thrown into the sea and killed through injection. (Respondent 67, Female refugee)

> They (Rohingyas) believe that if they die while being locked there (isolation center), they will not be released. They think they (patients) are locked (isolated) for stigma. (Respondent 2, Male humanitarian worker, Swiss Red Cross)

> Being afraid people took treatment from Rohingya doctors (Quacks) instead of going to the hospital. They did not go to the hospital for testing since they anticipated that they would be sent to other places if identified with corona. (Respondent 68, Male refugee)

10.4.2 Vulnerabilities of Rohingya Refugees to COVID-19

Lockdown, entry restrictions to refugee camps, and cutdown of non-emergency services increased the plight of the refugees. The humanitarian workers were largely unable to address the vulnerabilities resulting from the COVID pandemic.

> We usually provide snacks for one time to the adolescent girl center. We could not organize any sessions during COVID time. The girls did not get the food. (Respondent 6, Female humanitarian worker, Partners in Health and Development)

Though there is no official permission for refugees to work, the agencies engage them in camp-based activities like road reconstruction, house repairing, food distribution, etc. as paid volunteers. Due to the cutoff of non-emergency activities in camps, the refugees lost their income opportunities and failed to purchase some food items.

> I am a carpenter. When there is construction work in the block, I get a job. I was unemployed during the Corona period. We are suffering. What we get from WFP is not enough to survive a whole month. The amount is enough for a small family, but not for a big family. (Respondent 65, Male refugee)

Due to the school closure, all children were deprived of education and related services offered by humanitarian agencies. Children were only allowed to learn Arabic in *Moktob* (an Islamic institution) when the lockdown was withdrawn. Due to the shutdown of schools, the number of child laborers also increased at refugee camps.

> As the schools are closed, children are not getting an education. They are playing in dirty places with garbage (Respondent 47, Male Rohingya *Majhi*)

> All centers like education or games were closed. We observed a sharp increase in child labor in the camps. They were employed in small shops. Because they were free. (Respondent 3, Male humanitarian worker, Danish Refugee Council)

The elderly parents, pregnant mothers, and persons with disabilities or health conditions faced some problems, such as difficulties in movement and food collection, shortages of medicines, growing fear or distrust of hospital services, and obstacles in getting treatment from outside.

> The doctors keep us in the hospital suspecting corona if we have a little cough. Therefore, we did not send our ill mother to the hospital. Her treatment is ongoing by bringing medicines from outside. (Respondent 57, Male refugee)

> My mother has a health problem. We consulted a doctor in Chittagong (150km distance), and she advised us to meet her every two months. But we could not go on lockdown. (Respondent 53, Male Rohingya volunteer, Save the Children)

10.4.3 Training Refugees for Capacity Development

The humanitarian agencies executed multifarious activities in collaboration with refugee communities and other stakeholders. Community engagement was adopted as a core strategy to protect the Rohingya refugees. Training, awareness sessions, building infrastructure, and distribution of resources and protective equipment were the core approaches adopted for pandemic management. The agencies provided infrastructure such as handwashing facilities to increase health awareness, extended facilities for COVID-19 tests, isolation, quarantine, and treatment, utilized existing agency resources for COVID-19-related services, distributed masks, soap, and hand sanitizer, and developed a strong community-agency partnership through sharing information and resources, and coordination. The agencies executed these actions with the active involvement of the Rohingya leaders, teachers, religious leaders, and volunteers of NGOs. Through training and motivation, the refugees were capable of doing activities related to pandemic management.

> Under the shelter unit, we established some temporary structures for quarantine and isolation. We built many temporary hospitals inside or near the camps to provide services to a larger number of infected refugees. (Respondent 13, Male humanitarian worker, IOM)

> I learned how to make people aware involving the *Majhi*, different committees, and guardians. (Respondent 80, Male Rohingya volunteer, World Vision)

The Rohingya volunteers and other Rohingyas were trained to identify COVID-19 symptoms, what they should do when a person suffers from symptoms and when they should go for COVID-19 testing, and how the Rohingya volunteers could help the infected persons access treatment and other services. The volunteers were encouraged to facilitate agency activities and take responsibility during the absence of humanitarian workers at the refugee camps. Their main duties were to develop community capacity and resilience, help refugees understand the severity of COVID-19, and develop a sense of collective responsibility. NGO workers, with the help of volunteers, arranged meetings across the camps to increase community awareness and participation.

> I took part in three pieces of training for our NGO. They gave us two dustbins, one red for collecting disposable things and another green for dried things. COVID-19 has three medicines: masks, washing hands for twenty seconds, and social distancing meaning keeping away by three feet. Gathering at a shop and more gatherings at the mosque should be avoided. (Respondent 76, Male Rohingya volunteer, World Vision)

> Different NGOs taught us from where it (COVID-19) came, how it spread, by whom it spread, and how we can save ourselves from the virus. (Respondent 45, Male Rohingya *Imam*)

10.4.4 Volunteers Involved in Community Awareness Activities

The Rohingya volunteers were taught, guided, encouraged, motivated, and influenced to disseminate updated information, transfer knowledge, make people understand COVID-19 and agency interventions, teach the refugees about health safety rules and required actions for COVID-19 infection, distribute health safety equipment, and provide welfare services to the affected families.

> I got training about how to survive the corona. We took several awareness sessions about COVID-19. We made people understand how we can protect ourselves. Such as, being clean, remaining three feet away, using a mask outside, and washing hands three times inside and three times outside. Inside means washing before taking food, before cooking food, and before feeding the baby. Outside means washing before using the toilet, before cleaning the baby, and after sneezing. (Respondent 77, Male Rohingya volunteer, World Vision)

Being trained all Rohingya refugees voluntarily acted for community awareness, knowledge dissemination, and volunteering and facilitating COVID-19-related health services. They played leading roles in civic engagement through risk communication and information sharing. They visited door to door, disseminated scientific information about COVID-19 and health services, and organized community awareness meetings to make people understand about COVID-19, how it can spread from one person to another, and what the Rohingyas should do for individual and community protection. They encouraged other refugees for community participation in agency-led services and intervention.

> I made people aware. To stay away, not handshake, and wash hands while coming from outside. If anyone has a fever, cold, or cough he needs to be taken to the hospital after keeping in a separate room. I took one woman to the hospital. (Respondent 88, Male refugee and Guard, Save the Children)

> After being trained we took training sessions in the blocks. I also made people aware through an individual session. I also helped in maintaining social distancing during food distribution. (Respondent 51, Male Rohingya teacher)

> The volunteers came to the blocks and made us understand how to wash hands, use a mask, wash hands before taking food, and avoid a crowded environment. They gave us masks and soap. (Respondent 62, Male refugee)

10.4.5 Changing Public Health Behavior

Rohingya volunteers targeted Rohingya families to change their health behavior, stereotyped beliefs, and misconceptions that were risky for COVID-19. They counseled people with scientific and logical information and real-life experiences. They motivated and encouraged those people who were indifferent about COVID-19 despite the symptoms or confirmed COVID-19 patients to receive hospital services.

> I referred many people with the symptoms of fever, cold, and cough to hospitals. I made them aware after taking several sessions. I made those people understand who told that the lockdown had been imposed only to deprive the children of being educated. (Respondent 51, Male Rohingya teacher)

> Initially, people did not go to the hospital fearing corona. They thought that they would be kept in hospital for 14 days even if they had not been infected with corona. We arranged several awareness sessions with those people. (Respondent 79, Male Rohingya volunteer, Dhaka Ahsania Mission)

> Initially, people said, "Allah has given us disease, and he will recover us. Corona affects only Christians." I said that the disease came from Allah, but it does not know Christian. They believed it after making them understand repeatedly. (Respondent 82, Male Rohingya volunteer, Oparojeyo Bangladesh)

10.4.6 Building Public Trust

The volunteers strived to tackle rumors, misconceptions, stereotyped beliefs, negligence, and non-cooperation by providing updated and scientific information to the refugees. The awareness meetings, information sharing, distribution of safety equipment, and helping infected persons and their families by the Rohingya volunteers in collaboration with agencies were helpful to refute rumors, tackle misconceptions, and build community trust in protective and preventive actions performed by the volunteers and other stakeholders.

> People initially believed that corona originated from the Mog (Rakhine) and Hindu. But it did not infect the Muslims. After making them understand through home visits again and again, they begin to believe that disease can infect people of any religion. (Respondent 80, Male Rohingya volunteer, World Vision)

> There were many misconceptions and rumors. I told people that Corona was a disease from Allah. It was a *Sunnat* of our Prophet (speech of the Prophet Muhammad) to remain clean. I made them understand through those to whom they listened. The government and NGOs are helping us. (Respondent 51, Male Rohingya teacher)

> For those who had a fever, cold, and cough, I sent them to MSF (hospital). I made people aware of COVID-19. People listened to us. The community people helped us. (Respondent 91, Male Rohingya volunteer, HEX)

10.4.7 Facilitating Agency Services

The Rohingyas led by the volunteers and community leaders helped the agencies in service delivery, distribution, and facilitating agency services at the refugee camps. They closely worked with the healthcare workers in COVID-dedicated hospitals and isolation centers. They encouraged and motivated refugees and patients to follow COVID-19-related health safety rules.

> I helped many patients in isolation centers. We take all cases. If someone comes for shelter, we refer him. If someone has symptoms of fever and cold, we send him/her to the hospital. We submit case follow-up. (Respondent 79, Male Rohingya volunteer, Dhaka Ahsania Mission)

> Some people did not go to the hospital fearing corona. I send them to the hospital after talking. We also looked after Corona patients in the hospital. (Respondent 85, Male Rohingya volunteer, Concern Worldwide)

The volunteers helped vulnerable groups, such as pregnant mothers and elderly people, to access agency services and medical treatment. Some volunteers taught children voluntarily and inspired other parents to continue educating their children at home.

> Some pregnant women visited hospitals with the help of volunteers. I took one pregnant woman to MSF hospital. I helped old men carry rice bags during lockdown (Respondent 75, Male Rohingya volunteer, Good Neighbor)

> I helped some elderly people to reach the hospital. Some could not identify the prescribed medicines. I helped them use medicines. (Respondent 44, Male Rohingya volunteer, BRAC)

10.4.8 Bridging Community with Agency Services

The Rohingya volunteers acted as a bridge between community and agency services, and they linked the refugees with the available agency services. Thus, they worked for active community participation in agency intervention.

> Being afraid none was interested in visiting the hospital initially. We organized a program named "Pregnant Care." Now all go. We let the positive patients know about the reports (Respondent 72, Male Rohingya volunteer)

> People did not want to go to isolation centers fearing that they would be killed. I made them realize the matter. (Respondent 45, Male Rohingya *Imam*)

> I sent many people to NGOs to collect masks and soap. I could not help the poor. Here the rich and poor are the same. (Respondent 89, Male Rohingya volunteer, Solidarites International)

10.4.9 Outcome of Community Engagement Through Volunteers

The Rohingyas received scientific information about COVID-19 through the coordinated and collaborative actions of multiple stakeholders involved in risk communication and awareness programs. Community engagement activities through volunteers and refugee leaders significantly reduced rumor, prejudice, and misconception, changed public health behavior, raised awareness, built public trust in pandemic-related public health programs and medical services, developed civic responsibilities, and encouraged community participation and cooperation in programs and services introduced to protect the refugees. For example, due to the awareness activities, the refugees now believe that COVID-19 exists, and it can infect any person from any religion. After receiving scientific information from the volunteers and humanitarian workers, the refugees, who feared visiting the hospital earlier, now go to health centers for treatment.

> Around ten percent believe that they would not be infected with corona. They say, "The foreigners (people from outside Bangladesh) will be infected." We took several sessions with them. Now they know it (COVID-19). (Respondent 83, Male Rohingya volunteer, JCF)

> Corona is a big disease. It can spread quickly from one to another. There will be a fever, cold, and cough. We must wash our hands for 20 seconds and keep away from others by three feet. If I am infected, I need to stay outside of the home. (Respondent 66, Female refugee)

> People are obeying COVID-19 rules. Only two to three percent do not follow. (Respondent 48, Male Rohingya *Majhi*)

Community engagement activities led by the volunteers were helpful in the development of a sense of community among many refugees. This bond encouraged them to work collaboratively with different stakeholders to reduce the potential risks of COVID-19 and to come forward to help or serve fellow refugees within their capacity and limited resources. For example, volunteers and Rohingya leaders came forward helping poor and vulnerable groups through fundraising and by facilitating their access to emergency services.

> I helped patients from other blocks to send them to the hospital. I could not help them with money. For those who did not have rice and lentils, I managed them. (Respondent 56, Male Rohingya *Majhi*)

> We could not help people by violating lockdown rules. We sent some people outside for treatment by collecting money from the community. (Respondent 46, Male Rohingya *Imam*)

> The *Majhis* were requested to engage the volunteers in collecting relief for the elderly people. I also collected relief for old people. (Respondent 49, Male Rohingya teacher)

> We struggled to bring the elderly to MSF (hospital) as these are located far away from the residence. We three volunteers jointly bring one for health service. (Respondent 58, Male refugee)

The Rohingya volunteers and other Rohingyas believe that the agency-community collaborative actions led by the Rohingya volunteers and humanitarian workers significantly lowered the infection and death rates in refugee camps.

> People became aware because of the activities of NGO workers. All practice cleanliness. They use masks. They wash their hands with soap. They got the required medicine. People were made aware through the *miking* (Announcing awareness messages using a mobile loud speaker) of government and NGOs. That is why Corona patients were not found in our camp. (Respondent 89, Male Rohingya volunteer, Solidarites International)

> The awareness activities of the government and others were beneficial for us. People obeyed the rules and restrictions. So, people did not die in our camps, though many died in other countries. (Respondent 71, Male refugee)

Conversely, some Rohingyas explained the causes of low infection and the death rate from a religious point of view, though they acknowledge the contributions of agency efforts led by the volunteers and humanitarian workers.

> The spread of corona in the block is little because of the wishes of Allah. We became aware because of the government and NGOs. The government of Bangladesh helped us as they are Muslims. (Respondent 47, Male Rohingya *Majhi*)

> It is a miracle of Allah. But obeying some rules is good. We counseled and modified the behavior of those who did not follow health rules. (Respondent 85, Male Rohingya volunteer, Concern Worldwide)

The humanitarian workers also argued that the Rohingyas might have strong immunity, but the joint and collaborative activities of all stakeholders and agencies contributed to reducing the spread and controlling the death rate in Rohingya camps.

> We did not get many patients in the case of primary prevention. There were fewer patients. Since the number of patients was less, we presumed that our awareness programs were successful. (Respondent 1, Male humanitarian worker, Relief International)

10.5 Discussion

The primary focus of the study was to explain how Rohingya refugee volunteers were engaged in volunteering RCCE (Risk communication and community engagement) activities at refugee camps of Cox's Bazar, Bangladesh, and what they did to protect the refugee population from the pandemic. Similarly, in response to COVID-19, community-based organizations also mobilized volunteers for tracing, collecting supplies for epidemic control, providing community services, and building collaboration with different stakeholders in Zhejiang province of China (Cheng et al. 2020). The World Health Organization also focused on RCCE to control COVID-19 transmission. RCCE is a people-centered and community-led approach that builds trust and social cohesion, enables community-led response, provides information, reinforces community capacity, increases efforts to reduce stigma and discrimination, tackles misinformation, and establishes concerted and coordinated efforts of organizations—which are vital for arresting the spread of COVID-19 (World Health Organization 2020b). Recent empirical studies also highlighted the contributions of volunteers (Ekzayez et al. 2020; Irandoost et al. 2022; Miao et al. 2021) to RCCE and the importance of community engagement to manage a pandemic (Ha et al. 2021; Larmar et al. 2021; Tam et al. 2022).

After the influx of Rohingya refugees in 2017, different humanitarian agencies established and supported volunteer groups, and trained and incentivized them to volunteer and facilitate camp-based services in Cox's Bazar district of Bangladesh (Ergül 2020a). The refugees struggled to communicate with the agencies due to illiteracy and language barriers. The volunteers played dynamic roles in bridging community-agency services (Ergül 2020a). Similarly, Rohingya religious leaders were also engaged in community-based programs and community mobilization (Ergül 2020b). In fact, humanitarian agencies depended on Rohingya leaders and volunteers to ensure community participation in all camp-based activities and services. Following the working experience with the volunteers and refugee leaders, the Government of Bangladesh, the UN, and other humanitarian agencies emphasized community engagement activities through young Rohingya volunteers to manage the COVID-19 pandemic and its adverse effects. Moreover, resource crisis, absence of a large number of humanitarian workers due to lockdown and movement restrictions, Rohingyas' ignorance and illiteracy, perceived risks of COVID-19, and practical challenges of pandemic management at refugee camps made it essential to ensure local cooperation for the provision of some emergency services. Hence, the Rohingya volunteers were effectively used as a front-line workforce for RCCE activities, executing emergency services through collaboration with health workers, building public trust in agency intervention and services, raising civic responsibilities, and changing public health behavior.

Governments, particularly in resource-constrained countries, cannot manage a pandemic without citizen involvement. Therefore, community-based volunteer groups are involved in pandemic management. In rural Bangladesh, the local and central governments failed to manage the COVID-19-related crises, whereas collective efforts of the local community led by volunteers and community leaders were found helpful in addressing those crises (Ahmad et al. 2022). Despite the resource crisis and weak capacity of the health system in Syria, the local volunteers effectively worked for community awareness through information campaigns, information sharing, and resource mobilization during COVID-19 (Ekzayez et al. 2020). Thus, mobilizing volunteer groups through community-based organizations could be an effective strategy for pandemic management (Miao et al. 2021). Realizing the importance of volunteerism, humanitarian agencies in Cox's Bazar attempted to ensure community participation through the Rohingya volunteers at refugee camps. The agencies improved infrastructure and increased capacities for COVID-19 testing, treatment, isolation, and quarantine. However, the refugees were largely unaware of public health programs and treatment systems introduced to fight against COVID-19. The big challenge was to gain public trust and develop community solidarity so that the refugees would come forward and help the humanitarian agencies in executing COVID-19 programs and services. Furthermore, they needed to consider COVID-19 as a threat to the Rohingya community. In addition, lockdown and movement restrictions complicated the situation and exacerbated the vulnerabilities of the refugees to the pandemic. Against this backdrop, the Rohingya volunteers, Rohingya leaders (*Majhi*), religious leaders, and other refugees were trained in RCCE, and motivated and encouraged to organize awareness campaigns following health safety rules and to help other refugees understand COVID-19, and its prevention and control. After training, the Rohingya volunteers and other Rohingyas worked collaboratively with the humanitarian workers and played leading roles in raising community awareness, public trust in agency intervention and the services, civic responsibilities, and community participation in pandemic management. Likewise, the volunteers in Iran also engaged in training, distribution, social and mental health support, cooperation with government agencies, and encouraging and supporting people to fight against COVID-19 (Irandoost et al. 2022).

Face-to-face campaigns are more effective ways of changing public behavior than mass media campaigns during a pandemic (Ryan et al. 2020). Rohingya volunteers also acted for community engagement through counseling and guidance, door-to-door visits, teaching, knowledge dissemination, community-level meetings, helping, volunteering, individual-level motivation, distribution of safety equipment, tracing, bridging communities with agency services, and facilitating agency services. Conversely, engagement through mass and social media, the use of hotlines, and targeting groups were used as key RCCE strategies in Africa (Adebisi et al. 2021). Effective community engagement strengthens two-way communications and community participation and empowers communities (Ergül 2020a). Rohingya volunteers and other Rohingyas also adopted different working strategies to build public trust and community solidarity, strengthen community engagement, and overcome the challenges related to community-level non-cooperation and negligence, heightened risks of infection, religious misconception, rumors, stigma, and public fear about hospital and isolation services (Islam and Yeasir Yunus 2020). The results of this study also corroborate the findings of previous research in pandemic management (Galiatsatos et al. 2020; McElfish et al. 2021; O'Mara-Eves et al. 2015; Ryan et al. 2020; Tam et al. 2022).

Finally, research participants believe that the collaborative actions of agencies and Rohingya volunteers help build community trust and disseminate knowledge about COVID-19. Their activities encouraged people to follow health safety rules, significantly curbed the rate of infection, and lowered the death rate in Rohingya camps. However, the study suggests that multidisciplinary research is needed to assess the impact of RCCE activities on the rate of infection and death rates at refugee camps in Cox's Bazar during the pandemic. The study argues that Rohingya refugees gained scientific knowledge about COVID-19 and treatment measures, developed trust in agency activities related to pandemic management, changed their health behavior, followed health safety rules, and got benefits from agency services through the community engagement process. The Rohingya volunteers played dynamic roles in the whole process of pandemic management, especially during the lockdown.

10.6 Limitations of the Study

The generalizability of the findings is subject to some limitations. The samples may not represent the whole population since respondents were selected purposively. It is also difficult to generalize the findings in other contexts of pandemic management. The study might have missed the context related to planning and policy decisions as it did not include high-ranking officials. Furthermore, it did not use measurement tools for distinctly evaluating the effectiveness of community engagement activities performed by Rohingya volunteers, though the findings highlighted their contributions and explained the outcome of community-agency collaboration in pandemic management.

10.7 Conclusion and Policy Implications

This study has identified that civic engagement through community-based volunteers was the core strategy for pandemic management in the Rohingya refugee camps of Bangladesh. It shows how Rohingya volunteers developed people's civic responsibilities, changed public health behavior, strengthened people's participation in health programs, and encouraged the refugees to come forward to protect and serve the refugee population during the pandemic. The joint activities of volunteers and other refugees and humanitarian workers helped develop a sense of community harmony and strengthen social cohesion in the Rohingya community. Consequently, many refugees followed health safety rules and actively participated in health programs. Thus, the volunteers acted as an integral part of COVID-19-related programs and services introduced for Rohingya refugees.

The findings of the study clearly demonstrate that Rohingya volunteers were capable of delivering some emergency and non-emergency services at refugee camps in the absence of a large number of humanitarian workers during the first wave of COVID-19. Lockdown, movement restrictions, and suspension/contraction of non-emergency programs in camps affected the life and well-being of the refugee community. All agencies recruited local Rohingyas as volunteers and educated them about COVID-19 to overcome the problems of manpower shortage, resource constraints, community ignorance, misconception, rumors, panic, and heightened risks and uncertainty. Rohingya volunteers' engagement through training, continuous information flow, motivation, and encouragement helped develop their capabilities to work for community participation and execution of agency services. They disseminated information about COVID-19, its symptoms, protection, and treatment measures, and helped the refugees access available services. The Rohingya volunteers helped people understand rumors and misconceptions about COVID-19 and counseled the infected persons or people with symptoms for COVID-19 testing, treatment, isolation, and quarantine. Thus, the active engagement of Rohingya volunteers was crucial for risk communication and slowing the rate of infection, providing services to the patients, and executing emergency medical and non-medical services at refugee camps.

Overall, the findings of the study strengthen the idea that community-based young volunteers could be used as front-line workers during an emergency or pandemic like COVID-19. Civic engagement through young Rohingya volunteers was used successfully as an exemplary model of pandemic management at the refugee settlements of Cox's Bazar, Bangladesh. In fact, it is often difficult for humanitarian workers to develop social cohesion and solidarity and strengthen civic engagement, all of which are crucial for pandemic management in refugee communities. Since the Rohingya refugees have distinct culture, ethnic identity, and a common history of victimization, humanitarian agencies involved local volunteers to act as gatekeepers and facilitate people's participation in agency-led programs and services from the very beginning of the refugee crisis at Cox's Bazar (Ergül 2020a). Later, this idea of engaging community-based volunteers was effectively used under the guidance of humanitarian workers as a model of pandemic management during COVID-19.

The study lays the groundwork for future research into the role of community-based volunteers in protecting people from natural and man-made disasters in any location. A further study using a mixed methods approach could be carried out to assess the impacts of the actions performed by the Rohingya volunteers in strengthening community bonds and social cohesion, and encouraging civic engagement for pandemic management, and how those actions contributed to slowing the infection rate at refugee camps during the pandemic. Despite the study's limitations, the findings have several implications for future practice in refugee camps. Policymakers and international humanitarian agencies can mobilize local volunteers for active civic engagement and multistakeholder collaboration during an emergency.

Acknowledgments The study (Project ID: SS/2020/1/34) was funded by the University Research Center, Shahjalal University of Science and Technology (SUST), Sylhet, Bangladesh. It got ethical clearance from the SUST Research Ethics Board [Ref: SREB/EC/SSS02 (2022)]. The researcher acknowledges the contribution of the anonymous reviewers of the project and experts to developing the study protocol and the cooperation of the Rohingya refugees and volunteers and humanitarian workers during fieldwork. Finally, the researcher would like to thank the reviewers for their valuable comments and suggestions, which were significantly helpful in improving this paper.

References

Adebisi, Y.A., A. Rabe, and D.E. Lucero-Prisno Iii. 2021. Risk communication and community engagement strategies for COVID-19 in 13 African countries. *Health Promotion Perspective* 11 (2): 137–147. https://doi.org/10.34172/hpp.2021.18.

Ahmad, F., R. Chowdhury, B. Siedler, and W. Odek. 2022. Building community resilience during COVID-19: Learning from rural Bangladesh. *Journal of Contingencies and Crisis Management* 30 (3): 327–338. https://doi.org/10.1111/1468-5973.12405.

Al-Zaman, M.S. 2020. Healthcare crisis in Bangladesh during the COVID-19 pandemic. *The American Journal of Tropical Medicine and Hygiene* 103 (4): 1357–1359. https://doi.org/10.4269/ajtmh.20-0826.

Braun, V., and V. Clarke. 2006. Using thematic analysis in psychology. *Qualitative Research in Psychology* 3 (2): 77–101. https://doi.org/10.1191/1478088706qp063oa.

Campbell, S., M. Greenwood, S. Prior, T. Shearer, K. Walkem, S. Young, D. Bywaters, and K. Walker. 2020. Purposive sampling: Complex or simple? Research case examples. *Journal of Research in Nursing* 25 (8): 652–661. https://doi.org/10.1177/1744987120927206.

Cheng, Y., J. Yu, Y. Shen, and B. Huang. 2020. Coproducing responses to COVID-19 with community-based organizations: Lessons from Zhejiang province, China. *Public Administration Review* 80 (5): 866–873. https://doi.org/10.1111/puar.13244.

Creswell, J.W. 2013. *Qualitative inquiry and research design: Choosing among five approaches*. New Delhi: SAGE Publications.

den Broeder, L., J. South, A. Rothoff, A.-M. Bagnall, F. Azarhoosh, G. van der Linden, M. Bharadwa, and A. Wagemakers. 2021. Community engagement in deprived neighbourhoods during the COVID-19 crisis: Perspectives for more resilient and healthier communities. *Health Promotion International* 37 (2): daab098. https://doi.org/10.1093/heapro/daab098.

Ekzayez, A., M. al-Khalil, M. Jasiem, R. Al Saleh, Z. Alzoubi, K. Meagher, and P. Patel. 2020. COVID-19 response in Northwest Syria: Innovation and community engagement in a complex conflict. *Journal of Public Health* 42 (3): 504–509. https://doi.org/10.1093/pubmed/fdaa068.

Ergül, H. 2020a. *Mobilizing for change: Strengthening engagement through community mobilization volunteers in Cox's Bazar, Bangladesh*. https://www.unicef.org/bangladesh/en/reports/mobilizing-change. Accessed 10 Feb 2023.

———. 2020b. *The role of faith in the humanitarian response: Strengthening community participation and engagement through religious leaders in Rohingya camps in Cox's Bazar, Bangladesh*. https://www.unicef.org/bangladesh/en/reports/role-faith-humanitarian-response. Accessed 10 Feb 2023.

Galiatsatos, P., K. Monson, M. Oluyinka, D. Negro, N. Hughes, D. Maydan, S.H. Golden, P. Teague, and W.D. Hale. 2020. Community calls: Lessons and insights gained from a medical-religious community engagement during the COVID-19 pandemic. *Journal of Religion and Health* 59 (5): 2256–2262. https://doi.org/10.1007/s10943-020-01057-w.

Gautam, S., S. Setu, M.G. Quader Khan, and Md.B. Khan. 2022. Analysis of the health, economic and environmental impacts of COVID-19: The Bangladesh perspective. *Geosystems and Geoenvironment* 1 (1): 100011. https://doi.org/10.1016/j.geogeo.2021.100011.

Gilmore, B., R. Ndejjo, A. Tchetchia, V. de Claro, E. Mago, A.A. Diallo, C. Lopes, and S. Bhattacharyya. 2020. Community engagement for COVID-19 prevention and control: A rapid evidence synthesis. *BMJ Global Health* 5 (10): e003188. https://doi.org/10.1136/bmjgh-2020-003188.

Ha, B.T.T., L.N. Quang, P.Q. Thanh, D.M. Duc, T. Mirzoev, and T.M. Anh Bui. 2021. Community engagement in the prevention and control of COVID-19: Insights from Vietnam. *PLoS One* 16 (9): e0254432. https://doi.org/10.1371/journal.pone.0254432.

Hirani, S.A.A., and J. Wagner. 2022. Impact of COVID-19 on women who are refugees and mothering: A critical ethnographic study. *Global Qualitative Nursing Research* 9: 23333936221121335. https://doi.org/10.1177/23333936221121335.

Hu, G., and W. Qiu. 2020. From guidance to practice: Promoting risk communication and community engagement for prevention and control of coronavirus disease (COVID-19) outbreak in China. *Journal of Evidence-Based Medicine* 13 (2): 168–172. https://doi.org/10.1111/jebm.12387.

Irandoost, S.F., S. Sedighi, A. Sadat Hoseini, A. Ahmadi, H. Safari, F.E. Fard Azar, and J.Y. Lebni. 2022. Activities and challenges of volunteers in confrontation with COVID-19: A qualitative study in Iran. *International Journal of Disaster Risk Reduction* 82: 103314. https://doi.org/10.1016/j.ijdrr.2022.103314.

Islam, M.M., and M.D. Yeasir Yunus. 2020. Rohingya refugees at high risk of COVID-19 in Bangladesh. *The Lancet Global Health* 8 (8): e993–e994. https://doi.org/10.1016/S2214-109X(20)30282-5.

Johnston, D., J. Becker, and D. Paton. 2012. Multi-agency community engagement during disaster recovery. *Disaster Prevention and Management: An International Journal* 21 (2): 252–268. https://doi.org/10.1108/09653561211220034.

Jubayer, F., S. Kayshar, and T. Islam Limon. 2020. First COVID-19 case in the Rohingya camp in Bangladesh: Needs proper attention. *Public Health* 191: 20. https://doi.org/10.1016/j.puhe.2020.05.033.

Khan, Md.N., M. Mofizul Islam, and Md.M. Rahman. 2020. Risks of COVID19 outbreaks in Rohingya refugee camps in Bangladesh. *Public Health in Practice* 1: 100018. https://doi.org/10.1016/j.puhip.2020.100018.

Khan, S., J. Mishra, N. Ahmed, C.D. Onyige, K.E. Lin, R. Siew, and B.H. Lim. 2022. Risk communication and community engagement during COVID-19. *International Journal of Disaster Risk Reduction* 74: 102903. https://doi.org/10.1016/j.ijdrr.2022.102903.

Larmar, S., M. Sunuwar, H. Sherpa, R. Joshi, and L.P. Jordan. 2021. Strengthening community engagement in Nepal during COVID-19: Community-based training and development to reduce child labour. *Asia Pacific Journal of Social Work and Development* 31 (1–2): 23–30. https://doi.org/10.1080/02185385.2020.1833749.

Mackenzie, C., C. McDowell, and E. Pittaway. 2007. Beyond "do no harm": The challenge of constructing ethical relationships in refugee research. *Journal of Refugee Studies* 20 (2): 299–319. https://doi.org/10.1093/jrs/fem008.

Maher, R., and B. Murphet. 2020. Community engagement in Australia's COVID-19 communications response: Learning lessons from the humanitarian sector. *Media International Australia* 177 (1): 113–118. https://doi.org/10.1177/1329878x20948289.

Mboya, I.B., J.S. Ngocho, M. Mgongo, L.P. Samu, J.J. Pyuza, C. Amour, M.J. Mahande, B.J. Leyaro, J.M. George, R.N. Philemon, F. Muro, J. Renju, and S.E. Msuya. 2020. Community engagement in COVID-19 prevention: Experiences from Kilimanjaro region, Northern Tanzania. *Pan African Medical Journal* 35 (Suppl 2): 146. https://doi.org/10.11604/pamj.supp.2020.35.146.24473.

McElfish, P.A., A.B. Cleek, D.E. Willis, R.S. Purvis, and L.P. James. 2021. Leveraging community engagement capacity to address COVID-19 disparities among Pacific Islander and Latinx

communities in Arkansas. *Journal of Clinical and Translational Science* 5 (1): e81. https://doi.org/10.1017/cts.2020.562.
Mehta, M., H. Sarvaiya, and A. Chandani. 2022. Community engagement through responsible leadership in managing pandemic: Insight from India using netnography. *International Journal of Sociology and Social Policy* 42 (3/4): 248–261. https://doi.org/10.1108/IJSSP-06-2020-0214.
Miao, Q., S. Schwarz, and G. Schwarz. 2021. Responding to COVID-19: Community volunteerism and coproduction in China. *World Development* 137: 105128. https://doi.org/10.1016/j.worlddev.2020.105128.
Mondal, A. 2021. The importance of community engagement on COVID-19 vaccination strategy: Lessons from two California pilot programs. *EClinicalMedicine* 32: 100754. https://doi.org/10.1016/j.eclinm.2021.100754.
Mughal, R., L.J.M. Thomson, N. Daykin, and H.J. Chatterjee. 2022. Rapid evidence review of community engagement and resources in the UK during the COVID-19 pandemic: How can community assets redress health inequities? *International Journal of Environmental Research and Public Health* 19 (7): 4086. https://doi.org/10.3390/ijerph19074086.
Neely-Barnes, S., A. Hunter, J. Meiman, C. Malone, M. Hirschi, and E. Delavega. 2021. Leaning into the crisis: Managing COVID-19 in social services and behavioral health agencies. *Human Service Organizations: Management, Leadership & Governance* 45 (4): 293–306. https://doi.org/10.1080/23303131.2021.1915905.
O'Mara-Eves, A., G. Brunton, S. Oliver, J. Kavanagh, F. Jamal, and J. Thomas. 2015. The effectiveness of community engagement in public health interventions for disadvantaged groups: A meta-analysis. *BMC Public Health* 15 (1): 129. https://doi.org/10.1186/s12889-015-1352-y.
Ryan, B., K.A. Johnston, M. Taylor, and R. McAndrew. 2020. Community engagement for disaster preparedness: A systematic literature review. *International Journal of Disaster Risk Reduction* 49: 101655. https://doi.org/10.1016/j.ijdrr.2020.101655.
Sahana, M., S. Jahangir, and M.D. Anisujjaman. 2019. Forced migration and the expatriation of the Rohingya: A demographic assessment of their historical exclusions and statelessness. *Journal of Muslim Minority Affairs* 39 (1): 44–60. https://doi.org/10.1080/13602004.2019.1587952.
Satizábal, P., I. Cornes, M. de Lourdes Melo, and Zurita, and B.R. Cook. 2022. The power of connection: Navigating the constraints of community engagement for disaster risk reduction. *International Journal of Disaster Risk Reduction* 68: 102699. https://doi.org/10.1016/j.ijdrr.2021.102699.
Tam, W.J., N. Gobat, D. Hemavathi, and D. Fisher. 2022. Risk communication and community engagement during the migrant worker COVID-19 outbreak in Singapore. *Science Communication* 44 (2): 240–251. https://doi.org/10.1177/10755470211061513.
UNHCR. 2022. Global trends: Forced displacement in 2021. https://www.unhcr.org/62a9d1494/global-trends-report-2021. Accessed 20 Jan 2023.
World Health Organization. 2020a. *ApartTogether survey: Preliminary overview of refugees and migrants self-reported impact of COVID-19*. https://iris.who.int/bitstream/handle/10665/337931/9789240017924-eng.pdf?sequence=1. Accessed 10 Jan 2023.
———. 2020b. COVID-19 global risk communication and community engagement strategy, December 2020–May 2021: Interim guidance, 23 December 2020. https://apps.who.int/iris/handle/10665/338057. Accessed 08 Jan 2023.

Md. Fakhrul Alam is a faculty member in the Department of Social Work at Shahjalal University of Science and Technology (SUST), Sylhet, Bangladesh. He completed undergraduate and graduate degrees in Social Work at SUST. In 2017, he earned his Master of Public Policy degree from the Australian National University, Australia. Mr. Alam has profound research interests in gender-based violence and discrimination, refugees, street children, and poverty and marginalization. For a comprehensive overview of his notable contributions, including research projects and publications, one can explore his faculty profile on the SUST official website: https://www.sust.edu/d/scw/faculty-profile-detail/459.

Part IV
The Impact of COVID-19 on Children's Well-being

Chapter 11
Children's Well-being During COVID-19 Pandemic: An Exploratory Study Among 10–12 Year Old School Children in Bangladesh

Haridhan Goswami, Bijoy Krishna Banik, Gour Gobinda Goswami, and M. Ibrahim Khalil

11.1 Introduction

Research on children's well-being ("children's evaluations of their lives—the degree to which their thoughtful appraisals and affective reactions indicate that their lives are desirable and proceeding well," Diener et al. 2015, 234) is vital for evidence-based policies. That is why Grand Challenges such as the UN's Sustainable Development Goals (SDGs) consider well-being as one of the key policy goals (see Goal No. 3—ensure healthy lives and promote well-being for all at all ages). However, countries faced (and are still facing) enormous challenges to meet SDG targets because of the COVID-19 pandemic affecting billions of children globally. Researchers are gradually shedding light on the harmful effects of the pandemic on families and children. These studies are playing a vital role in formulating evidence-based policies. However, these studies were conducted predominantly in Western and economically developed countries. Even though these studies have significantly contributed to our knowledge and understanding of the impact of the COVID-19 pandemic on children's lives, we still know very little about the pandemic's influence on children's well-being in developing countries like Bangladesh, which has around 64 million children. This book chapter fills this gap by using the Children's

H. Goswami (✉)
Manchester Metropolitan University, Manchester, UK
e-mail: H.Goswami@mmu.ac.uk

B. K. Banik
University of Rajshahi, Rajshahi, Bangladesh

G. G. Goswami
North South University, Dhaka, Bangladesh

M. I. Khalil
Government Brojomohun College Barishal, Barishal, Bangladesh

C. Suter et al. (eds.), *Well-being During the Pandemic*, Social Indicators Research Series 90, https://doi.org/10.1007/978-3-031-63440-6_11

Worlds Special Survey on the COVID-19 pandemic completed in 2021. This book chapter deals with the identification of the impact of the COVID-19 pandemic on children's subjective well-being in Bangladesh, utilizing data gathered directly from children who assessed different domains of their lives during the pandemic. Key research questions are:

a) What was children's day-to-day life during the COVID-19 pandemic?
b) How did children assess different domains or aspects of their lives during the pandemic, and was there any difference in that assessment by their gender and rural-urban location?

The rest of the chapter is structured in the following way. Section 11.2 gives a short overview of Bangladesh during the COVID-19 pandemic. This contextual information will be helpful to understand the findings of the study. Section 11.3 discusses the methods used in this research. Section 11.4 presents the study's results, while Sect. 11.5 deals with the key findings in the context of different theories of subjective well-being and previous empirical studies. Section 11.6 draws policy messages for improving children's well-being in the post-pandemic recovery phase. Section 11.7 acknowledges some limitations and puts forward some suggestions for future studies. Section 11.8 contains a short conclusion.

11.2 Bangladesh

11.2.1 Macro-Level Context

Bangladesh, a relatively new country in South Asia, became independent in 1971. The country covers an area of 147,570 square kilometers with a massive population of above 161 million, making it one of the most densely populated (1077 people per square km) countries in the world. With almost 28% of people less than 15 years old and another 20% aged 15–24 years, Bangladesh can be characterized as a youth-populated country as nearly half of its population is less than 25 years old.

Most of the people are Muslims (around 89.35%), and the rest are Hindus (9.64%), Buddhists (0.57%), and Christians (0.27%), while other minorities constitute a small portion (0.17%). Although Bengali people constitute 98% of the population, the remaining 2% of the population comes from non-Bengali backgrounds. Around 34% of Bangladeshi people live in urban settings. The literacy rate, as defined by those who can read and write at the age of 15 years is approximately 61%.

Childhood inequality in Bangladesh is evident in crucial aspects of children's lives, and the key influencers are gender, location, region, wealth, ethnicity, and religion. In a recent report by Save the Children (Geoghegan 2018) Bangladesh scored 701 out of 1000 points, improving by 21 points primarily due to enhanced school-going behaviour. Nevertheless, her overall rank out of 175 countries is just 130th, which is disappointing due to poor performance in seven factors like school dropout rate, child labor, violence against children, under-5 mortality, child malnutrition, child marriage, and adolescent pregnancy. The same report also opines that 44% of the teenagers in Bangladesh get married before turning 20 years of age. Nearly 3.5% of the children fail to reach their fifth birthday. However, according to UNESCO, school dropout rates have significantly reduced by 36 percentage points over the last 5 years. Despite all the development in the primary education level, many children remain outside the formal schooling system in Bangladesh.

11.2.2 Context of the COVID-19 Pandemic

The timeline of COVID-19 in Bangladesh can be classified into six phases. In phase one, COVID-19 arrived in Bangladesh from January 2020 to March 2020, followed by the first wave and General Holiday or lockdown from March 2020 to May 2020 in phase two (IEDCR 2020). The third and the fourth phase continued from June 2020 to December 2020 and from December 2020 to March 2021. In the fifth phase, we had the second wave spanning from March 2021 to May 2021, followed by the third and the final wave from May 2021 to August 2021.

The COVID-19 outbreak, in general, and general holidays or lockdowns, in particular, harmed the lives of the most vulnerable and physically challenged children. This includes loss of family income, disruption of their access to healthcare services, education, and overall physical (free from physical violence and punishments) and mental (social interaction with friends, relatives, and well-wishers, free from fear, anxiety, and worry) well-being (Hussain and Al Mamun 2020; Islam et al. 2020; Save the Children n.d.).

The nature of the lockdown in Bangladesh was minimal, and it was limited to social distancing, wearing of masks, and closure of educational institutions and other offices, but only on a limited scale. The readymade garments industry went through lockdown only for a limited time, which paved the way for earning foreign exchanges through export. Apart from educational institutions, the lockdown was softer, which helped Bangladesh fight against recession and move towards recovery within the shortest possible time. Due to digital inequality, Bangladeshi children from lower-income families attached to the public school system were severely affected during school closures. Their education was not adequately replaced by online teaching as it was in English medium schools where students come from a relatively affluent part of society.

Like other developing countries, the coronavirus pandemic has significantly affected Bangladesh's economy. Many garment factories, mills, poultry industries, markets, and shopping malls were closed following the introduction of the social distance policy. The amount of remittance, the core of Bangladesh's economy, also decreased due to this catastrophe (Islam et al. 2020). Eighty-one of 121 children in a study reported in their telephone interviews that their family income stopped due to the COVID-19 pandemic. Sixty-four percent of the same group also mentioned a severe food crisis in their household during the coronavirus period (Save the

Children, n.d). According to another study, about 72% of respondents experienced decreased household income due to reduced informal work and unpaid leave (iMMAP 2022).

11.3 Methods

Initially, we planned to survey 1370 children of 10–12 years of age located in three regions or districts of Bangladesh. The districts were selected based on a convenient sampling procedure. However, these districts represent three zones: Barishal from the Southern part of Bangladesh, Rajshahi from the North-west and Moulvibazar from the North East. We used this approach to use the existing network of a previous survey (wave 3) carried out for Children's World, but the respondents were not necessarily the same. These three areas were close to the areas of our Co-investigators. This process facilitated the data collection during this catastrophic pandemic. However, we had to postpone the data collection at one stage and convert the survey to an online platform to avoid COVID-19 transmission. For paper-based versions, the professional network was used to locate school teachers to facilitate access to children. The three zones represent village, sub-urban, and city settings (Table 11.1).

Our original decision was to conduct the whole survey on a face-to-face basis. After completing some interviews, the second wave of COVID-19 hit Bangladesh, and the country went under lockdown for a considerable period. It was not clear when restrictions would be lifted. There was tremendous uncertainty about face-to-face data collection because of the lockdown, so it was decided to start data collection online during the lockdown period (2nd wave). Almost 2 weeks after launching the online survey, lockdown restrictions were gradually lifted, however, schools were still shut down. Taking help from school teachers, we conducted face-to-face interviews with some students when they visited schools to collect their homework on selected dates only.

Although some children from other regions in the country participated in the online survey, most of the children who took part in the online version came from large cities (mainly Dhaka—the capital city). The total number of children who

Table 11.1 Distribution of respondents by region and mode

	Data collection mode		
Region	Interviews	Online	Total
Barishal district (Southern part of Bangladesh)	350	0	350
Rajshahi district (North-West of Bangladesh)	360	0	360
Moulvibazar district (North-East of Bangladesh)	350	0	350
Dhaka city (and a few other regions)	0	310	310
Total	**1060**	**310**	**1370**

Source: Sample survey

Table 11.2 Distribution of children in the survey by their gender and age (%)

Gender	10 year-old	11 year-old	12 year-old	Total[a]
Girl	174 (54.0)	231 (51.0)	275 (48.0)	680 (50.0)
Boy	151 (46.0)	218 (49.0)	304 (52.0)	673 (50.0)
Total	**325 (100)**	**449 (100)**	**579 (100)**	**1353 (100)**

[a]Missing Cases = 17
Source: Sample survey

completed the online survey was 310 (22.6%). Active consent was sought from both children and their parents or guardians before data collection started.

Table 11.2 compiles the age and gender distribution of the children who took part in the survey. It is observed that an equal number of boys and girls participated in the survey. In a Bengali medium set-up, 10 year old children belong to class five, 11 year old children are in class six, and 12 year old children are in class seven. We tried to keep the distribution balanced across age groups and gender.

11.4 Results

11.4.1 Children's Daily Life During COVID-19 Pandemic

In response to the questions that describe children's situation during the COVID-19 pandemic, more than eight out of ten children reported that their local area (city/town/village) was under lockdown for many days (Table 11.3). Almost nine out of ten children acknowledged that they could not attend school for many days due to the COVID-19 pandemic. Around two-thirds of children reported having to stay home for many days during the pandemic. Almost one-third of the children reported being extra careful because they had someone at home who was at high risk of getting ill if they got infected with COVID-19. Regarding the spread of the disease, almost four out of ten children reported that they knew someone in their neighborhood or in their circle of friends who became infected with COVID-19. Just over one in ten children said that they or somebody at home had a COVID-19 infection.

The results presented in Table 11.4 suggest that almost all children (96%) reported that their school was closed during lockdown. Over two-thirds of children (68.5%) reported staying home all day because of the Coronavirus. Slightly fewer than one in five children (17.4%) indicated that at least one of their parents was forced to stop working and did not receive monetary assistance from the government. Almost half of the children (51.5%) reported that there were times when they were only allowed to leave their homes for a few hours during the day because of the fears of contracting the Coronavirus. Only a small number of children (4.1%) reported that their family had to move to another home during the pandemic.

Table 11.3 Children's responses to questions describing their situation during the pandemic (%)

Situation during the pandemic	Yes	No	Not sure
Everybody in my city/town/village was in lockdown for many days (N = 1353)	84.0	11.6	4.4
I or somebody in my home got infected with coronavirus (N = 1353)	12.5	84.7	2.8
Somebody in my family (not living with me) got infected with coronavirus (N = 1353)	12.5	82.6	4.9
Somebody I know got infected with coronavirus (e.g.: From my neighbourhood or in a friend's family) (N = 1353)	39.2	50.5	10.3
At home we had to be very careful because somebody was considered at high risk of getting very sick if they got infected with the coronavirus (N = 1353)	33.0	62.7	4.3
I had to stay at home for many days (N = 1353)	66.5	32.2	1.3
I could not attend school for many days (N = 1353)	91.6	7.9	0.5

Source: Sample survey

Table 11.4 Children's responses to questions describing their situation during the pandemic (%)

Statements describing the pandemic situation to the children	Yes	No	Not sure
My family had to move to another home	4.1	93.6	2.3
At least one of my parents was forced/had to stop working and receive money from the government	6.0	89.7	4.3
At least one of my parents was forced to stop working and did not receive money from the government	17.4	72.0	10.6
My school was closed during lockdown	96.1	3.8	0.1
There were times when I had to be in my home all day (including the garden, yard, or balcony, if you have) because of the coronavirus	68.5	29.6	1.8
There were times when I was only allowed to leave my home for a few hours during the day because of the coronavirus	51.5	45.3	3.2

Source: Sample survey

11.4.2 Children's Assessment of Different Domains of their Life During the Pandemic

In addition to asking children to evaluate their life as a whole (see Fig. 11.1), the survey asked questions about 12 specific aspects of their life—their satisfaction with (1) the people they live with, (2) the house they live in, (3) area they live, (4) feeling safe, (5) their friends, (6) time use, (7) appearance, (8) things they have or material possession, (9) freedom, (10) future, (11) how adults listen to them, and (12) their health. Children were asked to rate their happiness in each aspect of their life using an 11-point scale where ten represents "totally satisfied," and 0 means "not at all satisfied."

The mean scores in Fig. 11.1 suggest that children had the highest satisfaction (mean = 8.4) with the people they lived with, followed by the house they lived in (mean = 7.7), how safe they felt (mean = 7.6), the area they lived in (mean = 7.4), things they had (mean = 7.4), health (mean = 7.4). The aspect of their life in which

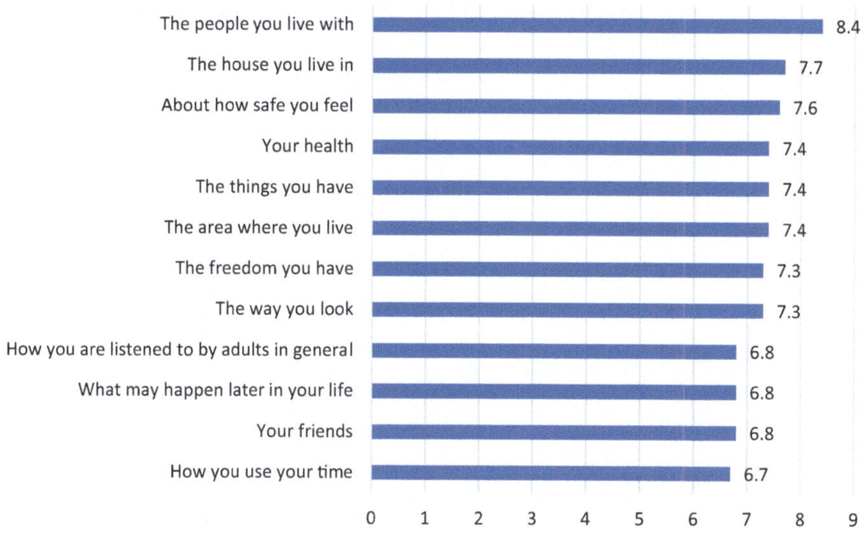

Fig. 11.1 Children's level of satisfaction (mean score) in different aspects of their lives. Source: Sample survey

they appeared to be less satisfied was the way they used their time (lowest mean score of 6.7), friends (mean score = 6.8), future prospect (mean = 6.8), and how adults listened to them (mean = 6.8). This simple analysis shows that although these children are happy with some aspects such as family relationships, house, etc., there are certain areas in their lives where they are less happy and require support.

11.4.2.1 Gender Difference in Children's Assessment of Different Domains of their Life During the Pandemic

Further analysis of the data in Table 11.5 revealed that out of the 12 domains covered in the study, there was no statistically significant gender difference in children's rating on nine aspects of their lives. However, a statistically significant gender difference was observed in three areas during the pandemic: the people the children lived with, the things children had, and how the children were listened to by adults. In all these three areas, girls reported to have significantly lower satisfaction than boys.

11.4.2.2 The Rural-Urban Difference in Children's Assessment of Different Domains of their Life During the Pandemic

Table 11.6 presents the results of the analysis of children's assessment of different domains of life by their area of living (rural-urban) during the pandemic. Out of 12 aspects of life, rural children were significantly less satisfied in seven areas. These

Table 11.5 Gender difference in self-assessed satisfaction with different domains of life during the COVID-19 pandemic

Domains (satisfaction with)	Gender (mean score, 0–10 scale)		T-test	Effect (Cohen's d)
	Girl	Boy		
The people you live with	8.24	8.49	−1.73*	2.62
The house you live in	7.72	7.79	−0.46	2.94
The area where you live	7.38	7.42	−0.23	3.00
About how safe you feel	7.58	7.55	0.13	2.91
Your friends	6.93	6.74	1.09	3.14
How do you use your time	6.75	6.69	0.33	3.13
The way you look	7.32	7.25	0.40	3.09
The things you have	7.27	7.6	−2.03*	2.95
The freedom you have	7.17	7.36	−1.17	3.07
What may happen later in your life	6.72	6.86	−0.78	3.21
How you are listened to by adults in general	6.63	6.99	−2.02*	3.21
Your health	7.46	7.39	0.46	3.02

Notes: * $p < 0.05$
Source: Sample survey

Table 11.6 Rural-urban difference in self-assessed satisfaction with different domains of life during the COVID-19 pandemic

Domains (satisfaction with)	Area of living (mean score, 0–10 scale)		T-test	Effect (Cohen's d)
	Urban	Rural		
The people you live with	8.49	8.23	1.78*	2.62
The house you live in	8.07	7.43	3.98***	2.92
The area where you live	7.64	7.15	3.01***	2.99
About how safe you feel	7.82	7.30	3.27***	2.90
Your friends	6.80	6.77	0.79	3.14
How you use your time	6.78	6.66	0.70	3.13
The way you look	7.38	7.19	1.15	3.09
The things you have	7.64	7.23	2.57**	2.95
The freedom you have	7.27	7.27	0.01	3.07
What may happen later in your life	7.05	6.52	3.08***	3.20
How you are listened to by adults in general	6.81	6.82	−0.05	3.22
Your health	7.52	7.28	1.79*	3.02

Notes: * $p < 0.05$; ** $p < 0.01$; *** $p < 0.001$ (one-tailed)
Source: Sample survey

were (a) people they lived with, (b) their home, (c) area of living, (d) safety, (e) learning at school, (f) future, and (g) health. The remaining five areas in which no significant difference was observed were (a) friends, (b) time use, (c) appearance, (d) freedom, and (e) listening by adults.

11.5 Discussion

The key aim of this chapter was to describe children's experiences during the COVID-19 pandemic and examine the impact of the pandemic on children's well-being in Bangladesh by surveying 10–12 year old school children who assessed different aspects of their lives during the pandemic in this international survey. This section discusses the key findings in the light of conventional theoretical underpinnings of well-being and other applied research in this area.

The preventive measures, such as lockdown of local areas and school closures undertaken to stop the virus spreading, affected almost all children who participated in the study. Their daily life was affected as they could not attend school and had to confine themselves at home for many days. One of the children's most significant challenges was to continue learning from home. The far-reaching negative impact of this on their future learning and development is yet to be assessed. Some studies found the disastrous effect of the pandemic on emotional development (Pearcey et al. 2020), mental health and physical development (Bento and Dias 2017), and readiness for school (Nicholls et al. 2020; Tracey et al. 2022).

Although not many children reported being infected by the virus in this research, the spread in their community was evident from their reporting of the virus among people in their neighborhood and circle of friends. This has also affected the daily life of some children, especially those with family members in the high-risk health category. These children had to be extra careful about the virus because of higher COVID-19 death rates among the high-risk groups. Previous studies revealed the risk of psychological burden (Rawal et al. 2017) and being stigmatized by others (Verberk et al. 2021) for family members living with COVID-19 patients and receiving care in the intensive care unit (ICU) or at home.

This study also found evidence of disruption in children's family economy. Many children (17%) reported that their parents lost their jobs, and these families did not get government support during the pandemic. Although developed countries adopted many policies, for example, the Furlough scheme in the UK to support families during the pandemic, children from lower and lower-middle-income countries, e.g., Bangladesh, went through economic hardship, which is likely to have a more prolonged negative impact on their well-being as they grow up. Choi et al.'s (2019) research demonstrated that children who experienced economic disadvantages and early childhood adversity had adverse behavioral outcomes during adulthood. Other studies, e.g., Walker et al. (2011) and Halfon (2014), provide evidence on the negative impact of living in poverty during childhood on adolescents' educational attainment and adult health.

In child well-being research, an argument is made for measuring subjective well-being in terms of life as a whole and concerning particular aspects or domains of life—such as satisfaction with personal relationships. Rees et al. (2010) argue that people make judgments of their satisfaction with various aspects of their lives and that their overall well-being consists of a summary of these judgments. They further add that this approach is beneficial as it can explore how well-being in particular domains contributes to a person's overall well-being. This can indicate aspects of people's lives requiring further attention to improve their overall well-being. When this framework was applied to evaluate children's satisfaction in 12 different aspects (people they live with, the house they live in, the area they live, feeling safe, their friends, time use, appearance, things they have or material possessions, freedom, future, how adults listen to them, and their health) during the pandemic, children were found to be distinctively less satisfied in four areas: time use, friends, future prospect, and how adults listened to them. This suggests that more attention is required in these four areas to improve children's overall well-being in the post-pandemic recovery phase.

A simulation study by Rahman and Sharma (2021) found that the fifth graders' reading proficiency is expected to decline significantly due to school closure. Although some research, e.g., Evans et al. (2020) reported that the COVID-19 pandemic brought positive outcomes for families in terms of relationships with family members during the pandemic, parents in Singapore reported a more significant impact of COVID-19 reflected in higher stress, harsher parenting, and less closeness to their children (Chung et al. 2022). The results of the longitudinal study shed further light on this complex relationship. Family chaos during that period was also associated with increased conflict between children, parents, and siblings (Cassinat et al. 2021).

One of the significant areas of impact of the pandemic in this research was found to be on children's relationships with friends. In Larivière-Bastien et al.'s (2022) research, children missed their friends more than anything else during the pandemic. Evaluating children's perspectives, they argued that friendships cannot be replaced by family relationships, fun leisure activities at home, relationships with pets, or virtual communication. Research found that children's relationships with friends had the second highest effect (after family relationships) on their overall well-being (Goswami 2012). As children reach their mid-childhood, relations with friends become increasingly important. For children, friendship positively impacts social-emotional development (Pianta 2006). Getting on with friends is crucial for children because social reinforcement usually comes from peers, influencing their subjective well-being (Holder and Coleman 2009). Unlike adults, who have different platforms for interaction with friends, children have limited options, and these are mostly confined to school contexts and other settings arranged by adults. Extended closure of schools and other organized group activities meant these options were not available to most children, hindering their interaction with friends.

In this study, girls reported experiencing lower levels of satisfaction with time use and learning at home during the pandemic than boys. This finding supports the theories of subjective well-being and the well-established fact of gender inequalities. According to livability theory (Tay and Diener 2011; Veenhoven and Ehrhardt 1995), the societal system can either hinder or promote subjective well-being. Women would be less satisfied if they were in a disadvantaged position globally (Cassondra Batz-Barbarich et al. 2018).

Although the rural children in Bangladesh were significantly less satisfied with their homes, area of living, safety, learning at school, and future during the pandemic, the result may not be apparent in other countries because the definitions of rural and urban areas may not be the same in other countries. Rural residents have higher levels of subjective well-being (Cummins et al. 2003; Goswami et al. 2023). However, in other studies, urban residents have higher levels of subjective well-being than their rural counterparts (Goswami 2021; Millward and Spinney 2013; Murray et al. 2004). This happiness differential may result from rural-urban disparity in the level of economic development (Easterlin et al. 2011). The rural-urban divide in terms of road infrastructure, electric power availability, health care, transportation, and mobile phone signal strength all of which are limited to children living in rural areas in Bangladesh, and these might be considered as some reasons that explain why rural children reported lower levels of satisfaction.

11.6 Policy Implications

This chapter illustrated school children's lives during the COVID-19 pandemic in Bangladesh when they experienced minimum mobility even in their own neighborhood. To check their satisfaction level, we used their assessment by asking them directly about what happened to them during the crisis period. These lived experiences of children during the pandemic are vital for policies targeted to improve children's well-being in the post-pandemic recovery phase. Since children reported having the lowest level of satisfaction with how time was spent, relationships with friends, their future prospects, and how adults listened to them during the pandemic, these four aspects of children's lives require more attention (and investments). The needs of boys should also be addressed as they reported significantly lower satisfaction with their material possessions and how adults listened to them.

Further to this gender dimension, girls' requirements also need to be addressed especially since they reported a greater degree of reduction in satisfaction with the way they spent their time and their learning at home during the pandemic. Rural children's well-being also needs to be addressed by giving special attention to the areas where they reported being less satisfied: home, area of living, safety, learning at school, and future. These rural children also reported a more significant reduction in overall well-being during the pandemic. To sum up, any future policy initiative to improve children's well-being in Bangladesh must prioritize rural children and design gender-based interventions in children's material possessions, ways adults listen to children, how children spend time, and their learning at home.

11.7 Limitations and Future Directions

Despite many strengths, including a child-friendly questionnaire, asking children directly about their experience during the pandemic, a good sample size, and equal representation of children by gender, our study has the following limitations.

First, the convenience sampling method of collecting data only from four regions has its limitations of underrepresenting other areas of the country. Therefore, a comprehensive study covering all the diverse regions is desired. The online responses should not be treated equally with face-to-face methods in normal times. Second, this study only covered children within the age bracket of 10–12 so it is not representative of all children.

Third, the samples are drawn mainly from mainstream Bengali medium schools except for the online portion. Therefore, at least in the face-to-face part, a section of the student population from English medium schools and faith-based schools like Madrassas are not included. Future studies need to address the issues of those groups as well for a more comprehensive picture of factors associated with children's experiences and subjective well-being during the pandemic in Bangladesh. Finally, this study is based on a cross-sectional design. Therefore, it does not provide evidence of causal links between the pandemic and children's well-being. Longitudinal data is needed to test and establish the causal connections.

11.8 Conclusion

Promoting wellbeing is a key Sustainable Development Goal (Goal No. 3). However, the COVID-19 pandemic has seriously affected children's wellbeing and education worldwide. According to UNICEF, 37 million children in Bangladesh had their education disrupted by one of the world's longest pandemic school closures (543 days). Following the children's rights perspective, this research examined the lives of 10–12 years old children by allowing them to rate their lives during the pandemic. Among 12 different aspects of life i.e., their satisfaction with (1) the people they live with, (2) the house they live in, (3) the area they live, (4) feeling safe, (5) their friends, (6) time use, (7) appearance, (8) things they have or material possession, (9) freedom, (10) future, (11) how adults listen to them, and (12) their health examined in the study, the children were less satisfied in four specific areas during the pandemic. These were (a) time use (lowest mean score of 6.7), (b) friends (mean score = 6.8), (c) future prospects (mean = 6.8), and (d) how adults listened to them (mean = 6.8). Moreover, results of gender and rural-urban differential in children's quality of life during the pandemic provided crucial policy insights for addressing inequality in children's education and wellbeing in the post-pandemic phase in Bangladesh.

References

Bento, G., and G. Dias. 2017. The importance of outdoor play for young children's healthy development. *Porto Biomedical Journal* 2 (5): 157–160.

Cassinat, J.R., S.D. Whiteman, S. Serang, A.M. Dotterer, S.A. Mustillo, J.L. Maggs, and B.C. Kelly. 2021. Changes in family chaos and family relationships during the COVID-19 pandemic: Evidence from a longitudinal study. *Developmental Psychology* 57 (10): 1597–1610.

Cassondra Batz-Barbarich, C., L. Tay, L. Kuykendall, and H.K. Cheung. 2018. A meta-analysis of gender differences in subjective Well-being: Estimating effect sizes and associations with gender inequality. *Psychological Science* 29 (9): 1491–1503.

Choi, J.-K., D. Wang, and A.P. Jackson. 2019. Adverse experiences in early childhood and their longitudinal impact on later behavioural problems of children living in poverty. *Child Abuse and Neglect* 98 (Dec): 104181. https://doi.org/10.1016/j.chiabu.2019.104181.

Chung, G., P. Lanier, and P.W.Y. Ju. 2022. Mediating effects of parental stress on harsh parenting and parent-child relationship during coronavirus (COVID-19) pandemic in Singapore. *Journal of Family Violence* 5: 801–812.

Cummins, R.A., R. Eckersley, J. Pallantj, J. Van Vuht, and R. Misajon. 2003. Developing a national index of subjective Well-being: The Australian unity wellbeing index. *Social Indicators Research* 64: 159–190.

Diener, E., S. Oishi, and R. Lucas. 2015. National accounts of subjective Well-being. *American Psychologist* 70: 234–242.

Easterlin, R.A., L. Angelescu, and S. Zweigj. 2011. The impact of modern economic growth on urban–rural differences in subjective Well-being. *World Development* 39 (12): 2187–2198.

Evans, S., A. Mikocka-Walus, A. Klas, L. Olive, E. Sciberras, G. Karantzas, and E.M. Westrupp. 2020. From "it has stopped our lives" to "spending more time together has strengthened bonds": The varied experiences of Australian families during COVID-19. *Frontiers in Psychology* 11: 588–667. https://doi.org/10.3389/fpsyg.2020.58866.

Geoghegan, T. 2018. The many faces of exclusion. End of childhood report 2018. Connecticut: Save the Children. https://resourcecentre.savethechildren.net/pdf/endofchildhood_report_2018_english_0.pdf/. Accessed 13 Oct 2023.

Goswami, H. 2012. Social relationships and children's subjective Well-being. *Social Indicators Research* 107: 575–588.

———. 2021. Children's subjective Well-being in Bangladesh: Influence of socio-demographic and economic factors. *Population Review* 61 (1): 119–140.

Goswami, H., G.G. Goswami, B.K. Banik, and M.I. Khalil. 2023. Factors associated with children's subjective wellbeing during COVID-19 pandemic in Bangladesh. *Child Indicators Research* 16: 1889–1911. https://doi.org/10.1007/s12187-023-10044-y.

Halfon, N. 2014. Socioeconomic influences on child health: Building new ladders of social opportunity. *Journal of the American Medical Association (JAMA)* 311 (9): 915–917.

Holder, M.D., and B. Coleman. 2009. The contribution of social relationships to children's happiness. *Journal of Happiness Studies* 10: 329–349.

Hussain, M., and M.A. Al Mamun. 2020. COVID-19 in children in Bangladesh: Situation analysis. *Asia Pacific Journal of Pediatrics and Child Health* 3 (April–June): 59–65.

IEDCR. 2020. *Corona Info. Institute of Epidemiology, Disease Control and Research (IEDCR).* IEDCR. 9 April 2020.

iMMAP. 2022. *COVID-19 impacts in Bangladesh nationwide survey on livelihoods, nutrition, education and health.* https://immap.org/wpcontent/uploads/2016/12/iMMAP_Bangladesh_Nationwide_Survey_on_COVID_19_impacts_Survey_-analysis-full-report_Final-1.pdf. Accessed 19 May 2022.

Islam, K., S. Ali, S.Z.R. Akanda, S. Rahman, A.H.M. Kamruzzaman, S.A.P. Pavel, and J. Baki. 2020. COVID-19 pandemic and level of responses in Bangladesh. *International Journal of Rare Disease and Disorder* 3: 019. https://doi.org/10.23937/2643-4571/1710019.

Larivière-Bastien, D., O. Aubuchon, A. Blondin, D. Dupont, J. Libenstein, F. Séguin, A. Tremblay, H. Zarglayoun, C.M. Herba, and M.H. Beauchamp. 2022. Children's perspectives on friendships and socialization during the COVID-19 pandemic: A qualitative approach. *Child: Care, Health and Development* 48 (6): 1017–1030. https://doi.org/10.1111/cch.12998.

Millward, H., and J. Spinney. 2013. Urban-rural variation in satisfaction with life: Demographic, health, and geographic predictors in Halifax, Canada. *Applied Research in Quality of Life* 8: 279–297.

Murray, G., F. Judd, H. Jackson, C. Fra-Ser, A. Komiti, G. Hodgins, P. Pat-Tison, J. Humphreys, and G. Robins. 2004. Rurality and mental health: The role of accessibility. *Australian and New Zealand Journal of Psychiatry* 38: 629–634.

Nicholls, M., I. Neale, O. Joyner, and M. Sheikh. 2020. *Kindred—School readiness*. https://www.kindredsquared.org.uk/wp-content/uploads/2020/11/Kindred2-YouGov-School-Readiness.pdf. Accessed 19 July 2022.

Pearcey, S., A. Shum, H. Dodd, and P. Lawrence. 2020. Changes in preschool children's emotional and behavioural difficulties through lockdown. Report 3. https://cospaceoxford.org/wp-content/uploads/2020/08/Co-SPYCE-report_03.pdf. Accessed 19 July 2022.

Pianta, R.C. 2006. Schools, schooling, and developmental psychopathology. In *Developmental psychopathology, Vol. 1 theory and method*, ed. D. Ciccheti and D.J. Cohen, 494–529. Hoboken, NJ: Wiley.

Rahman, T., and U. Sharma. 2021. A simulation of COVID-19 school closure impact on student learning in Bangladesh. Working paper. Dhaka: The World Bank. https://openknowledge.worldbank.org/bitstream/handle/10986/35043/A-Simulation-of-COVID-19-School-Closure-Impact-on-Student-Learning-in-Bangladesh.pdf?sequence=5&isAllowed=y. Accessed 20 July 2022.

Rawal, G., S. Yadav, and R. Kumar. 2017. Post-intensive care syndrome: An overview. *Journal of Translational Internal Medicine* 5 (2): 90–92.

Rees, G., J. Bradshaw, and A. Keung. 2010. *Understanding children's Well-being: A national survey of young people's Well-being*. London: The Children's Society.

Save the Children. n.d. *Covid-19 Coronavirus: Impact on children*. https://bangladesh.savethechildren.net/sites/bangladesh.savethechildren.net/files/library/Children%20Perception%20Survey%20on%20COVID19.pdf. Accessed 15 May 2022.

Tay, L., and E. Diener. 2011. Needs and subjective Well-being around the world. *Journal of Personality and Social Psychology* 101: 354–365.

Tracey, L., C. Bowyer-Crane, S. Bonetti, D. Nielsen, K. D'Apice, and S. Compton. 2022. *The impact of the COVID-19 pandemic on children's socio-emotional wellbeing and attainment during the reception year*. London: The Education Endowment Foundation. https://educationendowmentfoundation.org.uk/projects-and-evaluation/projects/the-impact-of-the-COVID-19-pandemic-on-childrens-socioemotional-well-being-and-attainment-during-the-reception-year. Accessed 19 July 2022.

Veenhoven, R., and J. Ehrhardt. 1995. The cross-national pattern of happiness: Test of predictions implied in three theories of happiness. *Social Indicators Research* 34: 33–68.

Verberk, J.D.M., S.A. Anthierens, S. Tonkin-Crine, H. Goossens, J. Kinsman, M.L.A. de Hoog, J.A. Bielicki, P.C.J.L. Bruijning-Verhagen, and N.H. Gobat. 2021. Experiences and needs of persons living with a household member infected with SARS-CoV-2: A mixed method study. *PLoS One* 16 (3): e0249391. https://doi.org/10.1371/journal.pone.0249391.

Walker, S.P., T.D. Wachs, S. Grantham-McGregor, B. Maureen, N. Charles, L.H. Sandra, B.-H. Helen, M.C. Susan, H. Jena, L. Betsy, M.M.G. Jlie, P. Christine, R. Alif, and R. Linda. 2011. Inequality in early childhood: Risk and protective factors for early child development. *Lancet* 378 (9799): 1325–1338.

Haridhan Goswami is a Reader in Sociology at Manchester Metropolitan University, United Kingdom. He is a Quantitative Sociologist with an interest in measuring children's and young people's wellbeing. He has expertise in designing and developing reliable and valid survey instruments suitable for children and young people and cross-national comparative research. Haridhan is the coordinator of the South Asian Research Network for Childhood and Youth Studies (SARNCYS) which includes academics and researchers from Bangladesh, India, Nepal, Sri Lanka, and the UK. He is the country lead of the Children's Worlds survey in Bangladesh. He serves on the editorial board of Child Indicators Research.

Bijoy Krishna Banik is a Professor of Sociology at the University of Rajshahi in Bangladesh. He obtained a Post-Graduate Diploma and Master of Arts degree from the International Institute of Social Studies, The Hague, The Netherlands. He received his PhD degree in sociology from the University of New England, Australia. He has participated and presented papers at many national and international conferences and published papers in both national and international reputed journals. In addition, he is editing and reviewing articles in many reputed journals. His current research includes COVID-19, children and well-being, public health, public and social policy, and social media.

Gour Gobinda Goswami is a Professor in the Department of Economics, School of Business & Economics, and Director of Student Affairs at North South University, Dhaka 1229, Bangladesh. Dr. Gour has 31 years of experience in teaching, research, and consultancy. He received his Ph.D. in Economics from the University of Wisconsin-Milwaukee, USA, and published extensively in Economics, Business, and Social Sciences. He has received the Emerald Literati Award 2022 as an Outstanding Reviewer from the Journal of Economic Studies, University Grants Commission (UGC) Award 2003 and 2006 for his contribution to Social Sciences in Economics. His research interests range from International Trade, International Finance, COVID-19, the Rohingya Displacement Problem, Subjective Well-being, Economic Integration, Gravity Equation, Exchange Rates, Purchasing Power Parity, and Cryptocurrency.

M. Ibrahim Khalil is an Associate Professor of Sociology at Government Brojomohun College, Barishal, Bangladesh. He pursued his PhD from the Institute of Bangladesh Studies (IBS) in January 2013. He obtained his MA in Education from the University of Nottingham. Dr. Khalil completed both his Bachelor's and Master's in Sociology from the University of Dhaka. His research interests include poverty, disaster vulnerability, climate change adaptation, disaster management, gender and development, livelihood security of vulnerable people, climate refugees, etc. He carried out several research projects and published several articles in refereed journals. He has presented several papers in various national and regional seminars in Bangladesh. Dr. Khalil is a Co-Investigator of the Children's Worlds Survey in Bangladesh.

Chapter 12
Children's Profiles of Subjective Well-being Change During the COVID-19 Pandemic and Its Correlates: A Multi-national Study

Oliver Nahkur and Karoliine Zarina

12.1 Introduction

COVID-19 pandemic has impacted the lives of everyone, particularly children (Folostina and Iacob 2021). As a response to the COVID-19 pandemic, most countries in the world implemented social-distancing measures and ordered the lockdown of all residents—including school closures in approximately 114 countries affecting more than 1.2 billion children (Zhu et al. 2021)—to slow the rate of transmission, ease the pressure on the healthcare system, and protect at-risk populations (Armitage and Nellums 2020). It changed children's everyday lives completely and the sudden and unexpected situation disrupted their usual routines (Stoecklin et al. 2021), having an impact on children's well-being that are currently not well understood (Engel de Abreu et al. 2021). Current studies analyzing the impact of the COVID-19 pandemic on children mainly focus on their mental health, indicating that mental health problems have increased since the beginning of the pandemic (e.g., Loades et al. 2020). For example, anxiety, including Coronavirus anxiety, depression, and post-traumatic symptoms have been observed in children and adolescents (Mondragon et al. 2021; Zhu et al. 2021). There are also some studies assessing the impact on children's well-being via parent ratings (e.g., Neubauer et al. 2021), but there is less evidence on how the pandemic impacts were reflected in children's overall subjective well-being. Moreover, as the stringency of social-distancing measures varied between countries—e.g., in some countries, children could leave home for sports or walks with their parents or guardians, whilst in other countries these activities were prohibited (Garcia 2020)—it is important to study

O. Nahkur (✉)
Faculty of Social Sciences, Institute of Social Studies, University of Tartu, Tartu, Estonia
e-mail: oliver.nahkur@ut.ee

K. Zarina
Tallinn University, Tallinn, Estonia

C. Suter et al. (eds.), *Well-being During the Pandemic*, Social Indicators Research Series 90, https://doi.org/10.1007/978-3-031-63440-6_12

the change of children's overall subjective well-being multi-nationally. Previously, predominantly single country studies have been conducted, showing that children's subjective well-being during the COVID-19 pandemic decreased (Kirsch et al. 2020; Magson et al. 2021; Mitra et al. 2021; Steinmayr et al. 2022; von Soest et al. 2020) or did not change (Choi et al. 2021) during the first wave of the pandemic. To our knowledge, there is only one multi-national study (Savahl et al. 2022), briefly describing the change of children's overall subjective well-being during the COVID-19 pandemic based on country means. To understand the impacts of the pandemic on children's overall subjective well-being and its change more thoroughly, it is important to go further from "country means" analyses and use children's "profiles of change" approach (e.g., previously used by Nahkur and Kutsar 2022). According to this approach, some children may have had predominantly negative or positive experiences, while some had both, and overall, their subjective well-being decreased, increased, or did not change much, respectively.

Moreover, to better understand the impacts of the pandemic on children's subjective well-being and its change, it is important to explore the correlates of children's subjective well-being change. There are some single country studies showing that children's social distancing experience (Magson et al. 2021), pandemic-related anxiety (Magson et al. 2021; von Soest et al. 2020), but also fulfillment of their psychological needs (Kutsar and Kurvet-Käosaar 2021; Magson et al. 2021; Mitra et al. 2021) can be important factors contributing to the change of children's subjective well-being during the COVID-19 pandemic. In this paper, by taking the "profiles of change" approach, we aim to explore multi-nationally the change of children's overall subjective well-being during the COVID-19 pandemic, including the role of social distancing experience, pandemic-related anxiety, and psychological needs fulfillment in this. Similarly to Savahl et al. (2022), we use International Children's Worlds COVID-19 Supplement Survey data collected in 2021 from approximately 20,000 children primarily aged 9–13 years from 16 countries across four continents. To our knowledge, this is the first such quantitative study based on such a large-scale multi-national sample.

12.2 Children's Subjective Well-being and Its Determinants

12.2.1 The Concept of Children's Subjective Well-being

Children's subjective well-being is a multifaceted construct that includes hedonic and eudaimonic well-being (Diener 1984; Gröndal et al. 2021; Kesebir and Diener 2008; Soffia and Turner 2021). Hedonic well-being is based on children's experiences, perceptions, and evaluations of those experiences, comprising children's longer-term cognitive evaluations of their lives as a whole (e.g., overall life satisfaction) and reports on affective well-being such as frequent experience of positive emotions and infrequent occurrence of negative emotions (Diener 1984). Eudaimonic well-being is not an outcome but a process of fulfilling one's true self, which can be associated with one's sense of meaning and purpose (Soffia and Turner 2021). Thus, subjective well-being is measured multidimensionally. In this paper, we focus on the pandemic impact on the hedonic component of children's subjective well-being by analyzing their overall happiness change before and during the COVID-19 pandemic. We argue that overall happiness—e.g., "Thinking about your life now during the Coronavirus, how happy are you with your life as whole?"—is not a pure affective nor cognitive measure. Although "happy" refers to affective well-being, in this question children evaluate their life as whole in a longer-term perspective, making it more similar to cognitive well-being measures.

12.2.2 Previous Evidence About the Change of Children's Overall Subjective Well-being During the COVID-19 Pandemic

There is little previous research on the change of children's overall subjective well-being during the COVID-19 pandemic. Mainly the change of children's overall subjective well-being has been explored during the first wave of COVID-19 pandemic in single country studies, e.g., longitudinally in Norway (von Soest et al. 2020), Germany (Steinmayr et al. 2022), Australia (Magson et al. 2021), South Korea (cross-cohort study by Choi et al. 2021), and cross-sectionally in Luxembourg (Kirsch et al. 2020) and Canada (Mitra et al. 2021). Some of these studies have focused on overall cognitive (Choi et al. 2021; Magson et al. 2021) or affective (Mitra et al. 2021) subjective well-being, but some on both (Kirsch et al. 2020; von Soest et al. 2020; Steinmayr et al. 2022). *Overall cognitive subjective well-being* decreased during the first wave of pandemic among children in Oslo, Norway (von Soest et al. 2020); 13–16 years-old adolescents in urban area of New South Wales, Australia (Magson et al. 2021); 6–16 years-old children in Luxembourg (Kirsch et al. 2020). For example, before the arrival of COVID-19, 96% of Luxembourg children were satisfied or very satisfied with their lives but it dropped to 67% during the pandemic. Among elementary school (Grades 2 to 4) children in Germany (Steinmayr et al. 2022), overall life satisfaction decreased but not on statistically significant level. However, a study by Choi et al. (2021) revealed that the life satisfaction of 9 to 10-year-old South Korean children has not changed compared to the time before the COVID-19 pandemic. *Overall affective subjective well-being* decreased during the first wave of pandemic among elementary school (Grades 2 to 4) children in Germany (Steinmayr et al. 2022) and 9–15 years-old children in Canada (Mitra et al. 2021).

Also, children's overall *cognitive and affective subjective well-being* decreased between second and third wave of the pandemic in twenty countries across four continents (Savahl et al. 2022), including in Estonia (Kutsar et al. 2022). To our knowledge, the study by Savahl et al. (2022) is only multi-national study exploring the change of children's overall subjective well-being during the COVID-19 pandemic. Based on country means on overall happiness in 2021, overall subjective well-being decreased the most in countries such as Bangladesh, Germany, or South Africa, while least in Russia, Spain, and South Korea.

Although Engel de Abreu et al. (2021) suggested that girls—supported by the findings of Magson et al. (2021) and Kutsar et al. (2022)—and adolescents from low-income homes may be especially vulnerable to negative indirect effects of COVID-19, Steinmayr et al. (2022) could not confirm gender or socio-economic status as a consistent moderator regarding the decrease in subjective well-being.

12.2.3 Children's Overall Subjective Well-being and Its Change During the COVID-19 Pandemic—What Matters?

There is some previous evidence showing that social distancing experience and pandemic-related anxiety can be important factors contributing to the change of children's subjective well-being during the COVID-19 pandemic. According to Magson et al. (2021), children in Australia reporting greater adherence to the stay-at-home rules reported lower declines in life satisfaction compared to those who continued to leave their homes more frequently. Moreover, Australian children with high and moderate levels of COVID-19 related distress experienced significantly greater decreases in life satisfaction, over time than those with low levels of COVID-19 related distress (Magson et al. 2021). Also in Norway, reduced life satisfaction during the COVID-19 restriction period was found to be linked with "concerns about illness and infection" (von Soest et al. 2020). We are not aware of any evidence showing the importance of pandemic-related school anxiety in children's subjective well-being change during the COVID-19 pandemic.

Moreover, the needs of relatedness, autonomy and competence—basic psychological needs that are the foundation of people's subjective well-being [self-determination theory by Ryan and Deci (2000)]—were probably not met due to the social-distancing measures, e.g., school, cultural and sports facilities closures, social contact restrictions and the need to stay at home during the COVID-19 pandemic, resulting in a possible decrease in children's subjective well-being. There is some empirical evidence showing the importance of relatedness in children's subjective well-being change during the COVID-19 pandemic. According to the longitudinal study by Magson et al. (2021), children from New South Wales, Australia perceiving high levels of social connection during COVID-19 reported significantly higher life satisfaction increase than those feeling socially disconnected during the lockdown period. Mitra et al. (2021) found that having a friend to share feelings with reduced the likelihood to have low affective well-being for Canadian 9–15 years-old children. There is also some evidence showing the importance of autonomy in children's subjective well-being change during the COVID-19 pandemic. The study by Kutsar and Kurvet-Käosaar (2021) revealed that although the children understood the seriousness of the situation, they blamed the rules resulting from the pandemic for taking away their freedom and worsening their life satisfaction. We are not aware of any evidence showing the importance of competence in children's subjective well-being change during the COVID-19 pandemic.

12.3 Gaps in Previous Research: Aim and Hypotheses

Children's subjective well-being change during the COVID-19 pandemic has been explored in single country studies (Choi et al. 2021; Kirsch et al. 2020; Kutsar et al. 2022; Magson et al. 2021; Mitra et al. 2021; von Soest et al. 2020; Steinmayr et al. 2022). There is only one such multi-national study (Savahl et al. 2022). Based on the same data we are using, Savahl et al. (2022) have shown that children's mean overall subjective well-being has decreased in twenty countries across four continents. However, to understand the impacts of the pandemic on children's overall subjective well-being and its' change more thoroughly, it is important to go further from "country means" analyses and use children's "profiles of change" approach (e.g., previously used by Nahkur and Kutsar 2022). More specifically, first, we are interested in how do children's 'profiles of change' vary across countries. Based on the results of Savahl et al. (2022), our first hypothesis is:

H1: compared to other countries, "decliners" was most common profile of subjective well-being change during pandemic in Bangladesh, Germany, and Turkey, and 'no changers' and "gainers" were most common profiles in South Korea, Albania, and Estonia.

Second, we are interested in how do children's "profiles of change" vary by their gender and socio-economic status. Based on the previous evidence (e.g., Engel de Abreu et al. 2021; Magson et al. 2021; Kutsar et al. 2022) described in Sect. 12.2.2, the next hypotheses are:

H2a: among girls, "decliners" was more, "no changers" and "gainers" less common profile of subjective well-being change during pandemic compared to boys;
H2b: "decliners" was more, "no changers" and "gainers" less common profile of subjective well-being change during pandemic among children with low compared to high socio-economic status.

Third, we are interested in how do subjective well-being decliners, no changers and gainers differ by their social distancing experience, pandemic-related anxiety, and psychological needs fulfillment during pandemic. Based on the previous research evidence (e.g., Kutsar and Kurvet-Käosaar 2021; Magson et al. 2021; Mitra et al. 2021; von Soest et al. 2020) and self-determination theory (Ryan and Deci 2000) described in Sect. 12.2.3, we hypothesize the following:

H3a: "gainers" experienced social distancing more than "no changers" and "decliners";

H3b: "decliners" experienced more pandemic-related anxiety than "no changers" and "gainers";
H3c: decliners' psychological needs were less fulfilled during pandemic compared to "no changers" and "gainers".

Fourth, to offer a new insight to better support children in such exceptional times, we are interested if children's social distancing experience and/or pandemic-related anxiety and/or psychological needs fulfillment during pandemic help to explain children's belonging to subjective well-being decliners compared to no changers profile. We hypothesize the following:

H4: children's social distancing experience, pandemic-related anxiety and psychological needs fulfillment during pandemic help to explain children's belonging to subjective well-being "decliners" compared to "no changers" profile.

12.4 Data and Methods

12.4.1 Data Source and Sample

We include approximately 20,000 primarily 9–13-year old children's data from 16 countries across the globe collected in 2021 as part of the International Child Well-being COVID supplement Survey. The data was collected mostly between the peaks of the second and third wave of the pandemic. The first version of the database included children's data from the following 20 countries: Germany, Turkey, Bangladesh, Italy, Albania, Romania, Chile, Wales, Colombia, Taiwan, Belgium, Algeria, Israel, South Korea, Indonesia, and Estonia. We excluded South Africa, Russia, Finland, and Spain due to the absence of data on some measures that we considered important.

Data collection methods varied from country to country between pencil and/or web survey methods. Due to the difficulties in collecting data from children during the COVID-19 pandemic (and during the (semi)lockdown in many countries), in most cases representative samples were not achieved. Different sampling methods were used, i.e., stratified (in Belgium) or cluster (in South Korea) as representative, and convenience (e.g., in Taiwan, Bangladesh, Indonesia, Israel), purposive (in Chile) and snowball (in Germany) as non-representative sampling methods. In many cases, only country regions were captured. In addition, sample sizes varied broadly from 590 in Germany to 2422 in Belgium. The gender distributions were quite even, ranging from 46% girls in Wales to 55% girls in Albania. This is described in more detail in Appendix Table 12.6.

12.4.2 Measures

We measure the overall subjective well-being before the COVID-19 pandemic with children's subjective retrospective assessments—"Thinking about how your life was before the Coronavirus, how happy were you with your life as whole?"; and during the pandemic with "Thinking about your life now during the Coronavirus, how happy are you with your life as whole?". Eleven-point assessment scale was used, where 0 was "not happy at all" and 10 "completely happy." Change of overall subjective well-being (SWB) for each child were computed as follows: "SWB now"—"SWB before the Coronavirus." Social distancing experience is measured with the agreement of "There were times where I had to be in my home all day (including the garden, yard or balcony, if you have) because of the Coronavirus" and "I could not attend school for many days." Under pandemic-related anxiety we measure Coronavirus and school anxiety. Coronavirus anxiety is measured with the seven-item Fear of COVID-19 psychometric scale, adapted from the adult version (Ahorsu et al. 2022). These include the agreement of different statements—e.g., "I am afraid of losing my life because of the Coronavirus" and "I cannot sleep because I'm worrying about getting the Coronavirus"—using a five-item Likert-type scale ranging from 0 = "not at all agree" to 4 = "totally agree." For each child, the sum of the values of these statements were computed, ranging from 0 to 28. School anxiety is measured with the question "During the last month, how worried have you been about the following things in your life? The changes in my life as a student because of the Coronavirus situation," where 0 was "not at all" and 10 was "very much." Psychological needs fulfilment is measured with the agreement of "I feel alone" (relatedness), "I am good at managing my daily responsibilities" (competence), and satisfaction with the freedom (autonomy) child has.

12.4.3 Data Analysis

We analyze data to test the hypothesis in three steps. First, to answer the first and second hypotheses we examined the percentages of "decliners," "no changers" and "gainers" in subjective well-being by countries, including by gender and socio-economic status. To answer the third hypotheses, differences in children's social distancing experience, pandemic-related anxiety, and psychological needs fulfill-ment are assessed by countries using the Kruskal-Wallis test. When a significant difference is found, post-hoc tests are conducted using Mann-Whitney's U test to assess the differences between each pair of the profiles. We use nonparametric tests because our variables do not meet normal distribution criteria and the size of the profiles differ markedly. To answer the fourth hypothesis, logistic regression analy-sis by countries is used. Children's profiles of subjective well-being change—decliners vs no changers (reference group)—is used as a dependent variable. Gainers as least common profile was left out due to the low numbers in many coun-tries. We used child gender (1 = girls, 2 = boys, non-binary children are excluded due to low numbers) and assessment about family socio-economic situation (During the last month, how worried have you been about the following things in your life? The money my family has during the Coronavirus period; 0-not at all...10-very much) as controls. Age of the children were not included as a control as we had data mostly for 9–13 years-old children, and in some countries the age range varied only one (e.g, only 10-year-olds in South Korea) or two (e.g, only 10-and 12-year-olds in Colombia) years.

12.5 Results

12.5.1 Profiles of Subjective Well-being Change During the COVID-19 Pandemic

"Decliners" as the most common profile of subjective well-being change occurred in all countries, being most evident in Turkey (79%), Germany (78%) and Bangladesh (74%), but it was above the total mean (60%) also in Italy, Romania, and South Korea (Table 12.1). In all countries, "no changers" was the second most common profile of change, being most evident in Albania, Colombia and South Korea, but it was above the total mean (28%) also in Chile, Estonia, Indonesia, Israel, and Taiwan. Only in Algeria, the second most common profile of subjective well-being change was "gainers"—for 23% of Algerian children the overall subjective well-being increased during the COVID-19 pandemic. Additionally, compared to other countries, there were relatively more "gainers" in Israel (17%) and Belgium (16%), and the proportion of "gainers" was above the total mean (12%) also in Estonia, Wales, Colombia, Taiwan, and Chile. Thus, hypothesis 1—"decliners" was most common profile of subjective well-being change during pandemic in Bangladesh, Germany, and Turkey, and "no changers" and "gainers" were most common profiles in South Korea, Albania, and Estonia—is largely confirmed, except in the case of "gainers," as in South Korea and Albania, the proportion of "gainers" were not the highest but instead being below the total mean.

Children's profiles of subjective well-being change varied less by their gender and more by their socio-economic status. Hypothesis 2a—"decliners" was more, "no changers" and "gainers" less common profile of subjective well-being change during pandemic among girls compared to boys—is fully confirmed in Wales, partially confirmed in Algeria, Chile, Estonia, Germany, and Israel, and not confirmed in other countries. Among Welsh girls, the proportion of "decliners" was 16% higher, "no changers" 11% and "gainers" 5% lower, compared to Welsh boys. In Algeria, Chile, Estonia, Germany, and Israel, "decliners" was more and "no changers" less common profile of change among girls compared to boys. Interestingly, in Belgium, "decliners" was more and "no changers" less common among boys, in Chile and Colombia, "gainers" was less common among boys. In other countries, profiles of subjective well-being change did not vary by gender. Hypothesis 2b—"decliners" was more, "no changers" and "gainers" less common profile of subjective well-being change during pandemic among children with low compared to high socio-economic status—is fully confirmed in Algeria and Germany, partially confirmed in all other countries, except in Chile, Colombia, and South Korea. In Germany, where the socio-economic differences were most apparent, the proportion of "decliners" were 26% higher, "no changers" 21% and "gainers" 5% lower among children with low ("much worry") compared to high ("no worry") socio-economic status. In all other countries with socio-economic differences, except in Indonesia, Israel, and South Korea, "decliners" was more common and "no changers" less common profile of subjective well-being change among children with low

Table 12.1 Percent of decliners, no changers, and gainers by gender, socio-economic status, and in total

	Gender						Socio–economic status: worry the money my family has during the Coronavirus period									Total			
	Boys			Girls			No worry (0–3)			Little worry (4–6)			Much worry (7–10)						
	Dec. %	No ch %	Gain %	Dec. %	No ch %	Gain %	Dec. %	No ch %	Gain %	Dec. %	No ch %	Gain %	Dec. %	No ch %	Gain %	Dec. %	No ch %	Gain %	N
Albania	45.4	45.4	9.2	46	42.9	11.1	35.5	55.8	8.8	46	40.8	13.3	50.5	40	9.6	45.7	44.0	10.2	1006
Algeria	52.6	25.0	22.4	59.4	16.3	24.3	44.2	27.1	28.7	59.8	13.6	26.6	62	20.4	17.6	56.1	20.5	23.4	791
Bangladesh	75.4	17.1	7.5	72.8	18.1	9.1	68.2	22.2	9.5	73.5	16	10.5	77.5	15.5	7	74.1	17.6	8.3	1370
Belgium	61.1	22.9	16.0	53.7	29.9	16.4	55.1	28.7	16.3	59.8	22.2	18	60.5	23.5	15.9	57.2	26.4	16.4	2279
Chile	53.2	34.8	12.0	63.8	24.1	16.4	56.3	31.7	12	59.7	26.4	13.8	59.2	28.8	12	58.7	29.0	12.3	1659
Colombia	54.9	34.7	10.4	50.9	32.3	16.8	48.6	35.2	16.2	55.9	28.7	15.3	53.3	34.8	11.9	52.9	33.5	13.6	955
Estonia	47.6	38.0	14.4	55.9	28.0	16.1	48.4	36	15.6	54.8	31.1	14.2	60.8	24.2	15	51.9	32.9	15.2	1176
Germany	75.3	20.4	4.3	80.2	15.6	4.1	65.7	27.9	6.4	82.4	13.2	4.4	92	6.9	1.1	77.5	18.3	4.2	481
Indonesia	57.8	33.1	9.1	59.7	30.2	10.1	50.5	31.8	17.7	54.1	34.7	11.2	60.8	30.8	8.4	58.8	31.5	9.6	2222
Israel	47.7	33.5	18.8	58.3	26.2	15.6	49.4	33.1	17.5	58.6	20.7	20.7	55.4	30.5	14.2	52.6	30.4	17.1	896
Italy	62.6	28.1	9.4	64.1	25.8	10.1	57.7	31.3	11	62.9	26.5	10.6	68.1	23.3	8.6	63.4	26.8	9.8	835
Romania	65.7	24.0	10.3	66.7	22.2	11.1	64.1	27.3	8.6	69.3	15.3	15.3	69.5	18.6	11.9	66.2	23.0	10.7	1806
South Korea	60.4	33.1	6.5	60.2	33.2	6.6	66.3	29.6	4.1	61.9	31.8	6.3	57.5	35.1	7.4	60.3	33.1	6.5	1497
Taiwan	56.0	31.6	12.4	56.4	31.2	12.4	51.1	37	12	52	35.8	12.2	60.9	26.4	12.7	56.3	31.3	12.4	1155
Turkey	78.1	17.5	4.4	81.0	15.2	3.8	73.5	21.3	5.2	76	18.2	5.8	83.3	13.3	3.4	79.4	16.4	4.2	793
Wales	52.1	31.2	16.7	68.3	19.8	11.9	54.9	32.5	12.5	63.3	16.5	20.2	67.1	20.1	12.8	60.0	25.8	14.1	573
All countries	59.2	29.4	11.4	61.0	26.9	12.1	55.8	31.1	13.1	60.4	26.4	13.2	63.4	26.5	10.1	60.1	28.1	11.8	19,494

Notes: Gender: due to the small N, non-binary children are not included. Abbreviations: "Dec." = "Declincers," "No ch" = "No changers," "Gain" = "Gainers"
Source: International Children's Worlds COVID-19 Supplement Survey 2021 (ISCWeB 2023).

compared to high socio-economic status. Profiles of subjective well-being change did not vary by socio-economic status in Chile and Colombia.

12.5.2 Social Distancing Experience, Pandemic-related Anxiety, and Psychological Needs Fulfillment by Profiles of Subjective Well-being Change During the COVID-19 Pandemic

12.5.2.1 Social Distancing Experience by Profiles of Subjective Well-being Change During the COVID-19 Pandemic

In Albania, Chile, Colombia, Estonia, Germany, Romania, Taiwan and Wales, there were no significant differences in social distancing experience regarding staying home and not attending school between "decliners," "no changers," and "gainers" (Table 12.2).

However, in Algeria, and South Korea, there were significant differences between children with different profiles of change in social distancing experience regarding staying home and not attending school. In Algeria, for "decliners" it was significantly more likely that there were times where they had to be in their home all day because of the Coronavirus and they could not attend school for many days compared to "gainers". In South Korea, for "decliners" it was significantly more likely that there were times where they had to be in their home all day because of the Coronavirus compared to "gainers" and "no changers"; also for "no changers" compared to "gainers." Also, for "decliners" in South Korea it was significantly more likely that they could not attend school for many days compared to "no changers."

In Bangladesh, Belgium, and Israel, there were significant differences between children with different profiles of change in social distancing experience regarding staying home but not regarding not attending school. In Bangladesh, for "decliners" and "no changers" it was significantly more likely that there were times where they had to be in their home all day because of the Coronavirus compared to "gainers." In Belgium, for "decliners" it was significantly more likely that there were times where they had to be in their home all day because of the Coronavirus compared to "gainers" and "no changers." In Israel, for "decliners" it was significantly more likely that there were times where they had to be in their home all day because of the Coronavirus compared to "no changers."

In Indonesia, Italy, and Turkey, there were significant differences between children with different profiles of change in social distancing experience regarding not attending school but not regarding staying home. In Indonesia, for "decliners" and "no changers" it was significantly more likely that they could not attend school for many days compared to "gainers." In Italy, for "decliners" it was significantly more likely that they could not attend school for many days compared to "gainers." In Turkey, for "decliners" it was significantly more likely that they could not attend school for many days compared to "gainers" and "no changers."

Table 12.2 Means of social distancing experience (1 = yes, 2 = not sure, 3 = no) by profiles of subjective well-being change during the COVID-19 pandemic

	Staying home: There were times where I had to be in my home all day because of the Coronavirus				Not attending school: I could not attend school for many days			
	Decliners	No changers	Gainers	Kruskal–Wallis H	Decliners	No changers	Gainers	Kruskal–Wallis H
Albania	1.4	1.5	1.5	NS	1.3	1.3	1.4	NS
Algeria	1.5[G]	1.7	1.8	18.8***	1.5[G]	1.6	1.6	8.0*
Bangladesh	1.6[G]	1.6[G]	2.0	19.0***	1.2	1.2	1.3	NS
Belgium	1.4[G,NC]	1.5	1.5	9.3*	1.4	1.4	1.4	NS
Chile	1.4	1.5	1.5	NS	1.2	1.2	1.2	NS
Colombia	1.3	1.3	1.5	NS	1.2	1.2	1.2	NS
Estonia	1.5	1.6	1.6	NS	2.3	2.3	2.4	NS
Germany	1.9	2.2	2.1	NS	1.1	1.1	1.0	NS
Indonesia	1.7	1.7	1.7	NS	1.2[G]	1.2[G]	1.4	26.8***
Israel	1.4[NC]	1.6	1.5	7.0*	1.4	1.4	1.4	NS
Italy	1.8	1.9	1.9	NS	1.0[G]	1.0	1.1	7.8*
Romania	1.6	1.6	1.6	NS	1.4	1.4	1.5	NS
South Korea	1.7[G,NC]	2.0[G]	2.3	57.3***	2.4[NC]	2.6	2.4	13.6**
Taiwan	1.3	1.4	1.3	NS	2.4	2.4	2.3	NS
Turkey	1.2	1.3	1.5	NS	1.1[G,NC]	1.2	1.3	11.6**
Wales	1.3	1.3	1.4	NS	1.4	1.3	1.5	NS

Notes: [G] = significantly ($p < 0.05$; based on Mann-Whitney test) different from "gainers"; [NC] = significantly different from "no changers"

***p < 0,001; ** p < 0,01; * p < 0,05; NS = not significant

Source: International Children's Worlds COVID-19 Supplement Survey 2021 (ISCWeB 2023)

All in all, we can conclude that hypothesis 3a—"gainers" experienced social distancing more than "no changers" and "decliners"—is not confirmed in any of the countries.

12.5.2.2 Pandemic-related Anxiety by Profiles of Subjective Well-being Change During the COVID–19 Pandemic

In Estonia and Taiwan, "decliners" had significantly higher Coronavirus and school anxiety compared to "gainers" and "no changers" (Table 12.3). In many countries, for example in Germany, Israel, Algeria, Romania, Belgium, Wales and Turkey, "decliners" had significantly higher Coronavirus and school anxiety compared to "no changers." Also "gainers" had significantly higher Coronavirus anxiety compared to "no changers" in Algeria and Romania, and school anxiety in Wales. Surprisingly, in South Korea, "gainers" had significantly higher Coronavirus anxiety compared to "no changers" but also "decliners." For more detailed results, see Table 12.3. All in all, we can conclude that hypothesis 3b—"decliners" experienced

Table 12.3 Means of Coronavirus (0 lowest and 28 highest) and school anxiety (0 "not at all" and 10 "very much") by profiles of subjective well-being change during the COVID-19 pandemic

	Coronavirus anxiety				Pandemic-related school anxiety			
	Decliners	No changers	Gainers	Kruskal–Wallis H	Decliners	No changers	Gainers	Kruskal–Wallis H
Albania	10.4^{NC}	8.6	11.6^{NC}	27.5***	7.3	6.7	6.8	NS
Algeria	10.8^{NC}	8.7	10.8^{NC}	18.9***	5.8^{NC}	4.7	5.4	9.2*
Bangladesh	13.6	12.5	13.0	NS	7.4^{G}	6.6	6.7	9.7**
Belgium	6.3^{NC}	5.5	5.9	23.6***	$5.3^{G,NC}$	4.2	4.7	43.7***
Chile	7.1	6.2	6.4	NS	$7.1^{G,NC}$	6.3	6.3	24.8***
Colombia	10.5^{NC}	9.3	10.0	7.2*	7.0^{G}	6.8	6.1	7.2*
Estonia	$4.0^{G,NC}$	3.2	2.7	44.5***	$4.7^{G,NC}$	3.3	3.2	59.5***
Germany	6.2^{NC}	3.8	3.7	13.5**	$7.7^{G,NC}$	5.1	5.1	52.4***
Indonesia	12.2	12.7	12.3	NS	8.3^{G}	8.1^{G}	7.0	51.7***
Israel	6.0^{NC}	4.8	4.8	16.3***	5.7^{NC}	4.2	5.1	27.9***
Italy	$8.0^{G,NC}$	6.5	6.6	23.5***	6.7	6.2	5.7	NS
Romania	6.7^{NC}	5.1	6.2^{NC}	35.3***	6.2^{NC}	5.0	5.7	32.3***
South Korea	10.7	12.0^{D}	$15.0^{D,NC}$	42.7***	6.6	6.7	6.7	NS
Taiwan	$10.6^{G,NC}$	9.5	9.0	12.1**	$7.3^{G,NC}$	5.9	6.4	56.2***
Turkey	11.3^{NC}	9.6	11.6	7.3*	$7,7^{G,NC}$	6.3	5.8	23.8***
Wales	5.8^{NC}	5.0	4.4	9.7**	$5,5^{NC}$	3.9	5.3^{NC}	23.5***

Notes: ^{G} = significantly ($p < 0.05$; based on Mann-Whitney test) different from "gainers"; ^{NC} = significantly different from "no changers"; ^{D} = significantly different from "decliners"

***$p < 0{,}001$; ** $p < 0{,}01$; * $p < 0{,}05$; NS = not significant

Source: International Children's Worlds COVID-19 Supplement Survey 2021 (ISCWeB 2023)

more pandemic-related anxiety than "no changers" and "gainers"—is fully confirmed in Estonia and Taiwan, partially confirmed in all other countries, except in South Korea.

12.5.2.3 Psychological Needs Fulfillment by Profiles of Subjective Well-being Change During the COVID–19 Pandemic

Relatedness

In Bangladesh and Estonia, "decliners" significantly more than "gainers" and "no changers" agreed that they felt lonely (Table 12.4). In Indonesia and Turkey, "decliners" significantly more than "no changers" agreed that they felt lonely. In Belgium, Chile, Israel, and Wales, "decliners," but also "gainers" significantly more than "no changers" agreed that they felt lonely. However, in Algeria, "gainers" significantly more than "decliners" agreed that they felt lonely. Also in Romania, and South Korea, "gainers" significantly more than "decliners" and "no changers" agreed that they felt lonely. In Albania, Colombia, Germany, Italy, and Taiwan, no significant differences occurred in loneliness perception between children with different profiles of change.

Autonomy

In Colombia, Germany and Turkey, "decliners" were significantly less satisfied with the freedom they had compared to "no changers" (Table 12.4). In Chile, "decliners" were significantly less satisfied with the freedom they had compared to "gainers" and "no changers," but also "gainers" were less satisfied compared to "no changers." However, in Algeria and Romania, "gainers" were significantly less satisfied with the freedom they had compared to "decliners" and "no changers," but also "decliners" were less satisfied compared to "no changers." In Albania, Bangladesh, Belgium, Estonia, Indonesia, Israel, Italy, "decliners" and "gainers" were significantly less satisfied with the freedom they had compared to "no changers." In Wales, "gainers" were significantly less satisfied with the freedom they had compared to "no changers." In South Korea and Taiwan, no significant differences occurred in satisfaction with the freedom between children with different profiles of change.

Competence

Only in Colombia and South Korea, "decliners" significantly more disagreed that they are good at managing their daily responsibilities compared to "no changers" (Table 12.4). In Albania, Belgium, Chile, Estonia, Germany, Indonesia, Israel, Italy, Romania, and Wales, "decliners" and "gainers" significantly more disagreed that they are good at managing their daily responsibilities compared to "no changers."

Table 12.4 Means of psychological needs fulfillment (relatedness, autonomy, competence) by profiles of subjective well-being change during the COVID-19 pandemic

	Relatedness: I feel alone				Autonomy: satisfaction with the freedom you have				Competence: I am good at managing my daily responsibilities			
	Decliners	No changers	Gainers	Kruskal-Wallis H	Decliners	No changers	Gainers	Kruskal-Wallis H	Decliners	No changers	Gainers	Kruskal-Wallis H
Albania	0.6	0.6	0.7	NS	1.2^{NC}	0.8	1.9^{NC}	38.9***	1.4^{NC}	0.9	1.7^{NC}	46.5***
Algeria	1.0	1.3	1.3^{D}	8.8*	3.3^{NC}	2.4	4.4$^{D.NC}$	39.1***	2.6	2.6	4.0$^{D.NC}$	26.3***
Bangladesh	2.2$^{G.NC}$	1.8	1.8	16.7***	2.8^{NC}	2.2	3.5^{NC}	29.1***	2.8^{NC}	2.4	4.0$^{D.NC}$	26.0***
Belgium	0.8^{NC}	0.7	0.8^{NC}	16.6***	1.7^{NC}	1.4	1.9^{NC}	34.7***	2.8^{NC}	2.4	3.0^{NC}	27.3***
Chile	1.5^{NC}	0.7	1.4^{NC}	104.9***	2.8$^{G.NC}$	1.3	2.2^{NC}	118.5**	3.8^{NC}	2.6	3.5^{NC}	55.2***
Colombia	0.8	0.7	0.7	NS	2.2^{NC}	1.6	2.2	9.5**	1.8^{NC}	1.5	1.8	8.6*
Estonia	1.1$^{G.NC}$	0.8	0.9	19.9***	1.8^{NC}	1.1	2.1^{NC}	61.3***	2.6^{NC}	1.6	2.5^{NC}	66.2***
Germany	1.5	1.6	0.9	NS	2.5^{NC}	1.6	2.3	12.4**	3.4^{NC}	2.4	4.1^{NC}	15.9***
Indonesia	1.9^{NC}	1.7	1.9	8.6*	2.3^{NC}	2.0	2.9^{NC}	43.7***	2.4^{NC}	1.9	2.7^{NC}	47.1***
Israel	0.8^{NC}	0.5	0.9^{NC}	22.4***	1.7^{NC}	0.9	1.8^{NC}	36.3***	2.2^{NC}	1.5	2.5^{NC}	29.1***
Italy	0.8	0.8	0.8	NS	1.4^{NC}	0.8	1.7^{NC}	30.1***	2.1^{NC}	1.7	2.3^{NC}	17.2***
Romania	0.7	0.6	1.0$^{D.NC}$	21.2***	1.0^{NC}	0.5	1.4$^{D.NC}$	67.0***	2.0^{NC}	1.4	2.3^{NC}	32.2***
South Korea	1.5	1.5	2.1$^{D.NC}$	18.0***	2.9	2.8	3.0	NS	3.2^{NC}	2.9	3.2	16.3***
Taiwan	1.1	0.9	1.1	NS	2.5	2.4	2.4	NS	3.1	3.0	3.3	NS
Turkey	2.0^{NC}	1.4	1.7	25.2***	3.2^{NC}	2.1	2.9	24.0***	2.9	2.5	3.9^{NC}	10.4**
Wales	1.2^{NC}	0.8	1.1^{NC}	17.1***	1.7	1.5	1.9^{NC}	6.9*	2.7^{NC}	2.0	3.3^{NC}	26.1***

Notes: Relatedness: "I feel alone"; 0 = I do not agree, 1 = I agree a little, 2 = I agree somewhat, 3 = I agree a lot, 4 = I totally agree; Autonomy: "Satisfaction with: The freedom you have"; 0 = totally satisfied…10 = not satisfied at all; Competence: "I am good at managing my daily responsibilities"; 0 = totally agree…10 = not agree at all. ^{G} = significantly ($p < 0.05$; based on Mann-Whitney test) different from "gainers"; ^{NC} = significantly different from "no changers"; ^{D} = significantly different from "decliners"

***p < 0,001; ** p < 0,01; * p < 0,05; NS = not significant

Source: International Children's Worlds COVID-19 Supplement Survey 2021 (ISCWeB 2023)

However, in Algeria, "gainers" significantly more disagreed that they are good at managing their daily responsibilities compared to "decliners" and "no changers." In Bangladesh, "gainers" significantly more disagreed that they are good at managing their daily responsibilities compared to "decliners" and "no changers"; also "decliners" disagreed more than "no changers." In Turkey, "gainers" significantly more disagreed that they are good at managing their daily responsibilities compared to "no changers." In Taiwan, no significant differences occurred in competence perception between children with different profiles of change.

All in all, we can conclude that hypothesis 3c—decliners' psychological needs were less fulfilled during pandemic compared to "no changers" and "gainers"—is partially confirmed in Albania, Belgium, Chile, Colombia, Estonia, Germany, Indonesia, Israel, Italy, Bangladesh (except competence), Turkey (except competence), Wales (except autonomy), and not confirmed in Algeria, Romania, South Korea, and Taiwan.

12.5.3 *Correlates of Children's Subjective Well-being Decline: Regression Analysis*

Social distancing experience, pandemic-related anxiety, psychological needs fulfillment, but also gender and socio-economic status as control factors seems to help to explain children's belonging to "decliners" in subjective well-being profile compared to "no changers" the most (Nagelkerke $R^2 > 0.1$) in Germany, Chile, Israel, Algeria, Estonia, Wales and Turkey, and least (Nagelkerke $R^2 < 0.05$) in Colombia, Bangladesh and Indonesia (Table 12.5). Girls were more likely "decliners in subjective well-being" in Algeria, Chile, Estonia, and Israel; boys in Belgium. Children with more economic worry were more likely "decliners in subjective well-being" in Algeria and Germany, and less in Israel.

Regarding *social distancing experience* factors, Belgium, Israel, and South Korean children who had to be in home all day and South Korean children who could not attend school for many days were more likely to be "decliners in subjective well-being" compared to "no changers" (Table 12.5). In other countries, social distancing experience factors did not help to explain children's belonging to "decliners in subjective well-being" profile compared to "no changers."

Regarding pandemic-related *anxiety* factors, Albanian, Algeria, Colombian and Romanian children who had higher levels of Coronavirus anxiety were more likely to be "decliners in subjective well-being" compared to "no changers"; however, it was the opposite in Indonesia and South Korea. In other countries, Coronavirus anxiety did not help to explain children's belonging to "decliners in subjective well-being" profile compared to "no changers." School anxiety helped to explain children's belonging to "decliners in subjective well-being" profile compared to "no changers" in all countries—except in Albania, Bangladesh, Colombia, and Italy—children with higher levels of school anxiety were more likely to be "decliners in subjective well-being" compared to "no changers."

Table 12.5 Binary logistic regression model for predicting the likelihood to be "decliner" compared to "no changer" by countries (+ positive association; – negative association; NS = not significant)

		AL	DZ	BD	BE	CL	CO	EE	DE	ID	IL	IT	RO	KR	TW	TU	WA
Controls	Girls (ref: boys)	NS	+	NS	–	+	NS	+	NS	NS	+	NS	NS	NS	NS	NS	NS
	Socio–economic status	NS	+	NS	NS	NS	NS	NS	+	NS	–	NS	NS	NS	NS	NS	NS
Social distancing experience	Had to be in home all day (ref: had not to be)	NS	NS	NS	+	NS	NS	NS	NS	NS	+	NS	NS	+	NS	NS	NS
	Not sure if had to be in home all day (ref: had not to be)	NS	NS	NS	NS	NS	NS	NS	NS	NS	+	NS	NS	NS	NS	NS	NS
	Could not attend school for many days (ref: could attend)	NS	NS	NS	NS	NS	NS	NS	NS	NS	NS	NS	NS	+	NS	NS	NS
	Not sure if could attend school for many days (ref: could attend)	NS	NS	NS	NS	NS	NS	NS	NS	NS	NS	NS	NS	NS	NS	NS	NS
Pandemic-related anxiety	Coronavirus anxiety	+	+	NS	NS	NS	+	NS	NS	–	NS	NS	+	–	NS	NS	NS
	School anxiety	NS	+	NS	+	+	NS	+	+	+	+	NS	+	+	+	+	+
Psychological needs fulfillment	Relatedness	–	–	+	NS	+	NS	NS	NS	+	NS	NS	NS	NS	NS	+	NS
	Autonomy	+	+	+	NS	+	+	NS	NS	NS	NS	+	+	NS	NS	+	NS
	Competence	+	NS	NS	+	+	NS	+	NS	+	NS	NS	+	+	NS	NS	NS
N		816	505	1256	1358	1255	748	905	291	2008	523	723	1344	1399	1010	645	431
Nagelkerke R^2		0.085	0.144	0.042	0.065	0.185	0.035	0.127	0.284	0.037	0.148	0.075	0.083	0.069	0.078	0.113	0.125

Notes: AL-Albania, DZ-Algeria, BD-Bangladesh, BE-Belgium, CL-Chile, CO-Colombia, EE-Estonia, DE-Germany, ID-Indonesia, IL-Israel, IT-Italy, RO-Romania, KR-South Korea, TW-Taiwan, TU-Turkey, WA-Wales

Source: International Children's Worlds COVID-19 Supplement Survey 2021 (ISCWeB 2023)

Regarding *psychological needs fulfillment* factors, Bangladeshi, Chilean, Indonesian and Turkish children who agreed more that they felt lonely were more likely to be "decliners in subjective well-being" compared to "no changers"; however, it was the opposite in Albania, Algeria. In other countries, the perception of loneliness as the lack of fulfillment of relatedness need did not help to explain children's belonging to "decliners in subjective well-being" profile compared to "no changers." In Albania, Algeria, Bangladesh, Chile, Colombia, Italy, Romania and Turkey, children who were more dissatisfied with the freedom they had were more likely to be "decliners in subjective well-being" compared to "no changers." In other countries, dissatisfaction with the freedom as the lack of fulfillment of autonomy need did not help to explain children's belonging to "decliners in subjective well-being" profile compared to "no changers." In Albania, Belgium, Chile, Estonia, Indonesia, Romania and South Korea, children who disagreed more that they are good at managing their daily responsibilities were more likely to be "decliners in subjective well-being" compared to "no changers." In other countries, the perception of lack of fulfillment of competence need did not help to explain children's belonging to "decliners in subjective well-being" profile compared to "no changers."

All in all, we can conclude that hypothesis 4—children's social distancing experience, pandemic-related anxiety and psychological needs fulfillment during pandemic help to explain children's belonging to subjective well-being "decliners" compared to "no changers" profile—is partially confirmed in all countries.

12.6 Discussion and Conclusions

Previously, predominantly single country studies have been done, showing that children's subjective well-being during the COVID-19 pandemic decreased (Kirsch et al. 2020; von Soest et al. 2020; Magson et al. 2021; Mitra et al. 2021; Steinmayr et al. 2022) or did not change (Choi et al. 2021) during the first wave of the pandemic. To our knowledge, there is only one multi-national study (Savahl et al. 2022) exploring the change of children's subjective well-being during COVID-19 pandemic, and it showed that children's mean overall subjective well-being decreased in 20 countries across four continents. However, to understand the impacts of the pandemic on children's overall subjective well-being and its change more thoroughly, it is important to go further from "country means" analyses and use children's "profiles of change" approach (e.g., previously used by Nahkur and Kutsar 2022), and explore the correlates of children's subjective well-being change. Thus, by taking the "profiles of change" approach, present study aimed to explore the change of children's overall subjective well-being during the COVID-19 pandemic, including the role of social distancing experience, pandemic-related anxiety, and psychological needs fulfillment based on the data collected in 2021 from approximately 20,000 children primarily aged 9–13 years from 16 countries.

12.6.1 Decliners as Most Common Profile of Subjective Well-being Change

Although the changes accompanied by the COVID-19 pandemic suited some children, our study confirmed that in all countries, most children's overall subjective well-being decreased. However, the decline was of different sizes in different countries. Confirming hypothesis 1, the decrease was most notable in Turkey, Germany, and Bangladesh, where overall subjective well-being decreased for approximately 3 out of 4 children. Contrary to Savahl et al. (2022), the "profiles of change" approach allowed us to detect Turkey—having one of the most extended periods of school closures, being physically closed for almost 2 years (Müderrisoğlu et al. 2023)—as the country where children's overall subjective well-being decrease was most common. Although in Turkey, but also in Germany and Bangladesh, children reported most often that they could not attend school for many days (see Nahkur and Kutsar 2022), our regression analyses showed that in these countries social distancing experience factors did not help to explain children's belonging to the "decliners" compared to the "no changers" profile. However, school closures could influence children's subjective well-being indirectly through other factors. For example, we found that in Turkey and Germany, higher pandemic—related school anxiety, but in Turkey and Bangladesh, also lack of relatedness and autonomy perceptions helped to explain children's belonging to the "decliners" profile. Also, Müderrisoğlu et al. (2023) found that long duration of school closure in Turkey brought longing for school as a relational space where children interact with their peers and teachers, but also as a place of freedom from their families. Moreover, Nahkur and Kutsar (2022) found that in Turkey, Germany and Bangladesh, the decrease in satisfaction with relationships with family and friends during the pandemic were steepest.

12.6.2 Decliners' Characteristics

In accordance with Engel de Abreu et al. (2021), Magson et al. (2021) and Kutsar et al. (2022), we were able to confirm that "decliners" in subjective well-being were more commonly girls (hypothesis 2a) in Algeria, Chile, Estonia, Israel, Wales, and Germany. Also, recent Europe, Central Asia, and Canada country-pooled analysis by Cosma et al. (2023)—based on Health Behaviour in School-aged Children 2021/2022 survey—showed that overall subjective well-being decrease during pandemic was larger for girls than boys. Interestingly, we found that in Belgium "decliners" were more commonly boys. However, in other countries, in accordance with Steinmayr et al. (2022), we could not confirm the gender difference. In accordance with previous evidence (Engel de Abreu et al. 2021; Kutsar et al. 2022; Magson et al. 2021), our study confirmed that in almost all countries "decliners" were more commonly children with low socio-economic status (hypothesis 2b). In accordance with Steinmayr et al. (2022), no socio-economic differences were detected in Chile and Colombia. Interestingly, in South Korea, "decliners" were more commonly children with high socio-economic status.

Contrary to our hypothesis 3a—based on Magson et al. (2021)—"decliners" experienced social distancing more than "no changers" and/or "gainers" in Algeria, Belgium, Bangladesh, Indonesia, Israel, Italy, South Korea, and Turkey. In Albania, Chile, Colombia, Estonia, Germany, Romania, Taiwan, and Wales, the "decliners" did not experience more social distancing than the "no changers."

In accordance with hypothesis 3b based on Magson et al. (2021) and von Soest et al. (2020), "decliners" experienced more pandemic-related anxiety than "no changers" and/or "gainers" in all countries, except in South Korea. Interestingly, in South Korea, "decliners" experienced Coronavirus anxiety less than "no changers" and "gainers."

In accordance with hypothesis 3c based on previous research evidence (Kutsar and Kurvet-Käosaar 2021; Magson et al. 2021; Mitra et al. 2021), decliners' psychological needs were less fulfilled during pandemic compared to "no changers" and/or "gainers" in Albania, Belgium, Chile, Colombia, Estonia, Germany, Indonesia, Israel, Italy. It also applied to Bangladesh and Turkey, except in case of competence need, and Wales, except in case of autonomy need. It was not confirmed in Algeria, Romania, South Korea, and Taiwan. Interestingly, in Algeria, "decliners" psychological needs were more fulfilled than "gainers"; in Romania, "decliners" relatedness and autonomy needs were more fulfilled than "gainers"; in South Korea, decliners' relatedness need was more fulfilled than "gainers." In Taiwan, no differences were found.

12.6.3 Social Distancing Experience, Pandemic-related Anxiety, and Psychological Needs Fulfillment as Correlates of Children's Subjective Well-being Decline

Children's social distancing experience and/or pandemic-related anxiety and/or psychological needs fulfillment during pandemic helped to explain their subjective well-being decline in all countries, at least partially confirming hypothesis 4. Among different factors, higher pandemic-related school anxiety most consistently, almost in all countries, helped to explain children's belonging to the "decliners" profile. It is important new research evidence, expanding the Wu and Lee (2022) pre-pandemic evidence that school anxiety matters for overall cognitive subjective well-being in various world regions. Moreover, pandemic-related school anxiety mattered also in countries from Eastern European, Latin American and Confucian Asia region where Wu and Lee (2022) did not detect the association between school anxiety and overall cognitive subjective well-being. It is possible that "decliners" had lower self-efficacy, thus were less able to adapt to new normalcy of life as a student. Our regression analyses showed that school anxiety did not matter only in Albania, Bangladesh, Colombia, and Italy. Considering the effect of school anxiety, Coronavirus anxiety mattered in less than half of the countries. Moreover, only in Belgium, Israel, and South Korea, stricter social-distancing experience helped to explain children's belonging to the "decliners" profile when the effect of pandemic-related anxieties, psychological needs fulfillment, gender and socio-economic status were also considered.

Lack of psychological need(s) fulfillment was important in explaining children's belonging to the "decliners" profile in majority of countries. Concerning relatedness, we extended the evidence base from Australia (Magson et al. 2021) and Canada (Mitra et al. 2021) to Albania, Algeria, Bangladesh, Chile, Indonesia, and Turkey. Unexpectedly, in Albania and Algeria, children who were less likely to perceive a lack of relatedness, were more likely to be "decliners" rather than "no changers." Concerning autonomy, we extended the evidence base to Albania, Algeria, Bangladesh, Chile, Colombia, Italy, Romania, and Turkey. Contrary to Kutsar and Kurvet-Käosaar (2021), we did not find that in Estonia perceptions of lack of autonomy help to explain children's belonging to "decliners profile." As totally new research evidence, we found that lack of competence perceptions helped to explain children's belonging to "decliners" profile, especially in Albania, Belgium, Chile, Estonia, Indonesia, Romania, and South Korea. Regression analyses showed that children's perception of lack of relatedness, autonomy and competence did not matter in Germany, Israel, Taiwan, and Wales.

12.6.4 No Changers and Gainers

As totally new findings, the "profiles of change" approach allowed us to detect across countries the proportion of children whose subjective well-being did not change or even increased during the pandemic. Confirming hypothesis 1, our study showed that no change was most notable in Albania—for 44% of Albanian children the overall subjective well-being did not change during the COVID-19 pandemic. For "no changers," the negative and positive experiences probably offset each other. However, being not in accordance with Savahl's et al. (2022) country means'-based results, and not confirming hypothesis 1, overall subjective well-being increase was most notable in Algeria—23% of children the overall subjective well-being increased during the COVID-19 pandemic. For "gainers," sharing new circumstances could lead to increased closeness between family members, especially in cases of high pre-pandemic intra-familial closeness (Mariani et al. 2020) or due to new shared activities (Kutsar and Kurvet-Käosaar 2021; Stoecklin et al. 2021). These children may have benefitted also in the school context as Stoecklin et al. (2021) study showed that some children valued the opportunity to plan their own work, pace of activities and time. In further research, "gainers" should be examined in more detail.

12.6.5 Limitations of the Study and Directions for Future Research

There are several limitations to our study. First, the relevance of the retrospective "before the pandemic" assessments of overall subjective well-being can be debated. Unfortunately, we do not have so-called baseline data. However, we do not regard this as a serious limitation. Retrospective measures of pre-event outcomes measured simultaneously with post-event outcomes may be more effective than traditional pre-test/post-test methods at identifying how participants view the impact of an event (Levinson et al. 1990; Dollahite et al. 2022). Second, although our analyses are based on a novel multinational database with wide geographical coverage, most countries did not have representative samples, data sampling and collection methods varied between countries. However, exploring children's subjective well-being change and its correlates in 16 countries at the time between the second and third wave of COVID-19 offered us a unique opportunity to extend the evidence base of social-distancing measures impacts on children's well-being, especially on overall subjective well-being to different national contexts. Third, to include as many countries as possible, we did not control the effect of age in our study. A further separate study based on data from countries with bigger age-variation is needed.

In further research focusing on crises' impacts on children's subjective well-being, it is important to distinguish children with different "profiles of change." We consider it as a move towards still scarce research on children's subjective well-being using person-oriented approach (e.g., see Gierczyk et al. 2022). In order to find deeper explanations to changes in children's lives, more qualitative studies are needed (e.g., see recent *Children's Understandings of Wellbeing: Global and Local Contexts* (CUWB) project's Special Issue on the Covid-19 Pandemic and Children's Understandings of Well-being: International Perspectives on Social Contexts and Inequality; Barn et al. 2023).

12.6.6 Concluding Remarks

To conclude, our analyses revealed that children experienced social-distancing measures during the pandemic differently. However, in all countries, at least every second child's overall subjective well-being decreased during the COVID-19 pandemic. Among others, it increased the workload for psychologists, mental health practitioners, and other aid professionals working with children. Unfortunately, in many countries such professionals are lacking, possibly prolonging children's well-being recovery.

Our study confirmed the importance of keeping schools open not only with the aim of better educational outcomes but especially in terms of protecting overall subjective and mental well-being of children. Although social distancing experience was not an important correlate of children's subjective well-being decline in most of the countries, it influenced children's subjective well-being indirectly through other factors. Across countries, pandemic-related school anxiety was a most consistent correlate of children's subjective well-being decline, and in many countries the lack of psychological need(s) fulfillment also helped to explain the decline. Negative outcomes of school closures and the social distancing of the whole population outweigh its positive aspects.

Acknowledgements The research carried out for this publication was supported by a grant from the Estonian Research Council (Grant No. PRG700). Thanks are due to all children who kindly agreed to answer the questionnaire, to all principal investigators and to all research team members who participated in the data collection in the 16 countries included in the sample used here, to the coordinating team of the Children's Worlds project for kindly allowing us to use the database, and to the Jacobs Foundation for supporting the project.

Appendix

Table 12.6 Countries' sample representativeness, geographical coverage, data collection time and method (PPS-paper-pencil survey; WS-web survey), total number of children and gender distribution

	Represen-tative sample—yes or no	Geographical area covered by sampling strategy	Data collection time in 2021		Data collection method		Total number of children		Gender		
			Start	End	PPS (in person) %	WS (PC/tablet /mobile phone) %	N	%	Boys, %	Girls, %	Binary, %
Albania	No	The capital of Albania, Tirana in urban and rural areas	22.06	30.07	73.2	26.8	1034	5.1	54.5	45.5	0
Algeria	Yes	Province of Oran	2.11	16.12	100		816	4.0	52.3	47.7	0
Bangladesh	No	Mainly regions of Barishal, Moulvibazar, Rajshahi and Dhaka (capital)	10.08	31.08	78.0	22.0	1370	6.8	50.4	49.6	0
Belgium	Yes	Whole Flemish community in Belgium (Flemish region and the Dutch speaking population in Brussels)	25.05	29.06		100	2422	12.0	50.6	49.4	0
Chile	No	Metropolitan region of the cities of Santiago and Concepción (also Curicó, Quilpué and, Laja cities)	30.08	8.10	4.4	95.6	1682	8.3	47.8	49.2	3.1
Colombia	No	Whole country	1.08	31.08		100	976	4.8	49.3	50.7	0
Estonia	No	Whole country	21.04	7.06		100	1258	6.2	50.0	47.8	2.2
Germany	No	Whole country with a focus on Frankfurt/Hessen	25.10	29.11		100	590	2.9	51.2	48.1	0.7
Indonesia	No	West Java Province	17.07	14.09		100	2222	11.0	53.9	46.1	0

	Represen-tative sample—yes or no	Geographical area covered by sampling strategy	Data collection time in 2021		Data collection method		Total number of children		Gender		
			Start	End	PPS (in person) %	WS (PC/tablet /mobile phone) %	N	%	Boys, %	Girls, %	Binary, %
Israel	No	Whole country	Wave1: 30.05 Wave2: 30.09	Wave1: 27.06 Wave2: 20.10	100		930	4.6	47.0	50.7	2.3
Italy	No	Whole country but mainly the cities of Genoa and Rome and southern regions of Campania, Calabria, and Puglia.	End of May	30.09		100	919	4.5	49.6	50.4	0
Romania	Yes (mix between convenience and representative sample)	Whole country	20.05	15.06	100		1856	9.2	51.2	48.8	0
S Korea	Yes	Whole country	22.07	20.08		100	1497	7.4	48.9	51.1	0
Taiwan	No	Whole country	26.07	10.09		100	1155	5.7	54.4	45.5	0.2
Turkey	Yes (mix between purposive and representative sample)	Istanbul neighborhoods (for PPS)	8.06	30.08	50.5	49.5	804	4.0	49.8	49.2	1.0
Wales	No	Rural North, Rural Heartland, Metropolitan Wales, and Valleys	5.07	15.07		100	691	3.4	45.7	50.8	3.5
Total							20,222	100	50.4	48.8	0.8

References

Ahorsu, D.K., C.-Y. Lin, V. Imani, M. Saffari, M.D. Griffiths, and A.H. Pakpour. 2022. The fear of COVID-19 scale: Development and initial validation. *International Journal of Mental Health and Addiction* 20 (3): 1537–1545. https://doi.org/10.1007/s11469-020-00270-8.

Armitage, R., and L.B. Nellums. 2020. Considering inequalities in the school closure response to Covid-19. *Lancet Global Health* 8 (5): e644. https://doi.org/10.1016/S2214-109X(20)30116-9.

Barn, R., T. Fattore, and S. Fegter. 2023. Introduction to the special issue on the Covid-19 pandemic and children's understandings of well-being: International perspectives on social contexts and inequality. *International Journal on Child Maltreatment* 6: 353–365. https://doi.org/10.1007/s42448-023-00169-6.

Choi, J., Y. Park, H.-E. Kim, J. Song, D. Lee, E. Lee, H. Kang, J. Lee, J. Park, J.-W. Lee, S. Ye, S. Lee, S. Ryu, Y. Kim, Y.-R. Kim, Y.-J. Kim, and Y. Lee. 2021. Daily life changes and life satisfaction among Korean school-aged children in the COVID-19 pandemic. *International Journal of Environmental Research and Public Health* 18 (6): 1–17. https://doi.org/10.3390/ijerph18063324.

Cosma, A., S. Abdrakhmanova, D. Taut, K. Schrijvers, C. Catunda, and C. Schnohr. 2023. *A focus on adolescent mental health and wellbeing in Europe, Central Asia and Canada. Health behaviour in school-aged children international report from the 2021/2022 survey*. Vol. 1. Copenhagen: WHO Regional Office for Europe.

Diener, E. 1984. Subjective well-being. *Psychological Bulletin* 95 (3): 542–575. https://doi.org/10.1037/0033-2909.95.3.542.

Dollahite, D.C., H.H. Kelley, S. James, and L.D. Marks. 2022. Changes in home-centered religious practices and relational wellbeing following the initial onset of the Covid-19 pandemic. *Marriage & Family Review* 59 (2): 65–94. https://doi.org/10.1080/01494929.2022.2141942.

Engel de Abreu, P.M., S. Neumann, C. Wealer, N. Abreu, E. Coutinho Macedo, and C. Kirsch. 2021. Subjective well-being of adolescents in Luxembourg, Germany, and Brazil during the COVID-19 pandemic. *Journal of Adolescent Health* 69 (2): 211–218. https://doi.org/10.1016/j.jadohealth.2021.04.028.

Folostina, R., and C. Iacob. 2021. Impact of COVID-19 lockdown on children with developmental disabilities and their parents. *Cypriot Journal of Educational Science* 16 (4): 1878–1892. https://doi.org/10.18844/cjes.v16i4.6018.

García, C. 2020. Los psicologos insisten: "Si el estado de alarma es relajado, los ninos deberian ser los primeros en irse" [Psychologists insist: "If the state of alarm is relaxed, children should be the first to leave"]. El Pais. https://elpais.com/elpais/2020/04/14/mamas_papas/1586856472_075125.html. Accessed 13 Apr 2022.

Gierczyk, M., E. Charzyńska, and D. Dobosz. 2022. Subjective well-being of primary and secondary school students during the COVID-19 pandemic: A latent profile analysis. *Child Indicators Research* 15: 2115–2140. https://doi.org/10.1007/s12187-022-09952-2.

Gröndal, M., K. Ask, T.J. Luke, and S. Winblad. 2021. Self-reported impact of the COVID-19 pandemic, affective responding, and subjective well-being: A Swedish survey. *PlosOne* 16 (10): 1–15. https://doi.org/10.1371/journal.pone.0258778.

ISCWeB. 2023. International Survey of Children's Well-Being (ISCWeB). https://isciweb.org/the-data/wave-4-covid-19-reports/.

Kesebir, P., and E. Diener. 2008. In pursuit of happiness: Empirical answers to philosophical questions. *Perspectives on Psychological Science* 3 (2): 117–125. https://doi.org/10.1111/j.1745-6916.2008.00069.x.

Kirsch, C., P. Engel de Abreu, S. Neumann, C. Wealer, K. Brazas, and I. Hauffels. 2020. *Subjective well-being and stay-at-home-experiences of children aged 6–16 during the first wave of the COVID-19 pandemic in Luxembourg: A report of the project COVID-kids*. Luxembourg: University of Luxembourg.

Kutsar, D., and L. Kurvet-Käosaar. 2021. The impact of the COVID-19 pandemic on families: Young people's experiences in Estonia. *Frontiers in Sociology* 6: 1–12. https://doi.org/10.3389/fsoc.2021.732984.

Kutsar, D., M. Beilmann, K. Luhamaa, O. Nahkur, K. Soo, J. Strömpl, and M. Rebane. 2022. Laste heaolu tulevik. *Arenguseire keskus*. https://arenguseire.ee/pikksilm/laste–heaolu–tulevik/. Accessed 26 Feb 2022.

Levinson, W., G. Gordon, and K. Skeff. 1990. Retrospective versus actual pre-course self-assessments. *Evaluation & the Health Professions* 13 (4): 445–452. https://doi.org/10.1177/016327879001300406.

Loades, M.E., E. Chatburn, N. Higson-Sweeney, S. Reynolds, R. Shafran, A. Brigden, C. Linney, M. Niamh McManus, C. Borwick, and E. Crawley. 2020. Rapid systematic review: The impact of social isolation and loneliness on the mental health of children and adolescents in the context of COVID-19. *Journal of the American Academy of Child & Adolescent Psychiatry* 59 (11): 1218–1239. https://doi.org/10.1016/j.jaac.2020.05.009.

Magson, N.R., J.Y.A. Freeman, R.M. Rapee, C.E. Richardson, E.L. Oar, and J. Fardouly. 2021. Risk and protective factors for prospective changes in adolescent mental health during the COVID-19 pandemic. *Journal of Youth and Adolescence* 50: 44–57. https://doi.org/10.1007/s10964-020-01332-9.

Mariani, R., A. Renzi, M. Di Trani, G. Trabucchi, K. Danskin, and R. Tambelli. 2020. The impact of coping strategies and perceived family support on depressive and anxious symptomatology during the coronavirus pandemic (COVID-19) lockdown. *Frontiers in Psychiatry* 11: 1–9. https://doi.org/10.3389/fpsyt.2020.587724.

Mitra, R., E.O.D. Waygood, and J. Fullan. 2021. Subjective well-being of Canadian children and youth during the COVID-19 pandemic: The role of the social and physical environment and healthy movement behaviours. *Preventive Medicine Reports* 23 (4): 1–7. https://doi.org/10.1016/j.pmedr.2021.101404.

Mondragon, N.I., N. Berasategi Sancho, M. Dosil Santamaria, and A. Eiguren Munitis. 2021. Struggling to breathe: A qualitative study of children's well-being during lockdown in Spain. *Psychology & Health* 36 (2): 179–194. https://doi.org/10.1080/08870446.2020.1804570.

Müderrisoğlu, S., B. Akkan, and P.U. Semerci. 2023. Experiences of children during the pandemic: Scrutinizing increased vulnerabilities in education in the case of Turkey. *International Journal on Child Maltreatment* 6: 431–451. https://doi.org/10.1007/s42448-023-00152-1.

Nahkur, O., and D. Kutsar. 2022. The change in children's subjective relational social cohesion with family and friends during the COVID-19 pandemic: A multinational analysis. *Frontiers in Sociology* 7: 1–21. https://doi.org/10.3389/fsoc.2022.974543.

Neubauer, A.B., A. Schmidt, A.C. Kramer, and F. Schmiedek. 2021. A little autonomy support goes a long way: Daily autonomy-supportive parenting, child well-being, parental need fulfillment, and change in child, family, and parent adjustment across the adaptation to the COVID-19 pandemic. *Child Development* 92 (5): 1679–1697. https://doi.org/10.1111/cdev.13515.

Ryan, R.M., and E.L. Deci. 2000. Self-determination theory and the facilitation of intrinsic motivation, social development, and well-being. *American Psychologist* 55: 68–78. https://doi.org/10.1037/0003-066X.55.1.68.

Savahl, S., B.J. Lee, and F. Casas, eds. 2022. *Children's views on their lives and well-being during Covid-19: A report on the children's worlds project, 2020–2022*. Jerusalem, Israel: Children's Worlds Project (ISCWeB).

Soffia, M., and A. Turner. 2021. *Measuring children and young people's subjective wellbeing*. United Kingdom: What Works Centre for Wellbeing.

Steinmayr, R., P. Paschke, and L. Wirthwein. 2022. Elementary school students' subjective well-being before and during the COVID-19 pandemic: A longitudinal study. *Journal of Happiness Studies* 23: 2985–3005. https://doi.org/10.1007/s10902-022-00537-y.

Stoecklin, D., C. Gervais, D. Kutsar, and C. Heite. 2021. Lockdown and children's well-being: Experiences of children in Switzerland, Canada and Estonia. *Childhood Vulnerability Journal* 3: 41–59. https://doi.org/10.1007/s41255-021-00015-2.

von Soest, T., A. Bakken, W. Pedersen, and M.A. Sletten. 2020. Life satisfaction among adolescents before and during the COVID-19 pandemic [Livstilfredshet blant ungdom før og under covid-19-pandemien]. *Tidsskrift for den Norske Lægeforening* 140 (10). https://doi.org/10.4045/tidsskr.20.0437. Accessed 26 Feb 2022.

Wu, Y.-J., and J. Lee. 2022. The most salient global predictors of adolescents' subjective well-being: Parental support, peer support, and anxiety. *Child Indicators Research* 15 (2): 1–29. https://doi.org/10.1007/s12187-022-09937-1.

Zhu, S., Y. Zhuang, and P. Ip. 2021. Impacts on children and adolescents' lifestyle, social support and their association with negative impacts of the COVID-19 pandemic. *International Journal of Environmental Research and Public Health* 18 (9): 1–17. https://doi.org/10.3390/ijerph18094780.

Oliver Nahkur (PhD in Sociology) is a Research Fellow of Research of Social Well-Being in the Institute of Social Studies, University of Tartu, Estonia. Research interests include social indicators research (including from cross-national comparative studies perspective), well-being studies (including mental health), child well-being and vulnerability, violence and conflicts in society, inclusive disaster management (including volunteering), and healthcare. Published papers in *Social Indicators Research, Child Indicators Research, Comparative Sociology, Frontiers in Sociology, Social Sciences, Journal of Baltic Studies, International Journal of Disaster Risk Reduction, Vaccine*. Oliver is Secretary-Treasurer in ISA RC55 (social indicators) and Board Member of ISA WG11 (violence and society).

Karoliine Zarina is a freelance researcher in Estonia. At the moment, she studies Political Sciences at the MA level at Tallinn University. Karoliine's bachelor thesis (supervisor: Oliver Nahkur) defended in 2022 at the University of Tartu and entitled "Changes in children's overall satisfaction with life compared to the COVID-19 pandemic and the time before, corona anxiety and their interconnection," was focusing on Estonia.

Chapter 13
The Impact of COVID-19 on Young People's Levels of Subjective Well-being: Evidence from HILDA 2001–2020

Jenny Chesters

13.1 Introduction

In January 2020, the novel coronavirus labelled COVID-19 spread to Australia and by March, the national borders were closed. Governments across Australia enacted various measures to slow the spread of the virus closing internal borders between states and territories, closing workplaces and schools, and shutting down social and sporting activities. Schools and workplaces were closed for at least 6 weeks across Australia and for extended periods of time in some states. Consequently, young people spent a lot more time with their families, were isolated from their friends and missed out on school-based opportunities to develop social skills integral to their development (Wang et al. 2021). Although Australians of all ages experienced dramatic changes in their social, cultural and physical environments, young people may have been adversely impacted given that they have little control over their living arrangements and conditions. In particular, young people aged 15–17 years living with their parents and attending secondary school had little control over their ability to respond to the health, social and economic threats of the pandemic and the measures governments enacted to slow the spread of the COVID-19 virus.

For this study, a comparison of five cohorts of young people is conducted to examine whether the pandemic influenced levels of subjective well-being of young people. The restrictions associated with the COVID-19 pandemic is regarded as a period effect (see Callens 2017; Parker et al. 2016; Wong et al. 2017; Yang 2008 for discussion of age-cohort-period effects). To eliminate differences related to age, levels of subjective well-being of young people of the same age (15–17 years) at five different time points are examined. Period effects refer to differences associated with a specific period of time. For example, young people entering the labor market during an economic expansion (say, in 2006–2007) would have a very different

J. Chesters (✉)
University of Melbourne, Melbourne, Australia
e-mail: jenny.chesters@unimelb.edu.au

C. Suter et al. (eds.), *Well-being During the Pandemic*, Social Indicators Research Series 90, https://doi.org/10.1007/978-3-031-63440-6_13

experience compared to young people trying to enter the labor market during a period of economic contraction (say, in 2008–2009 during the Global Financial Crisis).

As other researchers (Bayliss et al. 2017; Carlquist et al. 2017; Easterlin 2001) have noted, the terms well-being, subjective well-being, life satisfaction and happiness essentially hold the same meaning therefore, these terms are used interchangeably throughout this paper. Measures of life satisfaction provide an indication of how much an individual "positively evaluates the overall quality of his/ her life" (Veenhoven 1996, 6) and in particular, with the ability to achieve one's life goals (Headey et al. 2013). As Hori and Kamo (2018) point out, subjective evaluations of life experiences are dependent upon the context within which the individual is embedded. Levels of subjective well-being are typically measured using a global life satisfaction indicator derived from survey questions asking respondents how satisfied they are with their life overall (Chesters et al. 2021; Clark et al. 2010; Manning et al. 2016).

The research question driving this study is: "How did the COVID-19 pandemic impact on levels of subjective well-being of secondary school students?" The remainder of this paper is structured as follows: after providing a brief overview of the context, theoretical perspectives and extant literature, the data are introduced and the analytical strategy is outlined. The results of the analysis are then presented followed by the discussion of the implications and directions for further research.

13.1.1 Context

In the first 12 months of the pandemic, Australia recorded just 910 deaths related to COVID-19 (Department of Health 2021). This comparatively low death toll was largely due to the national and regional lockdowns implemented to stop the spread of the virus. The Federal Government closed the national border in March 2020 and state and territory borders also closed. Given that health is a state/ territory responsibility, the Federal Government could not enact national laws. Consequently, a National Cabinet was formed so that the Federal Government and State and Territory Governments could coordinate their response to COVID-19 pandemic. An initial 6-week national lockdown was implemented from March 2020 through to May 2020. Schools and workplaces, except those deemed to be essential, were closed and Australians were urged to stay home as much as possible. Restrictions on movements within Australia, between states and territories and even within states were implemented. In July 2020, the state of Victoria entered another lockdown when breaches in the isolation of returning travellers generated another outbreak (Chesters 2021). Throughout 2020 and 2021, various states and territories entered, emerged and re-entered lockdowns until over 90% of the population had been vaccinated against the virus. Consequently, people were isolated from their extended families and friends for long periods of time.

Although lockdowns and restrictions implemented to contain the pandemic impacted all Australians, young people were particularly affected. Adolescence is the period when young people develop their own social networks, thus, peer relationships become increasingly more important (Plenty and Mood 2016; Yucel and Vogt Yuan 2016). Wong et al. (2017) posit that experiences during adolescence shape values and behaviors throughout the life course giving rise to generational differences. For young people making this adjustment during 2020, the COVID-19 pandemic further complicated an already complex process. Schools were closed and sporting and other social activities were curtailed leaving young people with few options to engage in the peer-to-peer activities required to develop their own social standing independent of their parents.

13.1.2 Theoretical Perspectives

Levels of subjective well-being are a combination of one's physical and social well-being (Ormel et al. 1999) which are influenced by personal, community and societal factors (Diener et al. 2013). The desire to achieve high levels of subjective well-being is universal and therefore, underpins human behavior (Hadjar and Samuel 2015; Steverink et al. 2020). Overall levels of subjective well-being are dependent upon comparisons between the individual and their peer groups and/or their own aspirations. For example, young people may experience lower levels of subjective well-being if members of their peer group appear to be more successful in achieving their goals than they are or if they cannot achieve their own goals (Hori and Kamo 2018; Scharf et al. 2019).

Social Production Function (SPF) theory posits that levels of subjective well-being are dependent upon the attainment of five goals: stimulation, comfort, status, behavioral confirmation, and affection (Ormel et al. 1999). Stimulation, defined as the motivation to engage in physical activity, and comfort, the attainment of physical needs, are elements of physical well-being. Social well-being is attained through status, that is, one's rank relative to others; behavioral confirmation, feeling that one has done well in the eyes of relevant others; and affection derived from caring relationships that provide love, friendship and emotional support (Ormel et al. 1999, 67). The ability to satisfy these needs is constrained by access to resources. Therefore, individuals may need to choose between competing needs. For example, young people seeking to leave home and live with friends may need to choose between their need for physical comfort and their need for affection if living with their parents provides food and shelter but not love and emotional support.

Hadjar and Samuel's (2015) research provided some support for Social Production Function theory with subjective well-being being positively associated with indicators of the achievement of the affection (being in a stable relationship) and comfort (having good health) goals. However, the results of their analysis show that their indicator of status (achieving social mobility) was not associated with levels of subjective well-being. Research conducted by Scharf et al. (2019)

confirmed that comfort was an important factor in achieving physical well-being and that status was important for achieving social well-being. Research conducted by Steverink et al. (2020) found evidence of a gender differential in the importance of each of the five needs. For example, men placed more emphasis on the need for status and women placed more emphasis on the need for affection.

One's ability to satisfy the five needs outlined by Social Production Function theory is constrained by one's access to resources and this is of particular relevance to this study. During the COVID-19 pandemic, young people were not able to spend time with their friends and members of their extended families and this may have impacted on their ability to satisfy their need for affection. The lockdowns implemented in various states for various periods of time impacted on their need for stimulation, the motivation to engage in activities. Their need for comfort may have been impacted if their family income declined and/ or they or members of their family became ill with the virus. Their need for behavioral confirmation was impacted by the rapid changes in societal expectations and the abrupt changes to daily routines due to the restrictions imposed during 2020.

13.1.3 Factors Associated with Levels of Subjective Well-being

Researchers examining variations in levels of subjective well-being have generally focussed on the influence of various economic, social and personal factors (Layard et al. 2014). According to Layard et al. (2014), economic factors include education, employment and income. Social factors include family status and personal factors include sex, age and health. Layard et al.'s analysis of British Cohort Study data indicates that family background, childhood experiences and development impact subjective well-being. Given that the focus of this paper is on levels of subjective well-being of secondary school students, the focus is on sex, age, health and family status.

The results of examinations of the association between sex and well-being are inconsistent: some researchers have found that males are happier than females (Ambrey and Fleming 2014; Goldbeck et al. 2007) whereas others have found that females are happier than males (Blanchflower and Oswald 2005; Chesters et al. 2021; Frijters et al. 2014; Hori and Kamo 2018). Researchers examining the association between subjective well-being and health have consistently found that being in poor health is associated with having lower levels of subjective well-being (Ambrey and Fleming 2014; Chesters et al. 2021; Fleche et al. 2021; Manning et al. 2016). Family status is also consistently associated with the levels of subjective well-being of young people. Researchers generally find that living with two parents is associated with higher levels of subjective well-being (Fleche et al. 2021; Yucel and Vogt Yuan 2016). There is general agreement that levels of well-being decline during adolescence (Goldbeck et al. 2007; Gonzalez-Carrasco et al. 2017). For example, Goldbeck et al. (2007) found that those aged 16 years reported lower levels of well-being than their younger peers.

13.2 Methods

13.2.1 Data

To answer the research question, "How did the COVID-19 pandemic impact on levels of subjective well-being of secondary school students?", analyses of data collected by the Housing and Income Dynamics in Australia (HILDA) project are conducted. The HILDA project surveyed a representative sample of Australian households in 2001 (Summerfield et al. 2018). Every household member aged 15 years or older was invited to participate. Households are surveyed every year, thus, a new cohort of 15 year olds enter the project every year. For this study, five cohorts of young people aged 15–17 years living at home with their parent/ parents and attending secondary school in 2001, 2005, 2010, 2015 and 2020 were selected.

13.2.2 Variables

In the first phase of the analysis, levels of subjective well-being of the five cohorts of young people are examined. The dependent variable, levels of subjective well-being, was derived from a question asking: overall, how satisfied are you with your life and measured on a scale from 0 (extremely dissatisfied) to 10 (extremely satisfied). Several researchers have also used this question (Ambrey and Fleming 2014; Bellis et al. 2012; Chesters 2021; Clark et al. 2010; Clark and Oswald 1996; Headey et al. 2013; Headey and Muffels 2018; Manning et al. 2016).

The independent variables are derived from Social Production Function theory and include indicators of comfort needs and affection needs. Indicators of comfort needs include family income and health and the indicator of affection is family type. Family income is derived from the household disposable income variable by dividing the distribution into five equal groups. Households located in Quintile 1 have the lowest level of income; and households in Quintile 5 have the highest level of income. For the self-assessed health variable, the response options ranged from poor to excellent. These options were recoded into a dummy variable with 1 signifying good/excellent health; 0 signifying poor health. Family type is coded 0 for two-parent families and 1 for lone parent families. Young people living with one parent tend to have lower levels of life satisfaction than those living with two parents (Yucel and Vogt Yuan 2016). Age, sex, state/territory and migrant status are included as control variables as previous research (Callens 2017; Carlquist et al. 2017; Gonzalez-Carrasco et al. 2017; Hori and Kamo 2018; Wong et al. 2017) shows that these demographic factors influence levels of subjective well-being. The age variable has three categories: 15, 16, and 17. The state/territory variable has six categories: New South Wales/Australian Capital Territory (NSW/ ACT); Victoria (VIC); Queensland (QLD); Tasmania (TAS); South Australia (SA); Western Australia/ Northern Territory (WA/NT). Migrant status is coded 1 if the participant and/ or at least one of their parents were born overseas. Given that all of our participants were attending secondary school, level of education is not included in the models. Sex is coded 1 for female and 0 for male. Although researchers generally find that the effect of sex is either non-significant or very small (Gerling and Diener 2020), Frijters et al. (2014) argue that it is important to include sex in studies examining levels of subjective well-being during adolescence on the basis that girls and boys may experience adolescence differently.

The descriptive statistics for the Phase 1 variables for each of the 5 cohorts are presented in Table 13.6 in the Appendix. Roughly, half of the participants in each cohort were female and one-third were migrants. However, there are some notable differences between the cohorts. For example, the percentage of participants aged 17 varies from 23 to 31%; and the percentage of participants living in one parent families varies from 20 to 26%. The means and standard deviations for the outcome variable, subjective well-being, are presented in Table 13.1 and show that, on average, levels of subjective well-being varied little between the five cohorts.

In the second phase of the analysis, the focus is on differences in levels of subjective well-being within the 2020 cohort. As Bayliss et al. (2017) note, differences between groups are masked in aggregate analysis. Although the 2020 survey included a range of relevant variables, one variable measuring their concern for being infected with the COVID-19 virus and one variable measuring the impact of the pandemic on their ability to stay in contact with friends and family living outside their family home were selected. Participants were asked to nominate the percent chance that they may become infected with COVID-19. Responses ranged from 0 to 90%. Given that 14% nominated no chance and almost 60% nominated between a 1 and 25% chance, the distribution was divided into three categories: 0 = no chance; 1 = low chance (1–25%); 2 = high chance (>25%). The "staying in contact" variable options ranged from much less, a little less, about the same, a little more, much more. These options were recoded into a dummy variable: 0 = less contact/ no change; 1 = more contact.

Preliminary analysis indicated that students in Victoria experienced the longest lockdowns and consequently, a greater period of time away from school (see Table 13.7 in the Appendix). During the lockdowns, schools were closed and students were prevented from engaging in other social activities such as sport, dancing and generally spending time with their friends. To examine whether the extended lockdowns impacted more heavily on secondary school students in Victoria than in

Table 13.1 Summary statistics of the subjective well-being variable: 2001–2020

	N	Mean	Std. dev.
2001	617	8.33	1.38
2005	584	8.35	1.27
2010	647	8.45	1.20
2015	718	8.43	1.33
2020	623	8.42	1.33
Total	3189	8.40	1.30

Source: Housing and Income Dynamics in Australia (HILDA) Survey

Table 13.2 Summary statistics for the 2020 cohort

	Other	Victoria	p-value
Subjective well-being	8.39	8.48	0.4585
% chance of getting COVID-19	16.8	21.2	0.0072

Source: Housing and Income Dynamics in Australia (HILDA) Survey

other jurisdictions, the state/territory variable was recoded into a dummy variable: 1 = Victoria; and 0 = all other states/territories (New South Wales, Queensland, Tasmania, South Australia, Western Australia, Australian Capital Territory, Northern Territory).

The descriptive statistics for these variables for the 2020 cohort are presented in Table 13.8 in the Appendix. Almost three-quarters of the participants were living outside of Victoria, 86% thought that they had some chance of being infected with COVID-19, and 27% indicated that they had been able to spend more time with their friends and family members who were not living in the family home. The summary statistics presented in Table 13.2 indicate that there was no difference between students in Victoria and those in other state/territories in terms of subjective well-being, however, participants from Victoria were significantly more likely than their peers to be concerned about being infected with the COVID-19 virus.

13.2.3 *Analytical Strategy*

For the first step in phase 1 of the analyses, a series of multiple regression models were developed to examine the association between levels of subjective well-being and family type, sex, migrant status, age, health, location and family income quintile individually for each cohort. Family type is selected as the key explanatory variable due to the consistency of the findings generated by other researchers (Fleche et al. 2021; Yucel and Vogt Yuan 2016). In the second step, the five datasets were merged (n = 3189) to examine whether participants aged 15–17 years during the coronavirus crisis of 2020 were less satisfied with their lives than young people in the 2001, 2005, 2010, and 2015 cohorts. In the final step, an examination of the impact of changes in lifestyles and access to schools, friends and extended families associated with the coronavirus. All of the analyses were conducted using Stata14 (StataCorp 2015).

13.3 Results

The results for the regression analysis for each cohort are presented in Table 13.3. Being in good health is consistently associated with higher levels of subjective well-being. Apart from participants in the 2001 cohort, living in Western Australia is negatively associated with levels of well-being. Living in a one-parent family appears to be negatively associated with levels of well-being for each cohort, however only the results for 2001, 2015 and 2020 are statistically significant.

Table 13.3 Regression results for subjective well-being for each cohort

	2001	2005	2010	2015	2020
	Coeff. (Std. err.)	Coeff. (Std. err.)	Coeff. (Std. err.)	Coeff. (Std. err.)	Coeff. (Std. err.)
One parent =1	−0.38** (0.15)	−0.25 (0.13)	−0.12 (0.13)	−0.36** (0.13)	−0.39** (0.15)
Household income (ref. = Quintile 1)					
Quintile 2	−0.07 (0.18)	−0.12 (0.17)	−0.06 (0.15)	−0.14 (0.16)	0.17 (0.17)
Quintile 3	−0.04 (0.18)	0.36* (0.17)	−0.26 (0.15)	−0.11 (0.16)	−0.04 (0.18)
Quintile 4	0.17 (0.18)	0.30 (0.18)	−0.04 (0.16)	0.11 (0.17)	0.06 (0.19)
Quintile 5	0.23 (0.19)	0.19 (0.18)	0.13 (0.16)	0.01 (0.17)	0.10 (0.19)
Good health =1	0.77** (0.26)	1.03*** (0.23)	1.06*** (0.26)	1.07*** (0.26)	1.22*** (0.24)
Female =1	−0.22* (0.11)	−0.03 (0.10)	−0.13 (0.09)	−0.16 (0.10)	−0.21* (0.10)
Age (ref. = 15)					
16	−0.15 (0.13)	−0.002 (0.12)	−0.21 (0.11)	−0.20 (0.11)	−0.30* (0.13)
17	−0.31* (0.14)	−0.25 (0.14)	−0.37** (0.12)	−0.31* (0.12)	−0.21 (0.13)
State (ref. = VIC)					
NSW/ACT	0.03 (0.14)	−0.06 (0.14)	0.18 (0.12)	−0.18 (0.13)	0.02 (0.14)
QLD	−0.01 (0.17)	−0.23 (0.15)	−0.11 (0.14)	0.003 (0.15)	−0.06 (0.15)
SA	0.63** (0.20)	−0.30 (0.21)	−0.34* (0.17)	−0.16 (0.19)	−0.30 (0.20)
WA/NT	0.05 (0.24)	−0.40* (0.20)	−0.55** (0.19)	−0.47** (0.19)	−0.51** (0.20)
TAS	0.50 (0.30)	−0.44 (0.30)	0.05 (0.25)	−0.07 (0.26)	0.22 (0.28)
Constant	7.77*** (0.31)	7.54*** (0.29)	7.75*** (0.29)	7.90*** (0.31)	7.63*** (0.31)
N=	617	584	649	718	623
Adj. R-squared	0.0431	0.0700	0.0696	0.0521	0.0780

Notes: NSW=New South Wales; ACT = Australian Capital Territory; QLD = Queensland; SA = South Australia; WA = Western Australia; NT = Northern Territory; TAS = Tasmania
***p < 001; **p < 0.01; *p < 0.05
Source: Housing and Income Dynamics in Australia (HILDA) Survey

To answer the research question, the five individual datasets were merged to examine whether the cohort of participants from 2020 reported lower or higher levels of subjective well-being. The results of the regression models are reported in Table 13.4. The first model includes sex, family type, health status, age, and

Table 13.4 Regression results for levels of subjective well-being across the five cohorts

	Model 1	Model 2	Model 3
	Coeff. (Std. err.)	Coeff. (Std. err.)	Coeff. (Std. err.)
One parent =1	−0.34*** (0.05)	−0.29*** (0.06)	−0.29*** (0.06)
Household income (ref. = Quintile 1)			
Quintile 2		−0.06 (0.07)	−0.06 (0.07)
Quintile 3		−0.03 (0.08)	−0.03 (0.08)
Quintile 4		0.12 (0.08)	0.11 (0.08)
Quintile 5		0.13 (0.08)	0.13 (0.09)
Good health =1	1.04** (0.11)	1.03*** (0.11)	1.03*** (0.11)
Female =1	−0.14** (0.04)	−0.14** (0.04)	−0.14** (0.05)
Age (ref. = 15)			
16	−0.16** (0.05)	−0.17** (0.05)	−0.17** (0.05)
17	−0.27*** (0.06)	−0.29** (0.06)	−0.29*** (0.06)
State (ref. = VIC)			
NSW/ ACT	−0.001 (0.06)	−0.001 (0.06)	−0.01 (0.06)
QLD	−0.07 (0.07)	−0.07 (0.07)	−0.07 (0.07)
SA	0.09 (0.09)	−0.08 (0.09)	−0.08 (0.09)
WA/NT	−0.38*** (0.09)	−0.39*** (0.09)	−0.40*** (0.09)
TAS	0.08 (0.12)	0.10 (0.12)	0.10 (0.12)
Cohort (ref. = 2020)			
2001			−0.12 (0.07)
2005			−0.08 (0.07)
2010			−0.01 (0.07)
2015			−0.01 (0.07)
Constant	7.74*** (0.12)	7.70*** (0.13)	7.75*** (0.14)
N=	3189	3189	3189

(continued)

Table 13.4 (continued)

	Model 1	Model 2	Model 3
	Coeff. (Std. err.)	Coeff. (Std. err.)	Coeff. (Std. err.)
Adj. R-squared	0.0545	0.0565	0.0567

Note: NSW=New South Wales; ACT = Australian Capital Territory; QLD = Queensland; SA = South Australia; WA = Western Australia; NT = Northern Territory; TAS = Tasmania
***p < 001; **p < 0.01; *p < 0.05
Source: Housing and Income Dynamics in Australia (HILDA) Survey

location. As suggested by the results presented in Table 13.3, being in good health is positively associated with levels of subjective well-being. Being female and living in a one-parent family is negatively associated with subjective well-being as is living in Western Australia or the Northern Territory. These results hold when family income is added into Model 2. Family income is not independently associated with levels of subjective well-being. In the final model, these results remain when cohort is included (Model 3). The 2020 cohort is the reference category. The coefficients for the 2001, 2005, 2010, and 2015 cohorts are not statistically significant indicating that the 2020 cohort participants reported similar levels of well-being as their counterparts in earlier cohorts. This may be related to the timing of the data collection in 2020. The first round of lockdowns was national and lasted for just 6 weeks. During the first lockdown, there was a collective sense of "we are all in this together". However, the lockdowns implemented during late 2020 and throughout 2021 were state- and/or region-specific and thus, may have impacted on levels of subjective well-being for those who experienced the harshest and longest lockdowns.

In the next phase of the analysis, an examination of differences between groups within the 2020 cohort is conducted. To examine if the extended lockdowns in Victoria had an effect, a variable distinguishing between participants living in Victoria and those living elsewhere in Australia is included in the models. As indicated in Table 13.7, students in Victoria spent longer periods of time studying at home with almost three-quarters being locked out of school for more than 6 weeks. Participants from Victoria were also more likely than their peers to believe that they would become infected with the COVID-19 virus. The results of Model 1, presented in Table 13.5, indicate that students who were concerned about catching COVID-19 were less satisfied with their lives than their peers who were not concerned about catching it. The results for Model 2 presented in Table 13.5 indicate that students who spent more time with their friends and members of their extended families reported higher levels of subjective well-being than those who spent less time or the same amount of time with their friends and members of their extended families. When Models 1 and 2 are combined into Model 3, being able to spend more time with friends and family members not living in the family home was associated with higher levels of subjective well-being. Furthermore, the results indicate living in a one-parent family was associated with lower levels of subjective well-being.

Table 13.5 Regression results for subjective well-being in 2020 according to fear of contracting COVID-19 and ability to spend time with friends and members of extended family

	Model 1		Model 2		Model 3	
	Coeff.	Std. err.	Coeff.	Std. err.	Coeff.	Std. err.
One parent =1	−0.43***	0.12	−0.44***	0.12	−0.46***	0.12
Good health =1	1.23***	0.24	1.24***	0.24	1.19***	0.23
Female =1	−0.25*	0.10	−0.23*	0.10	−0.27*	0.10
Age (ref. = 15)						
16	−0.32*	0.12	−0.32**	0.12	−0.32**	0.12
17	−0.24	0.13	−0.23	0.13	−0.23	0.13
Victoria =1	0.13	0.12	0.09	0.12	0.12	0.12
Chance to get COVID (ref. = no chance)						
Low [<50%]	−0.49**	0.15			−0.49**	0.15
High [>50%]	−0.42*	0.17			−0.43*	0.17
More time with friends = 1			0.31**	0.12	0.31**	0.12
Constant	8.03***	0.29	7.52***	0.25	7.98***	0.29
N=	623		623		623	
Adj. R-squared	0.0825		0.0807		0.0916	

Note: ***p < 001; **p < 0.01; *p < 0.05
Source: Housing and Income Dynamics in Australia (HILDA) Survey

13.4 Discussion

Given the dramatic social changes that occurred during 2020 due to the outbreak of the COVID-19 pandemic, levels of subjective well-being of young people aged 15–17 years were expected to be lower for the 2020 cohort than those of the other four cohorts. Interestingly, despite having to abruptly adapt to changing social and economic conditions, the 2020 cohort of young people were no less satisfied than their counterparts in 2001, 2005, 2010 and 2015. Thus, it would appear that there is no evidence that, in the early stages of the pandemic, this cohort of young Australians were no less happy with their lives than their counterparts in previous cohorts. This may be due to their physical and social needs being met. During the early phase of the pandemic, being locked out of school was probably not too much of an issue given that they could use social media to keep in touch with their friends. Case numbers were very low so the expected impact on their health did not materialize. Family incomes may not have been affected in the early stages of the pandemic as employees were encouraged to work from home unless they were essential workers. To buffer families from the damage that the rapid shutdown of the economy may have generated, the Federal Government introduced JobKeeper payments (the Treasury 2023) for employees who were made redundant. Bayliss et al. (2017) also found that levels of well-being were largely unaffected by the 2007/2008 recession in Britain. They argue that it may take some time for changes in lived conditions to impact levels of life satisfaction. The national lockdown lasted for 6 weeks from mid-March to May 2020 during which there was a collective sense of "we are all in this together". That said, ensuing rounds of lockdowns in various states and regions may have impacted on levels of subjective well-being for those who experienced the harshest and longest lockdowns.

Despite the absence of an impact on the 2020 cohort overall, there were some notable variations within the cohort. As predicted by Social Production Function theory, young people who were suffering from poor health reported having lower levels of subjective well-being than their healthy peers. Research examining the impact of health on levels of happiness invariably finds that those experiencing poor health are less happy than their healthy peers (Chesters et al. 2021; Headey et al. 2013; Headey and Muffels 2018; Manning et al. 2016). Young people who rated their chance of contracting COVID-19 as being high also reported lower levels of subjective well-being. The ability of young people to satisfy their need for affection was also associated with levels of subjective well-being. Those who were able to spend more time with their friends and members of their extended families reported higher levels of subjective well-being.

The effect of age also aligns with previous research (Goldbeck et al. 2007; Gonzalez-Carrasco et al. 2017). Goldbeck et al. (2007) found a clear pattern of declining levels of life satisfaction between the ages of 11 and 16 years in Germany. The finding that female students enjoyed lower levels of subjective well-being than male students aligns with the findings of Goldbeck et al. (2007) but contradicts research conducted by Chesters et al. (2021), Frijters et al. (2014), Gonzalez-Carrasco et al. (2017), and Yucel and Vogt Yuan (2016). The finding that young people living with one parent reported having lower levels of well-being than their peers living with two parents aligns with the findings of Yucel and Vogt Yuan (2016) who suggested that adolescents in lone parent families may experience higher levels of stress than their peers living in two parent families.

With regards to Social Production Function theory, the findings presented here provide further evidence of the salience of satisfying physical and social needs for subjective well-being. Young people who were unable to satisfy their need for comfort in terms of being healthy reported lower levels of well-being. Living with one parent rather than two may be associated with a lower likelihood of satisfying one's need for affection and therefore, lower levels of subjective well-being (Steverink et al. 2020). Young people who indicated that they had been able to spend more time with their friends and members of their extended families reported having higher levels of well-being suggesting that their need for affection was satisfied. Hori and Kamo (2018) posit that support from family and friends is especially important during adolescence. Goldbeck et al. (2007) found that peer friendships were a consistently important factor contributing to levels of well-being during adolescence.

The focus of this paper was to examine whether COVID-19 pandemic and its associated restrictions impacted on average levels of subjective well-being of young Australians in the early stages of the COVID-19 pandemic. The HILDA project collects data from the same participants every year, therefore, it is possible to track individual trajectories and compare levels of life satisfaction before and during the COVID-19 pandemic for older cohorts. Furthermore, as further waves of data are collected and become available, an examination of levels of subjective well-being between 2020 and 2023 will be possible. Therefore, there is scope for further research in this field.

The contribution of this chapter is that it examines the effect of the initial national pandemic-related lockdown on a cohort of young Australians aged between 15 and 17 years in the first part of 2020. By comparing the average levels of subjective well-being of this cohort with their counterparts in 2001, 2005, 2010 and 2015, it provides an insight into how levels of subjective well-being at particular points in the life course are consistent over time. Young people attending secondary school were somewhat cushioned from the economic disruptions related to the pandemic as they focused on their need for affection at home and within their social networks and their need for validation from their peers by conforming with the behavioral expectations of their peer group. According to Social Production Function theory, the need for affection and the need for validation are integral factors associated with levels of subjective well-being (Ormel et al. 1999).

13.5 Conclusion

During 2020, the COVID-19 pandemic disrupted the social and economic lives of Australians. Young people, in particular, had to quickly adjust to restrictions that impeded their ability to attend school, participate in sporting and other organized social activities and spend time with their friends and family members who did not live in the family home. Given that adolescence is the period during which young people seek to develop their own social networks and become less reliant on their families for support, these rapidly implemented changes were expected to impact on levels of well-being. The findings presented here indicate that in the early stages of the pandemic, levels of subjective well-being were unaffected. There were, however, some notable results that give insight into the importance of friendships. Young people who were able to increase their contact with friends and members of their extended families reported having higher levels of subjective well-being compared to their counterparts who either maintained or decreased their levels of contact. Furthermore, young people who believed that they had a higher chance of contracting COVID-19 held lower levels of subjective well-being than their peers who were less concerned. These findings have important implications for how crises should be handled in the future. Calming concerns about being infected and enhancing opportunities for young people to engage in social activities with their friends and peers are central to the subjective well-being of young people.

Acknowledgements The paper uses unit record data from the Household, Income and Labour Dynamics in Australia (HILDA) Survey. The HILDA Project was initiated and is funded by the Australian Government Department of Social Services (DSS) and is managed by the Melbourne Institute of Applied Economic and Social Research (MIAESR). The findings and views reported in this paper, however, are those of the authors and should not be attributed to either DSS or MIAESR.

Appendix

Table 13.6 Descriptive statistics for the Phase 1 variables for each of the 5 cohorts

	2001	2005	2010	2015	2020
	%	%	%	%	%
Sex					
Male	49	51	48	52	50
Female	51	49	52	48	50
Age					
15	39	40	36	38	34
16	38	37	36	35	35
17	24	23	28	27	31
State					
NSW	31	31	31	31	26
VIC	29	25	28	26	27
QLD	16	22	19	19	23
SA	10	8	10	9	9
WA	6	8	7	9	8
TAS	4	3	4	4	4
NT	0.3	1	0.3	1	1
ACT	4	2	1	2	2
Migrant status					
Australian	62	69	68	66	68
Migrant	38	31	32	34	32
Family type					
Two parents	80	74	78	74	78
One parent	20	26	22	26	22
Employment status					
Employed	40	44	39	36	38
Not employed	60	56	61	64	62
Health status					
Good/ excellent	88	86	86	85	86
Poor/ fair	5	5	3	4	5
Missing	7	9	10	11	9

Note: NSW=New South Wales; QLD = Queensland; SA = South Australia; WA = Western Australia; TAS = Tasmania; NT = Northern Territory; ACT = Australian Capital Territory
Source: Housing and Income Dynamics in Australia (HILDA) Survey

Table 13.7 Descriptive statistics for the Phase 2 variables for the 2020 cohort

	2020 n = 623
	%
Location	
Victoria	27
Other state/ territory	73
% chance had/get COVID-19	.
None	14
Low	58
High	26
Missing	2
Change in time staying in contact with friend/ family	
More time	27
Less / same time	73

Source: Housing and Income Dynamics in Australia (HILDA) Survey

Table 13.8 reported number of weeks that schools impacted by COVID-19 by State/ Territory of residence

	n=	0	1–6	7–12	13–28
NSW	164	23.8	56.7	18.9	0.6
VIC	168	20.2	7.1	30.4	42.3
QLD	144	13.9	77.1	8.3	0.7
SA	53	34.0	60.4	3.8	1.9
WA	52	17.3	78.9	3.9	0
TAS	24	29.2	50.0	20.9	0
NT	5	60.0	40.0	0	0
ACT	13	15.4	69.2	15.4	0

Note: NSW=New South Wales; QLD = Queensland; SA = South Australia; WA = Western Australia; TAS = Tasmania; NT = Northern Territory; ACT = Australian Capital Territory
Source: Housing and Income Dynamics in Australia (HILDA) Survey

References

Ambrey, C.L., and C.M. Fleming. 2014. Life satisfaction in Australia: Evidence from ten years of the HILDA survey. *Social Indicators Research* 115: 691–714.

Bayliss, D., W. Olsen, and P. Walthery. 2017. Well-being during recession in the UK. *Applied Research in Quality of Life* 12: 369–387.

Bellis, M.A., H. Lowey, K. Hughes, L. Deacon, J. Stansfield, and C. Perkins. 2012. Variations in risk and protective factors for life satisfaction and mental wellbeing with deprivation: A cross-sectional study. *BMC Public Health* 12 (492): 1–17.

Blanchflower, D.G., and A.J. Oswald. 2005. Happiness and the human development index: The paradox of Australia. *Australian Economic Review* 38 (3): 307–318.

Callens, M. 2017. Long term trends in life satisfaction, 1973-2012: Flanders in Europe. *Social Indicators Research* 130: 107–127.

Carlquist, E., P. Ulleberg, A. Delle Fave, H. Nafsted, and R.M. Blakar. 2017. Everyday understandings of happiness, good life, and satisfaction: Three different facets of wellbeing. *Applied Research in Quality of Life* 12: 481–505.

Chesters, J. 2021. *Life satisfaction during the 2020 pandemic in Australia*. ISBN 978 0 7340 5676 4. Melbourne: YRC. https://education.unimelb.edu.au/__data/assets/pdf_file/0020/3806021/Life-satisfaction-during-the-2020-pandemic-in-Australia.pdf.

Chesters, J., J. Simona, and C. Suter. 2021. Cross-national comparison of age and period effects on levels of subjective Well-being in Australia and Switzerland during volatile economic times (2001-2016). *Social Indicators Research* 154 (1): 361–391.

Clark, A.E., and A.J. Oswald. 1996. Satisfaction and comparison income. *Journal of Public Economics* 61: 359–381.

Clark, A., A. Knabe, and S. Ratzel. 2010. Boon or bane? Others' unemployment, Well-being and job security. *Labour Economics* 17: 52–61.

Department of Health 2021. *COVID-19 summary statistics*. https://www.health.gov.au/news/health-alerts/novel-coronavirus-2019-ncov-health-alert/coronavirus-covid-19-current-situation-and-case-numbers. Accessed 26 Sep 2023.

Diener, E., R. Inglehart, and L. Tay. 2013. Theory and validity of life satisfaction scales. *Social Indicators Research* 112 (3): 497–527.

Easterlin, R.A. 2001. Income and happiness: Towards a unified theory. *The Economic Journal* 111: 465–484.

Fleche, S., W.N. Lekfuangfu, and A.E. Clark. 2021. The long-lasting effects of family and childhood on adult wellbeing: Evidence from British cohort data. *Journal of Economic Behaviour and Organization* 181: 290–311.

Frijters, P., D.W. Johnston, and M.A. Shields. 2014. Does childhood predict adult life satisfaction? Evidence from British cohort surveys. *The Economic Journal* 124: F688–F718.

Gerling, D.M., and E. Diener. 2020. Effect size strengths in subjective Well-being research. *Applied Research in Quality of Life* 15: 167–185.

Goldbeck, L., T.G. Schmitz, T. Besir, P. Herschbach, and G. Henrich. 2007. Life satisfaction decreases during adolescence. *Quality Life Research* 16: 969–979.

Gonzalez-Carrasco, M., F. Casas, S. Malo, F. Vinas, and T. Dinisman. 2017. Changes with age in subjective Well-being through the adolescent years: Differences by gender. *Journal of Happiness Studies* 18: 63–88.

Hadjar, A., and R. Samuel. 2015. Does upward social mobility increase life satisfaction? A longitudinal analysis using British and Swiss panel data. *Research in Social Stratification and Mobility* 39: 48–58.

Headey, B., and R. Muffels. 2018. A theory of life satisfaction dynamics: Stability, change and volatility in 25-year life trajectories in Germany. *Social Indicators Research* 140: 837–866.

Headey, B., R. Muffels, and G.G. Wagner. 2013. Choices which change life satisfaction: Similar results for Australia, Britain and Germany. *Social Indicators Research* 112: 725–748.

Hori, M., and Y. Kamo. 2018. Gender differences in happiness: The effects of marriage, social roles, and social support in East Asia. *Applied Research in Quality of Life* 13: 839–857.

Layard, R., A. Clark, F. Cornaglia, N. Powdthavee, and J. Vernoit. 2014. What predicts a successful life? A life-course model of wellbeing. *The Economic Journal* 124: 720–738.

Manning, M., C.L. Ambrey, and C.M. Fleming. 2016. A longitudinal study of indigenous wellbeing in Australia. *Journal of Happiness Studies* 17: 2503–2525.

Ormel, J., S. Lindenberg, and L.M. Verbrugge. 1999. Subjective well-being and social production functions. *Social Indicators Research* 46: 61–90.

Parker, P.D., J. Jerrim, and J. Andres. 2016. What effect did the global financial crisis have upon youth wellbeing? Evidence from four Australian cohorts. *Developmental Psychology* 52 (4): 640–651.

Plenty, S., and C. Mood. 2016. Money, peers and parents: Social and economic aspects of inequality in youth wellbeing. *Journal of Youth Adolescence* 45: 1294–1308.

Scharf, J., A. Hadjar, and A. Grecu. 2019. Applying social production function theory to benefits of schooling: The concept of values of education. *British Journal of Sociology of Education* 40 (7): 847–867.

StataCorp. 2015. *Stata statistical software: Release 14*. College Station, TX: StataCorp LP.

Steverink, N., S. Lindenberg, T. Spiegel, and A.P. Nieboer. 2020. The associations of different social needs with psychological strengths and subjective Well-being: An empirical investigation based on social production theory. *Journal of Happiness Studies* 21: 799–824.

Summerfield. M., A. Bevitt, K. Fok, M. Hahn, N. La, N. Macalalad, M. O'Shea, N. Watson, R. Wilkins, and M. Wooden. 2018. HILDA user manual-release 17. Melbourne: Melbourne Institute of Applied Economic and Social Research, University of Melbourne. HILDA-User-Manual-Release-17.1.pdf (unimelb.edu.au). Accessed 10 Dec 2019.

The Treasury (Australian Government) 2023. *JobKeeper payment*. https://treasury.gov.au/coronavirus/jobkeeper. Accessed 26 Sep 2023.

Veenhoven, R. 1996. Developments in satisfaction-research. *Social Indicators Research* 37 (1): 1–46.

Wang, L., T. Su, L. Tian, and E.S. Huebner. 2021. Prosocial behaviour and subjective Well-being in school among elementary school students: The mediating roles of the satisfaction of relatedness needs at school and self-esteem. *Applied Research in Quality of Life* 16: 1439–1459.

Wong, K.T., V. Zheng, and P. Wan. 2017. A dissatisfied generation? An age-period-cohort analysis of the political satisfaction of youth in Hong Kong from 1997 to 2014. *Social Indicators Research* 130: 253–276.

Yang, Y. 2008. Social inequalities in happiness in the United States, 1972 to 2004: An age-period-cohort analysis. *American Sociological Review* 73 (2): 204–226.

Yucel, D., and A.S. Vogt Yuan. 2016. Parents, siblings or friends? Exploring life satisfaction among early adolescents. *Applied Research in Quality of Life* 11: 1399–1423.

Jenny Chesters is Associate Professor Faculty of Education, at the University of Melbourne, Australia. She is a CI on the Life Patterns Research Project—a longitudinal mixed methods study tracking 3 cohorts of school leavers over time. Her research interests focus on transitions between education and employment throughout the life course and inequality in educational attainment. She is a Board member for the RC55 of the ISA. Her recent publications include the *Research Handbook on Transitions into Adulthood* (Edward Elgar 2024).

The manufacturer's authorised representative in the EU is Springer Nature Customer Service Centre GmbH, Europaplatz 3, 69115 Heidelberg, Germany. If you have any concerns regarding our products, please contact ProductSafety@springernature.com

Printed and bound by CPI Group (UK) Ltd, Croydon, CR0 4YY
01/10/2026
02225904-0007